系统解剖学 彩色图谱

Colour Atlas of Systematic Anatomy

（解剖学教材配套图谱）

主　编　段坤昌　王振宇　佟晓杰

主　审　柏树令　应大君

人民卫生出版社

图书在版编目（CIP）数据

系统解剖学彩色图谱/段坤昌等主编. —北京：人民
卫生出版社，2013.3
ISBN 978 - 7 - 117 - 16007 - 0

Ⅰ.①系⋯ Ⅱ.①段⋯ Ⅲ.①系统解剖学–图谱
Ⅳ.①R322-64

中国版本图书馆 CIP 数据核字（2012）第 103091 号

人卫社官网　www. pmph. com	出版物查询，在线购书
人卫医学网　www. ipmph. com	医学考试辅导，医学数
	据库服务，医学教育资
	源，大众健康资讯

系统解剖学彩色图谱

主　　编：段坤昌　王振宇　佟晓杰
出版发行：人民卫生出版社（中继线 010-59780011）
地　　址：北京市朝阳区潘家园南里 19 号
邮　　编：100021
E - mail：pmph @ pmph. com
购书热线：010-59787592　010-59787584　010-65264830
印　　刷：三河市宏达印刷有限公司（胜利）
经　　销：新华书店
开　　本：889×1194　1/16　印张：23
字　　数：728 千字
版　　次：2013 年 3 月第 1 版　　2022 年 8 月第 1 版第 6 次印刷
标准书号：ISBN 978-7-117-16007-0/R · 16008
定　　价：179.00 元

打击盗版举报电话：**010-59787491　E - mail：WQ @ pmph. com**
（凡属印装质量问题请与本社市场营销中心联系退换）

编 者 名 单

主　编　段坤昌　王振宇　佟晓杰

主　审　柏树令　应大君

副主编　潘　峰　初国良　齐亚力

编　者（以姓氏笔画为序）

丁　炯　南京医科大学　　　　　　　　　李德华　辽宁医学院

丁文龙　上海交通大学医学院　　　　　　杨伯宁　广西医科大学

王　玮　福建医科大学　　　　　　　　　佟晓杰　中国医科大学

王　洋　中国医科大学　　　　　　　　　沈若武　青岛大学医学院

王振宇　中国医科大学　　　　　　　　　初国良　中山大学医学院

王海杰　复旦大学上海医学院　　　　　　邵旭建　青岛大学医学院

王维晰　西安交通大学医学院　　　　　　易西南　海南医学院

文小军　新乡医学院　　　　　　　　　　罗学港　中南大学湘雅医学院

甘子明　新疆医科大学　　　　　　　　　段坤昌　中国医科大学

田国忠　佳木斯大学医学院　　　　　　　段维轶　中国医科大学

冯克俭　牡丹江医学院　　　　　　　　　凌树才　浙江大学基础医学院

刘仁刚　华中科技大学同济医学院　　　　高秀来　首都医科大学

刘学政　辽宁医学院　　　　　　　　　　高振平　吉林大学白求恩医学院

刘宝全　哈尔滨医科大学　　　　　　　　郭开华　中山大学医学院

刘绍壮　大连医科大学　　　　　　　　　黄学应　安徽医科大学

齐亚力　中国医科大学　　　　　　　　　宿宝贵　暨南大学医学院

孙晋浩　山东大学医学院　　　　　　　　富长海　中国医科大学

李　巍　中国医科大学　　　　　　　　　廖　华　南方医科大学

李志军　内蒙古医科大学　　　　　　　　潘　峰　中国医科大学

李洪鹏　中国医科大学　　　　　　　　　戴冀斌　武汉大学医学院

摄　影　段坤昌　齐亚力

前　　言

人体解剖学是阐述正常人体形态结构的科学,属于形态科学范畴,是建立在人体形态结构基础上的知识体系。因此,学习和研究人体解剖学理论知识与掌握客观存在的人体形态结构是同等重要。获取人体结构最有效的方式是对人体实物标本或其图像的直接观察。直观的图像配合适当的文字说明便于读者快捷、有效地学习和掌握人体解剖学知识。

该图谱是以国家级规划教材临床医学专业八年制《系统解剖学》(第1～2版)和临床医学专业五年制《系统解剖学》(第1～7版)为基础,由具有丰富解剖学教学经验的一线教师编著完成。其内容丰富、结构真实、容易理解、便于记忆,适合临床医学专业学生和临床医生学习和认识人体结构的一本工具书。

本图谱以教学大纲及全国规划教材为依据,遵循医学院校长学制的系统解剖学教学深度和高等医学院校五年制系统解剖学教学的精度。在精心设计和制作的实物标本的基础上,共拍摄图像735幅,并通过融入多媒体技术将其中的45幅实物标本图像制作成模式图。图谱内容在与教材各章节内容相呼应的基础上,延伸了教材的内容,以便于满足读者进一步学习的需要。如:教材中只有"尺神经深支分布于小鱼际、拇收肌、骨间掌侧肌、骨间背侧肌及第3、4蚓状肌"的简单叙述,缺少对尺神经深支走行及分布描述和示意。该图谱通过手的神经标本图像,真实地显示了尺神经深支支配上述各肌肉肌支的走行及入肌部位,结构清晰,一目了然,可加深读者对尺神经损伤引起手内在肌瘫痪,导致手功能障碍而形成"爪形手"的理解和认识。此外,本图谱还收集了一些罕见的畸形和异常结构的实物标本图像,如:异位肾、马蹄肾、双输尿管、双上腔静脉和双下腔静脉等。以增加学生学习的兴趣、拓展学生的知识面。

该图谱所采用的标本都是人体实物标本。在图谱的编著过程中,作者为了精雕细刻每一个标本花费了大量的时间和精力,并将标本的动脉染红色、静脉染兰色、神经染黄色、淋巴染绿色,以使得图像中的结构更突出,层次更分明。尽管如此,由于受到标本色泽、质地、体姿和肌肉丰满度的影响,与人工绘制(艺术加工)图谱相比,还显得不够"艳丽美观",但实物标本拍摄的图片能给读者更为真实的认识。

图谱初稿完成后,编委会进行了认真的审校和修改。书中的名词以全国自然科学名词审定委员会1991年公布《人体解剖学名词》为准,并进行中英文双语标注,便于学生对主要英语词汇的掌握和记忆。

最后我们期望该图谱能够符合全国医学院校教改的要求,适合教学实际的需要,为提高解剖学教学质量起到推动作用。但是,由于我们的水平有限,错误疏漏之处在所难免,敬请解剖界同仁、医务工作者和医学生提出宝贵意见。

段坤昌　王振宇　佟晓杰

二零一二年五月

目　　录

第一章　绪论 Introduction ·· 1

    图 1　人体解剖学姿势(前面观)Anatomical position. Anterior aspect ···················· 1

    图 2　人体侧面观 Lateral aspect of human body ··· 1

    图 3　人体的轴和面 Body axes and planes ·· 2

    图 4　人体的方向术语 Directional terms ··· 2

    图 5　躯干的标志线(前面观)Reference lines of trunk. Anterior aspect ·············· 3

    图 6　躯干的标志线(后面观)Reference lines of trunk. Posterior aspect ············· 3

    图 7　躯干的标志线(侧面观)Reference lines of trunk. Lateral aspect ··············· 4

    图 8　躯干的标志线(水平线)Horizontal reference lines of trunk ······················ 4

    图 9　人体的体表分区(前面观)Body regions. Anterior aspect ························· 5

    图 10　人体的体表分区(后面观)Body regions. Posterior aspect ······················ 5

    图 11　头面部的分区 Regions of head and face ··· 6

    图 12　颈部的分区 Regions of neck ··· 6

    图 13　胸部的分区 Thoracic regions ··· 7

    图 14　腹部的分区 Abdominal regions ··· 7

    图 15　背部和上肢的分区 Regions of back and upper limb ····························· 8

    图 16　下肢的分区(前面观)Regions of lower limb. Anterior aspect ·················· 8

第二章　骨学 Osteology ··· 9

    图 17　全身骨骼 Skeleton ··· 9

    图 18　骨的分类 Classification of bones ·· 10

    图 19　骨的内部构造 Interior of different bones ·· 10

    图 20　长骨的构造 Structure of long bone ··· 11

    图 21　骺软骨 Epiphysial cartilage ·· 11

    图 22　脊柱 Vertebral column ··· 12

    图 23　寰椎(上面观)Atlas. Superior aspect ·· 13

    图 24　寰椎(下面观)Atlas. Inferior aspect ·· 13

    图 25　枢椎(上面观)Axis. Superior aspect ·· 13

    图 26　枢椎(侧面观)Axis. Lateral aspect ·· 13

    图 27　颈椎(上面观)Cervical vertebra. Superior aspect ································· 13

    图 28　颈椎(侧面观)Cervical vertebra. Lateral aspect ··································· 13

    图 29　胸椎(上面观)Thoracic vertebra. Superior aspect ································ 14

    图 30　胸椎(侧面观)Thoracic vertebra. Lateral aspect ·································· 14

    图 31　腰椎(上面观)Lumbar vertebra. Superior aspect ································· 14

    图 32　腰椎(侧面观)Lumbar vertebra. Lateral aspect ··································· 14

图 33　骶骨（前面观）Sacrum. Anterior aspect …………………………………… 15

图 34　骶骨（后面观）Sacrum. Posterior aspect …………………………………… 15

图 35　尾骨（前面观）Coccyx. Anterior aspect …………………………………… 15

图 36　胸骨（前面观）Sternum. Anterior aspect …………………………………… 16

图 37　胸骨（侧面观）Sternum. Lateral aspect …………………………………… 16

图 38　肋骨 Costal bones …………………………………………………………… 16

图 39　额骨（前面观）Frontal bone. Anterior aspect …………………………… 17

图 40　顶骨（内面观）Parietal bone. Internal aspect …………………………… 17

图 41　枕骨（内面观）Occipital bone. Internal aspect ………………………… 18

图 42　筛骨（前面观）Ethmoid bone. Anterior aspect ………………………… 18

图 43　筛骨（侧面观）Ethmoid bone. Lateral aspect …………………………… 18

图 44　蝶骨（前面观）Sphenoid bone. Anterior aspect ……………………… 19

图 45　蝶骨（上面观）Sphenoid bone. Superior aspect ……………………… 19

图 46　颞骨（外面观）Temporal bone. External aspect ……………………… 20

图 47　颞骨（内面观）Temporal bone. Internal aspect ……………………… 20

图 48　颧骨 Zygomatic bone ……………………………………………………… 21

图 49　犁骨 Vomer ………………………………………………………………… 21

图 50　下颌骨（外侧面观）Mandible. Lateral aspect …………………………… 21

图 51　下颌骨（内侧面观）Mandible. Medial aspect …………………………… 22

图 52　下颌骨（牙槽面观）Mandible. Dental alveoli aspect ………………… 22

图 53　下颌骨（老年）Mandible. Aged …………………………………………… 22

图 54　舌骨（前面观）Hyoid bone. Anterior aspect …………………………… 23

图 55　舌骨（侧面观）Hyoid bone. Lateral aspect …………………………… 23

图 56　上颌骨（外侧面观）Maxilla. Lateral aspect …………………………… 23

图 57　上颌骨（内侧面观）Maxilla. Medial aspect …………………………… 24

图 58　上颌骨（后面观）Maxilla. Posterior aspect …………………………… 24

图 59　腭骨（后面观）Palatine bone. Posterior aspect ……………………… 25

图 60　腭骨（内侧面观）Palatine bone. Medial aspect ……………………… 25

图 61　颅底（内面观）Internal surface of the base of skull ………………… 26

图 62　颅底（外面观）External surface of the base of skull ………………… 27

图 63　颅（前面观）Skull. Anterior aspect …………………………………… 28

图 64　颅（外侧面观）Skull. Lateral aspect …………………………………… 29

图 65　翼腭窝 Pterygopalatine fossa ………………………………………… 30

图 66　颅冠状切面（经过第二磨牙）Coronal section of skull through the second molar ……… 30

图 67　鼻腔外侧壁（1）Lateral wall of nasal cavity（1） ……………………… 31

图 68　鼻腔外侧壁（2）Lateral wall of nasal cavity（2） ……………………… 31

图 69　婴儿颅（侧面观）Skull of infant. Lateral aspect ……………………… 32

图 70　婴儿颅（上面观）Skull of infant. Superior aspect ………………… 32

图 71　上肢骨 Bones of upper limb …………………………………………… 33

图 72　锁骨（上面观）Clavicle. Superior aspect ……………………………… 34

图 73　锁骨（下面观）Clavicle. Inferior aspect ……………………………… 34

图 74　肩胛骨（外侧面观）Scapular. Lateral aspect ………………………… 34

图 75　肩胛骨（前面观）Scapular. Anterior aspect ………………………… 35

图 76　肩胛骨（后面观）Scapular. Posterior aspect ⋯⋯⋯⋯⋯⋯⋯⋯⋯⋯⋯⋯⋯⋯⋯ 35

图 77　肱骨（前面观）Humerus. Anterior aspect ⋯⋯⋯⋯⋯⋯⋯⋯⋯⋯⋯⋯⋯⋯⋯⋯ 36

图 78　肱骨（后面观）Humerus. Posterior aspect ⋯⋯⋯⋯⋯⋯⋯⋯⋯⋯⋯⋯⋯⋯⋯⋯ 36

图 79　桡骨和尺骨（前面观）Radius and ulna. Anterior aspect ⋯⋯⋯⋯⋯⋯⋯⋯⋯ 37

图 80　桡骨和尺骨（后面观）Radius and ulna. Posterior aspect ⋯⋯⋯⋯⋯⋯⋯⋯ 37

图 81　桡骨和尺骨 Radius and ulna ⋯⋯⋯⋯⋯⋯⋯⋯⋯⋯⋯⋯⋯⋯⋯⋯⋯⋯⋯⋯⋯⋯ 38

图 82　手骨（前面观）Bones of hand. Anterior aspect ⋯⋯⋯⋯⋯⋯⋯⋯⋯⋯⋯⋯⋯ 39

图 83　手骨（后面观）Bones of hand. Posterior aspect ⋯⋯⋯⋯⋯⋯⋯⋯⋯⋯⋯⋯⋯ 39

图 84　下肢骨 Bones of lower limb ⋯⋯⋯⋯⋯⋯⋯⋯⋯⋯⋯⋯⋯⋯⋯⋯⋯⋯⋯⋯⋯⋯⋯ 40

图 85　髋骨（内面观）Hip bone. Internal aspect ⋯⋯⋯⋯⋯⋯⋯⋯⋯⋯⋯⋯⋯⋯⋯⋯ 41

图 86　髋骨（外面观）Hip bone. External aspect ⋯⋯⋯⋯⋯⋯⋯⋯⋯⋯⋯⋯⋯⋯⋯⋯ 41

图 87　髋骨（前面观）Hip bone. Anterior aspect ⋯⋯⋯⋯⋯⋯⋯⋯⋯⋯⋯⋯⋯⋯⋯⋯ 42

图 88　幼儿髋骨 Hip bone of infant ⋯⋯⋯⋯⋯⋯⋯⋯⋯⋯⋯⋯⋯⋯⋯⋯⋯⋯⋯⋯⋯⋯ 42

图 89　股骨（前面观）Femur. Anterior aspect ⋯⋯⋯⋯⋯⋯⋯⋯⋯⋯⋯⋯⋯⋯⋯⋯⋯ 43

图 90　股骨（后面观）Femur. Posterior aspect ⋯⋯⋯⋯⋯⋯⋯⋯⋯⋯⋯⋯⋯⋯⋯⋯⋯ 43

图 91　髌骨 Patella ⋯⋯⋯⋯⋯⋯⋯⋯⋯⋯⋯⋯⋯⋯⋯⋯⋯⋯⋯⋯⋯⋯⋯⋯⋯⋯⋯⋯⋯⋯ 44

图 92　胫骨和腓骨（前面观）Tibia and fibula. Anterior aspect ⋯⋯⋯⋯⋯⋯⋯⋯ 44

图 93　胫骨和腓骨（后面观）Tibia and fibula. Posterior aspect ⋯⋯⋯⋯⋯⋯⋯ 44

图 94　足骨（上面观）Bones of foot. Superior aspect ⋯⋯⋯⋯⋯⋯⋯⋯⋯⋯⋯⋯⋯ 45

图 95　足骨（下面观）Bones of foot. Inferior aspect ⋯⋯⋯⋯⋯⋯⋯⋯⋯⋯⋯⋯⋯⋯ 45

第三章　关节学 Arthrology ⋯⋯⋯⋯⋯⋯⋯⋯⋯⋯⋯⋯⋯⋯⋯⋯⋯⋯⋯⋯⋯⋯⋯⋯⋯ **46**

图 96　骨连结分类 Joint classification ⋯⋯⋯⋯⋯⋯⋯⋯⋯⋯⋯⋯⋯⋯⋯⋯⋯⋯⋯⋯ 46

图 97　骨性结合 Synosteosis ⋯⋯⋯⋯⋯⋯⋯⋯⋯⋯⋯⋯⋯⋯⋯⋯⋯⋯⋯⋯⋯⋯⋯⋯⋯ 47

图 98　椎骨间连结 Joints between vertebrae ⋯⋯⋯⋯⋯⋯⋯⋯⋯⋯⋯⋯⋯⋯⋯⋯⋯⋯ 47

图 99　椎间盘和关节突关节 Intervertebral disc and zygapophyseal joint ⋯⋯⋯⋯ 48

图 100　椎间盘 Intervertebral disc ⋯⋯⋯⋯⋯⋯⋯⋯⋯⋯⋯⋯⋯⋯⋯⋯⋯⋯⋯⋯⋯⋯ 48

图 101　黄韧带 Ligamenta flava ⋯⋯⋯⋯⋯⋯⋯⋯⋯⋯⋯⋯⋯⋯⋯⋯⋯⋯⋯⋯⋯⋯⋯ 49

图 102　项韧带 Ligamentum nuchae ⋯⋯⋯⋯⋯⋯⋯⋯⋯⋯⋯⋯⋯⋯⋯⋯⋯⋯⋯⋯⋯ 49

图 103　寰枢关节（水平切面）Atlantoaxial joint. Horizontal section ⋯⋯⋯⋯⋯⋯ 50

图 104　寰枕寰枢关节（矢状切面）Atlantooccipital joint and atlantoaxial joint. Sagittal section ⋯⋯⋯ 50

图 105　寰枕、寰枢关节（后面观）Atlantooccipital joint and atlantoaxial joint. Posterior aspect ⋯⋯⋯ 51

图 106　肋椎关节（上面观）Costovertebral joint. Superior aspect ⋯⋯⋯⋯⋯⋯⋯ 51

图 107　肋椎关节（后面观）Costovertebral joint. Posterior aspect ⋯⋯⋯⋯⋯⋯⋯ 52

图 108　胸肋关节和胸锁关节 Sternocostal joint and sternoclavicular joint ⋯⋯⋯ 52

图 109　胸廓（前面观）Thorax. Anterior aspect ⋯⋯⋯⋯⋯⋯⋯⋯⋯⋯⋯⋯⋯⋯⋯⋯ 53

图 110　颞下颌关节（外侧面观）Temporomandibular joint. Lateral aspect ⋯⋯⋯ 54

图 111　颞下颌关节（矢状切面）Temporomandibular joint. Sagittal section ⋯⋯⋯ 54

图 112　颞下颌关节（内侧面观）Temporomandibular joint. Medial aspect ⋯⋯⋯ 55

图 113　胸锁关节 Sternoclavicular joint ⋯⋯⋯⋯⋯⋯⋯⋯⋯⋯⋯⋯⋯⋯⋯⋯⋯⋯⋯⋯ 55

图 114　肩关节（前面观 1）Shoulder joint. Anterior aspect（1）⋯⋯⋯⋯⋯⋯⋯⋯ 56

图 115　肩关节（前面观 2）Shoulder joint. Anterior aspect（2）⋯⋯⋯⋯⋯⋯⋯⋯ 56

图 116　肩关节（冠状切面）Shoulder joint. Coronal section ⋯⋯⋯⋯⋯⋯⋯⋯⋯⋯ 57

图 117　肩关节腔（前面观）Cavity of shoulder joint. Anterior aspect ································· 57

图 118　肩关节腔（后面观）Cavity of shoulder joint. Posterior aspect ································ 57

图 119　肘关节（前面观 1）Elbow joint. Anterior aspect（1）································· 58

图 120　肘关节（前面观 2）Elbow joint. Anterior aspect（2）································· 58

图 121　肘关节（内侧面观）Elbow joint. Medial aspect ································· 59

图 122　肘关节（外侧面观）Elbow joint. Lateral aspect ································· 59

图 123　桡骨环状韧带 Annular ligament of radius ································· 60

图 124　肘关节（矢状切面）Elbow joint. Sagittal section ································· 60

图 125　前臂骨间膜 Interosseous membrane of forearm ································· 60

图 126　手关节（背面观）Joints of hand. Dorsal aspect ································· 61

图 127　手关节（掌面观）Joints of hand. Palmar aspect ································· 61

图 128　手关节（冠状切面）Joints of hand. Coronal section ································· 62

图 129　指骨间关节（侧面观）Interphalangeal joints of hand. Lateral aspect ································· 62

图 130　骨盆的韧带（前面观）Ligaments of pelvis. Anterior aspect ································· 63

图 131　骨盆的韧带（后面观）Ligaments of pelvis. Posterior aspect ································· 63

图 132　耻骨联合（冠状切面）Pubic symphysis. Coronal section ································· 64

图 133　骨盆的力传导弓 Arcus of mechanotransduction of pelvis ································· 64

图 134　骨盆径线（上面观）Diameter of pelvis. Superior aspect ································· 65

图 135　骨盆径线（侧面观）Diameter of pelvis. Lateral aspect ································· 65

图 136　女性骨盆（前面观）Pelvis of female. Anterior aspect ································· 66

图 137　男性骨盆（前面观）Pelvis of male. Anterior aspect ································· 66

图 138　髋关节（前面观）Hip joint. Anterior aspect ································· 67

图 139　髋关节冠状切面 Coronal section through hip joint ································· 67

图 140　髋关节（后面观 1）Hip joint. Posterior aspect（1）································· 68

图 141　髋关节（后面观 2）Hip joint. Posterior aspect（2）································· 68

图 142　膝关节（前面观）Knee joint. Anterior aspect ································· 69

图 143　膝关节（后面观）Knee joint. Posterior aspect ································· 69

图 144　膝关节（囊切开前面观）Opened knee joint. Anterior aspect ································· 70

图 145　膝关节（囊切开后面观）Opened knee joint. Posterior aspect ································· 70

图 146　膝关节半月板（上面观）Menici of knee joint. Superior aspect ································· 71

图 147　膝关节腔（前面观）Cavity of knee joint. Anterior aspect ································· 71

图 148　膝关节腔（内侧面观）Cavity of knee joint. Medial aspect ································· 71

图 149　足的关节韧带（内侧面观）Joints and ligaments of foot. Medial aspect ································· 72

图 150　足的关节韧带（外侧面观）Joints and ligaments of foot. Lateral aspect ································· 72

图 151　足的关节韧带（足底面观）Joints and ligaments of foot. Plantar aspect ································· 73

图 152　足的关节（水平切面）Joints of foot. Horizontal section ································· 73

图 153　足的关节（矢状切面）Joints of foot. Sagittal section ································· 74

图 154　足弓 Arch of foot ································· 74

第四章　肌学 Myology ································· 75

图 155　肌的形态 Various shapes of muscles ································· 75

图 156　大腿中部横切面（示筋膜）Transverse section through middle of thigh. Showing fasciae ································· 76

图 157　头肌（前面观）Muscles of head. Anterior aspect ································· 77

图 158　头肌（侧面观 1）Muscles of head. Lateral aspect（1）... 78

图 159　头肌（侧面观 2）Muscles of head. Lateral aspect（2）... 78

图 160　眼轮匝肌泪部与泪囊的关系 Relationship of lacrimal part of orbicularis oculi
　　　　and lacrimal sac 79

图 161　颈阔肌 Platysma 79

图 162　颈肌（前面观 1）Muscles of neck. Anterior aspect（1）.. 80

图 163　颈肌（前面观 2）Muscles of neck. Anterior aspect（2）.. 80

图 164　颈肌（前面观 3）Muscles of neck. Anterior aspect（3）.. 81

图 165　颈肌（侧面观）Muscles of neck. Lateral aspect 81

图 166　椎枕肌 Vertebrooccipital muscles 82

图 167　口底肌 Muscles of base of oral cavity 82

图 168　背肌（1）Muscles of back（1）.. 83

图 169　背肌（2）Muscles of back（2）.. 83

图 170　胸腰筋膜 Thoracolumbar fascia 84

图 171　颈部的屈和伸 Flexion and extension of neck 84

图 172　颈部的侧屈 Lateral flection of neck 84

图 173　胸肌 Muscles of thorax 85

图 174　前锯肌 Serratus anterior 85

图 175　肋间肌（前面观）Intercostales. Anterior aspect 86

图 176　胸横肌（后面观）Transverses thoracis. Posterior aspect 86

图 177　膈（下面观）Diaphragm. Inferior aspect 87

图 178　腹后壁肌 Muscles of posterior abdominal wall 87

图 179　腹前壁肌 Muscles of anterior abdominal wall 88

图 180　腹股沟区 Inguinal region 89

图 181　腹壁的横断面 Transverse sections of abdominal wall 89

图 182　上肢肌（前面观）Muscles of upper limb. Anterior aspect 90

图 183　上肢肌（后面观）Muscles of upper limb. Posterior aspect 90

图 184　肩、臂部肌（前面观 1）Muscles of shoulder and upper arm. Anterior aspect（1）............. 91

图 185　肩、臂部肌（前面观 2）Muscles of shoulder and upper arm. Anterior aspect（2）............. 91

图 186　肩、臂部肌（后面观）Muscles of shoulder and upper arm. Posterior aspect 92

图 187　肩的屈和伸 Flexion and extension of shoulder 92

图 188　肩的展和收 Abduction and adduction of shoulder 92

图 189　前臂肌（前面观 1）Muscles of forearm. Anterior aspect（1）.. 93

图 190　前臂肌（前面观 2）Muscles of forearm. Anterior aspect（2）.. 93

图 191　前臂肌（前面观 3）Muscles of forearm. Anterior aspect（3）.. 94

图 192　前臂肌（后面观 1）Muscles of forearm. Posterior aspect（1）... 94

图 193　前臂肌（后面观 2）Muscles of forearm. Posterior aspect（2）... 95

图 194　肘的屈和伸 Flexion and extension of elbow 95

图 195　手肌（前面观 1）Muscles of hand. Anterior aspect（1）... 96

图 196　手肌（前面观 2）Muscles of hand. Anterior aspect（2）... 96

图 197　手肌（前面观 3）Muscles of hand. Anterior aspect（3）... 97

图 198　手肌（后面观 1）Muscles of hand. Posterior aspect（1）... 97

图 199　手肌（后面观 2）Muscles of hand. Posterior aspect（2）... 98

图 200　骨间掌侧肌(前面观)Palmar interossei. Anterior aspect ·· 98

图 201　骨间背侧肌(前面观)Dorsal interossei. Anterior aspect ·· 99

图 202　腕的屈和伸 Flexion and extension of wrist ··· 99

图 203　腕的收和展 Adduction and abduction of wrist ·· 99

图 204　手指的收和展 Adduction and abduction of fingers ··· 100

图 205　拇指的收和展 Adduction and abduction of thumb ··· 100

图 206　指伸肌腱 Tendon of extensor digitorum ·· 100

图 207　骨间肌和蚓状肌的止点 Insertion of interosseus and lumbrical ······································· 101

图 208　屈肌腱和腱纽 Flexor tendons and vincula tendinum ·· 101

图 209　手腱鞘(前面观)Tendinous sheaths of hand. Anterior aspect ··· 102

图 210　手腱鞘(后面观)Tendinous sheaths of hand. Posterior aspect ·· 102

图 211　下肢肌(前面观)Muscles of lower limb. Anterior aspect ·· 103

图 212　下肢肌(后面观)Muscles of lower limb. Posterior aspect ··· 103

图 213　股部肌(前面观 1)Muscles of thigh. Anterior aspect(1) ··· 104

图 214　股部肌(前面观 2)Muscles of thigh. Anterior aspect(2) ··· 104

图 215　股部肌(后面观 1)Muscles of thigh. Posterior aspect(1) ·· 105

图 216　股部肌(后面观 2)Muscles of thigh. Posterior aspect(2) ·· 105

图 217　臀肌深层 Deep layer of gluteus ·· 106

图 218　盆壁肌(1)Muscles of pelvic wall(1) ·· 106

图 219　盆壁肌(2)Muscles of pelvic wall(2) ·· 106

图 220　股部肌(内侧面观)Muscles of thigh. Medial aspect ··· 107

图 221　大腿的收和展 Adduction and abduction of thigh ·· 107

图 222　髋关节的屈和伸 Flexion and extension of hip joint ·· 107

图 223　小腿肌(前面观)Muscles of leg. Anterior aspect ·· 108

图 224　小腿肌(外侧面观)Muscle of leg. Lateral aspect ··· 108

图 225　小腿肌(后面观 1)Muscles of leg. Posterior aspect(1) ·· 109

图 226　小腿肌(后面观 2)Muscles of leg. Posterior aspect(2) ·· 109

图 227　小腿肌(后面观 3)Muscles of leg. Posterior aspect(3) ·· 110

图 228　膝关节和大腿的屈和伸 Flexion and extension of knee and thigh ······································· 110

图 229　膝的屈和伸 Flexion and extension of knee ··· 110

图 230　足底肌(1)Plantar muscles(1) ·· 111

图 231　足底肌(2)Plantar muscles(2) ·· 111

图 232　足底肌(3)Plantar muscles(3) ·· 112

图 233　足底肌(4)Plantar muscles(4) ·· 112

图 234　足背肌 Muscles of dorsum of foot ·· 113

图 235　足的背屈和跖屈 Dorsiflexion and plantar flexion of foot ··· 113

图 236　足的内翻和外翻 Inversion and eversion of foot ·· 113

图 237　足腱鞘(前面观)Tendinous sheaths of foot. Anterior aspect ·· 114

图 238　足腱鞘(外侧面观)Tendinous sheaths of foot. Lateral aspect ··· 114

第五章　消化系统 Alimentary System ·· **115**

图 239　消化系统全貌 General arrangement of the alimentary system ·· 115

图 240　腭肌(前面观)Palatine muscles. Anterior aspect ·· 116

图 241　腭肌(侧面观)Palatine muscles. Lateral aspect ································· 116

图 242　乳牙的名称和符号 Name and notation of deciduous teeth ··················· 117

图 243　恒牙的名称和符号 Name and notation of permanent teeth ·················· 117

图 244　牙的切面 Section of teeth ·· 118

图 245　上颌窦与牙根的毗邻关系 Relations between the maxillary sinus and
root of teeth ··· 118

图 246　上颌恒牙 Maxillary permanent teeth ································· 119

图 247　下颌恒牙 Mandibular permanent teeth ································ 119

图 248　上颌乳牙 Maxillary deciduous teeth ································· 120

图 249　下颌乳牙 Mandibular deciduous teeth ································ 120

图 250　恒牙胚 Bud of permanent teeth ······································ 120

图 251　舌(背面观)Tongue. Dorsal aspect ··································· 121

图 252　舌下面 Inferior surface of tongue ···································· 121

图 253　舌肌(纵切面)Muscles of tongue. Longitudinal section ················· 122

图 254　舌肌(横切面)Muscles of tongue. Transverse section ·················· 122

图 255　舌外肌 Extrinsic muscles of tongue ·································· 123

图 256　口腔腺(外侧面观)Glands of oral cavity. Lateral aspect ················· 124

图 257　口腔腺(内侧面观)Gland of oral cavity. Medial aspect ················· 124

图 258　头部正中矢状切面 Median sagittal section of head ···················· 125

图 259　咽腔(后面观)Pharyngeal cavity. Posterior aspect ····················· 126

图 260　咽肌(后面观)Pharyngeal muscles. Posterior aspect ··················· 126

图 261　咽肌(外侧面观)Pharyngeal muscles. Lateral aspect ··················· 127

图 262　咽肌(内侧面观)Pharyngeal muscles. Medial aspect ··················· 127

图 263　食管的狭窄 Esophageal narrow ····································· 128

图 264　胃的形态 Shape of stomach ·· 129

图 265　胃的黏膜 Mucous membrane of stomach ······························ 129

图 266　胃的肌层 Muscular layer of stomach ·································· 130

图 267　胆道、十二指肠和胰 Biliary tract, duodenum and pancreas ·············· 130

图 268　空肠与回肠 Jejunum and ileum ····································· 131

图 269　结肠 Colon ·· 131

图 270　盲肠及阑尾 Cecum and vermiform appendix ··························· 132

图 271　直肠及肛管 Rectum and anal canal ··································· 132

图 272　直肠及肛管(冠状切面)Rectum and anal canal. Coronal section ··········· 133

图 273　肝的前面 Anterior surface of liver ···································· 133

图 274　肝的脏面 Visceral surface of liver ···································· 134

图 275　肝的膈面 Diaphragmatic surface of liver ······························ 134

图 276　肝门静脉 Hepatic portal vein ······································· 135

图 277　肝静脉(膈面观)Hepatic vein. Diaphragmatic aspect ··················· 135

图 278　肝脏管道铸型(脏面观)Cast of hepatic duct. Visceral aspect ············· 136

图 279　肝裂与肝段 Hepatic fissure and hepatic segments ····················· 136

图 280　胆囊与输胆管道(1)Gallbladder and biliary pore(1) ··················· 137

图 281　胆囊与输胆管道(2)Gallbladder and biliary pore(2) ··················· 137

第六章　呼吸系统 Respiratory System ································· **138**

图 282　呼吸系统全貌 General arrangement of respiratory system ·································· 138

图 283　鼻腔外侧壁（1）Lateral wall of nasal cavity（1）·································· 139

图 284　鼻腔外侧壁（2）Lateral wall of nasal cavity（2）·································· 139

图 285　鼻旁窦 Paranasal sinuses ·································· 140

图 286　喉软骨（前面观）Laryngeal cartilages. Anterior aspect ·································· 141

图 287　喉软骨（后面观）Laryngeal cartilages. Posterior aspect ·································· 141

图 288　喉软骨（侧面观）Larygeal cartilages. Lateral aspect ·································· 142

图 289　弹性圆锥和方形膜（侧面观）Elastic cone and quadrangular membrane.
　　　　Lateral aspect ·································· 142

图 290　弹性圆锥和方形膜（上面观）Elastic cone and quadrangular membrane.
　　　　Superior aspect ·································· 143

图 291　弹性圆锥（上面观）Elastic cone. Superior aspect ·································· 143

图 292　喉软骨及声韧带（上面观）Laryngeal cartilage and vocal ligament. Superior aspect ·································· 143

图 293　喉肌（前面观）Muscles of larynx. Anterior aspect ·································· 144

图 294　喉肌（后面观）Muscles of larynx. Posterior aspect ·································· 144

图 295　喉肌（侧面观）Muscles of larynx. Lateral aspect ·································· 145

图 296　喉的横切面（通过声门裂）Transverse section of larynx. Through the level
　　　　of fissure of glottis ·································· 145

图 297　喉口（上面观）Aperture of larynx. Superior aspect ·································· 145

图 298　喉冠状切（后面观）Coronal section of larynx. Posterior aspect ·································· 146

图 299　喉（矢状切面）Larynx. Sagittal section ·································· 146

图 300　气管与支气管（前面观）Trachea and bronchi. Anterior aspect ·································· 147

图 301　气管与支气管（后面观）Trachea and bronchi. Posterior aspect ·································· 147

图 302　喉、气管和肺 Larynx，trachea and lungs ·································· 148

图 303　肺门 Hilum of lung ·································· 149

图 304　肺根的结构 Structures of pedicle of lung ·································· 150

图 305　气管隆嵴 Carina of trachea ·································· 151

图 306　肺段支气管 Segmental bronchi ·································· 151

图 307　支气管肺段（外侧面观）Bronchopulmonary segments. Lateral aspect ·································· 152

图 308　胸膜顶的毗邻 Adjacent structures of cupula of pleura ·································· 152

图 309　胸膜与肺的体表投影 Body surface projection of pleura and lung ·································· 153

图 310　纵隔（右侧面观）Mediastinum. Right aspect ·································· 154

图 311　纵隔（左侧面观）Mediastinum. Left aspect ·································· 154

第七章　泌尿生殖系统 Urogenital System ································· **155**

图 312　男性泌尿生殖系统全貌 General arrangement of the male urogenital system ·································· 155

图 313　肾与输尿管 Kidney and ureter ·································· 156

图 314　腹后壁 Posterior abdominal wall ·································· 157

图 315　肾的体表投影（后面观）Body surface projection of kidney. Posterior aspect ·································· 158

图 316　肾周围的关系（前面观）Relation of kidney with peripheral organs. Anterior aspect ·································· 159

图 317　肾周围的关系（后面观）Relation of kidney with peripheral organs. Posterior aspect ·································· 159

图 318　肾的被膜（横切面）Coverings of kidney. Transverse section ·············· 160

图 319　肾的被膜（矢状切面）Coverings of kidney. Sagittal section ·············· 160

图 320　肾冠状切面 Coronal section of kidney ···················· 161

图 321　肾窦 Renal sinus ····························· 161

图 322　肾盂和肾盏 Renal pelvis and renal calices ·················· 161

图 323　肾动脉 Renal artery ·························· 162

图 324　肾段铸型（前面观）Cast of renal segments. Anterior aspect ············ 162

图 325　肾段铸型（后面观）Cast of renal segments. Posterior aspect ············ 162

图 326　马蹄肾 Horseshoe kidney. Anterior aspect ················ 163

图 327　不完全性重复肾 Incomplete renal duplication ··············· 163

图 328　不完全性重复肾（冠状切面）Incomplete renal duplication. Coronal section ········ 163

图 329　移位肾 Renal ectopia ························· 164

图 330　膀胱（侧面观）Urinary bladder. Lateral aspect ··············· 165

图 331　膀胱（前面观）Urinary bladder. Anterior aspect ·············· 165

图 332　男性盆腔正中矢状切面 Median sagittal section of the male pelvic cavity ······· 166

图 333　女性尿道 Female urethra ······················· 167

图 334　男性生殖系统 Male genital system ·················· 167

图 335　睾丸（外侧面观）Testis. Lateral aspect ················ 168

图 336　睾丸结构（模式图）Structures of testis. Diagram ············· 168

图 337　前列腺（前面观）Prostate. Anterior aspect ··············· 168

图 338　前列腺（后面观）Prostate. Posterior aspect ·············· 169

图 339　前列腺分区（矢状切面）Zonation of prostate. Sagittal section ········· 169

图 340　前列腺分区（横切面）Zonation of prostate. Transverse section ········· 169

图 341　阴囊的结构（模式图）Structure of scrotal. Diagram ············· 170

图 342　阴茎海绵体和尿道海绵体 Cavernous body of urethra and cavernous body of penis ··· 170

图 343　阴茎海绵体（背面观）Cavernous body of penis. Dorsal aspect ········· 171

图 344　尿道海绵体（背面观）Cavernous body of urethra. Dorsal aspect ········ 171

图 345　阴茎的横切面 Transverse section through the body of penis ··········· 172

图 346　阴茎正中矢状切面 Median sagittal section through penis ··········· 172

图 347　男性尿道（背面观）Male urethra. Dorsal aspect ············· 172

图 348　女性盆腔正中矢状切面 Median sagittal section of female pelvic cavity ······· 173

图 349　子宫、输卵管与卵巢（后面观）Uterus, uterine tube and ovary. Posterior aspect ···· 174

图 350　输卵管漏斗 Infundibulum of uterine tube ················ 174

图 351　女性内生殖器（前面观）Female internal genital organs. Anterior aspect ······ 175

图 352　子宫口的形态 Shapes of orifice of uterus ················· 175

图 353　子宫的分部（矢状切面）Distribution of uterus. Sagittal section ········· 176

图 354　子宫姿势的类型 Types of uterine attitude ··············· 176

图 355　子宫的血管 Blood vessels of uterus ················· 177

图 356　子宫的固定装置 Fixed structure of uterus ··············· 177

图 357　子宫阔韧带矢状切面（模式图）Sagittal section of broad ligament of uterus. Diagram ···· 178

图 358　阴蒂、前庭球和前庭大腺 Clitoris, bulb of vestibule and greater vestibular gland ····· 178

第八章　会阴和腹膜 Perineum and Peritoneum ·················· **179**

图 359　会阴的境界和分区（模式图）Perineal milien and zonation. Diagram ······· 179

图 360　女性外生殖器 Female external genital organs ································· 179

图 361　处女膜的类型 Type of hymen ·· 180

图 362　女性乳房 Mamma of female ··· 180

图 363　女性乳房（矢状切面）Mamma of female. Sagittal section ················· 180

图 364　女性盆底肌（上面观）Floor muscles of pelvis in the female. Superior aspect ········· 181

图 365　男性会阴肌 Muscles of male perineum ··· 181

图 366　女性会阴肌 Muscles of female perineum ·· 182

图 367　男性盆腔冠状切面（经直肠、肛管）Coronal section of male pelvic cavity. Through

rectum and anal canal ··· 182

图 368　男性盆腔冠状切面（示尿生殖膈和盆膈）Coronal section of male pelvic cavity. Showing

urogenital diaphragm and pelvic diaphragm ································· 183

图 369　女性盆腔冠状切面（通过子宫和阴道）Coronal section of female pelvis cavity. Through

uterus and vagina ··· 183

图 370　男性盆腔冠状切面（模式图）Coronal section of male pelvic cavity. Diagram ········· 184

图 371　右侧尿生殖膈矢状切面（模式图）Sagittal section of right urogenital diaphragm. Diagram ····· 184

图 372　腹膜与脏器的关系（下面观）Relationship between viscera and peritoneum. Inferior aspect ····· 184

图 373　小网膜及网膜孔 Lesser omentum and omental foramen ···················· 185

图 374　网膜囊及网膜孔（下面观）Omental bursa and omental foramen. Inferior aspect ········· 185

图 375　大网膜 Greater omentum ·· 186

图 376　腹前壁内面的皱襞和窝 Peritoneal folds and fossa on the inner surface of

anterior ventral wall ··· 186

图 377　腹膜形成的结构 Forming structures of peritoneum ··························· 187

图 378　结肠上区的间隙 Interspace of superior region of colon ····················· 187

第九章　心血管系统 Cardiovascular System ··· **188**

图 379　心肺的位置 Location of heart and lung ·· 188

图 380　冠状动脉（前面观）Coronary artery. Anterior aspect ························· 188

图 381　冠状动脉（膈面）Coronary arteries. Diaphragmatic surface ··············· 189

图 382　冠状动脉铸型 Cast of coronary arteries ·· 189

图 383　室间隔的血管 Blood vessels of interventricular septum ···················· 190

图 384　心脏的瓣膜（上面观）Cardiac valves. Superior aspect ······················ 190

图 385　右心房 Right atrium ··· 191

图 386　右心室 Right ventricle ·· 191

图 387　左心室和左心房 Left ventricle and atrium ······································· 192

图 388　室间隔和房间隔 Interventricular septum and interatrial septum ········· 192

图 389　心纤维支架（1）Fibrous framework of the heart（1）······················· 193

图 390　心纤维支架（2）Fibrous framework of the heart（2）······················· 193

图 391　心肌 Cardiac muscles ··· 194

图 392　心室横切面 Transverse section of ventricles ···································· 194

图 393　心传导系（1）Conduction system of the heart（1）·························· 195

图 394　心传导系（2）Conduction system of the heart（2）·························· 195

图 395　冠状动脉的分布类型 Distributional type of coronary artery ··············· 196

图 396　壁冠状动脉 Mural coronary artery ·· 196

图 397　心的静脉（前面观）Cardiac veins. Anterior aspect ……………………………………… 197

图 398　心的静脉（膈面）Cardiac veins. Diaphragmatic surface …………………………… 197

图 399　心包 Pericardium ………………………………………………………………………… 198

图 400　主动脉弓和胸主动脉 Aortic arch and thoracic aorta ………………………………… 199

图 401　胸廓内动脉 Internal thoracic artery …………………………………………………… 199

图 402　腹主动脉及其分支 Abdominal aorta and its branches ……………………………… 200

图 403　颈外动脉及其分支 External carotid artery and its branches ……………………… 201

图 404　颈内动脉和椎动脉 Internal carotid artery and vertebral artery …………………… 201

图 405　锁骨下动脉和腋动脉 Subclavian artery and axillary artery ……………………… 202

图 406　肩部的血管和神经（后面观）Blood vessels and nerves of the shoulder. Posterior aspect ……… 202

图 407　臂部的动脉（前面观）Arteries of arm. Anterior aspect …………………………… 203

图 408　前臂的动脉（前面观）Arteries of forearm. Anterior aspect ……………………… 203

图 409　前臂的动脉（后面观）Arteries of forearm. Posterior aspect ……………………… 204

图 410　手动脉铸型 Cast of arteries of hand …………………………………………………… 204

图 411　手的动脉（前面观 1）Arteries of hand. Anterior aspect（1）………………………… 205

图 412　手的动脉（前面观 2）Arteries of hand. Anterior aspect（2）………………………… 205

图 413　腹壁上动脉与腹壁下动脉 Superior epigastric artery and inferior epigastric artery ……… 206

图 414　腹腔干及其分支（1）Celiac trunk and its branches（1）…………………………… 207

图 415　腹腔干及其分支（2）Celiac trunk and its branches（2）…………………………… 207

图 416　肠系膜上动脉及其分支 Superior mesenteric artery and its branches ……………… 208

图 417　回结肠动脉及其分支 Ileocolic artery and its branches …………………………… 209

图 418　空、回肠动脉弓 Arterial arcades of ileum and jejunum …………………………… 209

图 419　肠系膜下动脉及其分支 Inferior mesenteric artery and its branches ……………… 210

图 420　直肠和肛管的动脉（前面观）Arteries of rectum and anal canal. Anterior aspect ……… 210

图 421　男性盆腔的动脉 Arteries of the male pelvic cavity ………………………………… 211

图 422　阴茎背动脉 Dorsal artery of penis …………………………………………………… 212

图 423　女性盆腔的动脉 Arteries of the female pelvic cavity ……………………………… 213

图 424　会阴部的动脉 Arteries of perineum …………………………………………………… 213

图 425　股部的动脉（前面观）Arteries of thigh. Anterior aspect ………………………… 214

图 426　臀部和股后部的动脉 Arteries of gluteal and posterior femoral regions …………… 215

图 427　小腿的动脉（前面观）Arteries of leg. Anterior aspect …………………………… 216

图 428　小腿的动脉（后面观）Arteries of leg. Posterior aspect …………………………… 216

图 429　足背的动脉 Arteries of the dorsum of foot …………………………………………… 217

图 430　足底的动脉 Plantar arteries …………………………………………………………… 217

图 431　足的动脉铸型（上面观）Cast of arteries of foot. Superior aspect ………………… 218

图 432　足的动脉铸型（下面观）Cast of arteries of foot. Inferior aspect ………………… 218

图 433　静脉瓣 Venous valve …………………………………………………………………… 219

图 434　板障管 Diploic canals ………………………………………………………………… 219

图 435　头颈部的静脉（侧面观）Veins of head and neck. Lateral aspect ………………… 220

图 436　面静脉 Facial vein ……………………………………………………………………… 221

图 437　翼静脉丛 Pterygoid venous plexus …………………………………………………… 221

图 438　上腔静脉及其属支 Superior vena cava and its tributaries ………………………… 222

图 439　双上腔静脉 Double superior vena cava ……………………………………………… 223

图 440　锁骨下静脉和腋静脉 Subclavian vein and axillary vein ················ 223

图 441　上肢浅静脉 Superficial veins of upper limb ················ 224

图 442　手背的浅静脉 Superficial veins of dorsum of hand ················ 224

图 443　椎外前静脉丛(前面观)Anterior external vertebral venous plexus. Anterior aspect ········ 225

图 444　椎外后静脉丛(后面观)Posterior external vertebral venous plexus. Posterior aspect ········ 225

图 445　下腔静脉及其属支 Inferior vena cava and its tributaries ················ 226

图 446　双下腔静脉 Double inferior vena cave ················ 227

图 447　盆部的静脉 Veins of pelvis ················ 228

图 448　肝门静脉及其属支 Hepatic portal vein and its tributaries ················ 229

图 449　大隐静脉及其属支 Great saphenous vein and its tributaries ················ 230

图 450　小隐静脉 Small saphenous vein ················ 231

图 451　足背静脉 Dorsal veins of foot ················ 231

第十章　淋巴系统 Lymphatic System ················ **232**

图 452　淋巴导管 Lymphatic ducts ················ 232

图 453　右位胸导管 Right thoracic duct ················ 232

图 454　颈部的淋巴管和淋巴结(1)Lymph vessels and nodes of neck(1) ················ 233

图 455　颈部的淋巴管和淋巴结(2)Lymph vessels and nodes of neck(2) ················ 233

图 456　颈深部淋巴管和淋巴结(前面观)Deep lymph vessels and nodes of neck. Anterior aspect ······ 234

图 457　喉的淋巴(矢状切面)Laryngeal lymph. Sagittal section ················ 234

图 458　喉部的淋巴(前面观)Laryngeal lymph. Anterior aspect ················ 234

图 459　腋淋巴结 Axillary lymph nodes ················ 235

图 460　胸骨旁淋巴结 Parasternal lymph nodes ················ 235

图 461　纵隔淋巴结(前面观)Mediastinal lymph nodes. Anterior aspect ················ 236

图 462　纵隔淋巴结(后面观)Mediastinal lymph nodes. Posterior aspect ················ 236

图 463　胃的淋巴管和淋巴结 Lymph vessels and nodes of stomach ················ 237

图 464　胆囊的淋巴管 Lymph vessels of gallbladder ················ 237

图 465　肠系膜上淋巴结 Superior mesenteric lymph nodes ················ 238

图 466　肠系膜下淋巴结 Inferior mesenteric lymph nodes ················ 238

图 467　腹膜后间隙的淋巴结 Lymph nodes of retroperitoneal space ················ 239

图 468　直肠旁淋巴结(后面观)Lymph nodes beside rectum. Posterior aspect ················ 239

图 469　男性盆腔淋巴管及淋巴结 Lymph vessels and nodes of male pelvic cavity ················ 240

图 470　女性盆腔淋巴管及淋巴结 Lymph vessels and nodes of female pelvic cavity ················ 240

图 471　腹股沟浅淋巴结 Superficial inguinal lymph nodes ················ 241

图 472　脾 Spleen ················ 241

图 473　下肢淋巴管造影 Lymphangiography of lower limb ················ 242

图 474　淋巴管瓣膜造影 Visualization of lymphatic valve ················ 242

第十一章　视器 Visual Organ ················ **243**

图 475　左眼(前面观)Left eye. Anterior aspect ················ 243

图 476　眶壁、眼球、视神经和视交叉 Orbital wall,eyeball,optic nerve and optic chiasma ················ 243

图 477　眼球水平切面 Horizontal section of the eyeball ················ 244

图 478　眶及眼球的冠状切面(后面观1)Coronal section of orbit and eyeball. Posterior aspect(1) ······ 244

图 479　眶及眼球的冠状切面(后面观 2)Coronal section of orbit and eyeball. Posterior aspect(2) ······ 244

图 480　虹膜和睫状体(后面观)Iris and ciliary body. Posterior aspect ···················· 245

图 481　角膜缘结构 Structures of limbus corneae ·························· 245

图 482　视网膜血管 Blood vessels of retina ···························· 245

图 483　眶及眼球的矢状切面 Sagittal section of orbit and eyeball ·············· 246

图 484　眶周围结构 Peripheral structures of orbit ························ 246

图 485　眼睑部的动脉 Arteries of eyelids ···························· 247

图 486　眼睑部的静脉 Veins of eyelids ···························· 247

图 487　泪器(1)Lacrimal apparatus(1) ·························· 248

图 488　泪器(2)Lacrimal apparatus(2) ·························· 248

图 489　眼外肌(外侧面观)Extraocular muscles. Lateral aspect ·············· 249

图 490　眼外肌(上面观)Extraocular muscles. Superior aspect ·············· 249

图 491　眼外肌(前面观)Extraocular muscles. Anterior aspect ·············· 250

图 492　眶腔的冠状切面 Coronal section of orbital cavity ·················· 250

图 493　眼球筋膜鞘(后面观 1)Sheath of eyeball. Posterior aspect(1) ·········· 251

图 494　眼球筋膜鞘(后面观 2)Sheath of eyeball. Posterior aspect(2) ·········· 251

图 495　眶腔内的血管和神经(上面观)Blood vessels and nerves in the orbital cavity.
　　　　Superior aspect ·································· 252

图 496　眼动脉及其分支(外侧面观)Ophthalmic artery and its branches. Lateral aspect ······ 252

图 497　虹膜的动脉和涡静脉 Arteries of iris and vorticose veins ·············· 253

图 498　眼球的血管 Blood vessels of eyeball ·························· 253

第十二章　前庭蜗器 Vestibulocochlear Organ ·························· **254**

图 499　耳廓 Auricle ···································· 254

图 500　咽鼓管和外耳道 Auditory tube and the external acoustic meatus ·········· 254

图 501　鼓膜(外侧面观)Tympanic membrane. Lateral aspect ·············· 254

图 502　鼓室鼓膜壁(内侧面观)Membranous wall of tympanic cavity. Medial aspect ······ 255

图 503　鼓室迷路壁(外侧面观)Labyrinthine wall of tympanic cavity. Lateral aspect ······ 255

图 504　鼓室(内侧面观)Tympanic cavity. Medial aspect ·················· 255

图 505　乳突、乙状窦和面神经的关系 Relations of the mastoid process,sigmoid sinus
　　　　and facial nerve ································ 256

图 506　听骨链 Chain of auditory ossicles ·························· 256

图 507　听小骨 Auditory ossicles ···························· 256

图 508　前庭蜗器 Vestibulocochlear organ ·························· 257

图 509　骨迷路 Bony labyrinth ···························· 257

图 510　膜迷路 Membranous labyrinth ·························· 258

图 511　骨迷路和膜迷路 Bony labyrinth and membranous labyrinth ·············· 258

图 512　耳蜗(剖面 1)Cochlea. Section(1) ···················· 258

图 513　耳蜗(剖面 2)Cochlea. Section(2) ···················· 259

图 514　声波的传导途径 Conducting pathway of sound wave ·············· 259

图 515　内耳道底 Fundus of internal acoustic meatus ·················· 259

第十三章　中枢神经系统 Central Nervous System ···················· **260**

图 516　脊髓外形 Shape of spinal cord ·························· 260

图 517　脊髓节段和脊神经与椎骨的关系 Relation of segment of spinal cord and spinal
　　　　nerve to the vertebrae ··· 260

图 518　脊髓的颈段（横切面）Cervical segment of spinal cord. Cross section ········· 261

图 519　脊髓的胸段（横切面）Thoracic segment of spinal cord. Cross section ········· 261

图 520　脊髓灰质主要核团 Principal gray nucleus ··· 261

图 521　脊髓与脊神经根 Spinal cord and roots of spinal nerves ··························· 262

图 522　薄束和楔束 Fasciculus gracilis and fasciculus cuneatus ························· 262

图 523　脊髓丘脑侧束和前束 Lateral spinothalamic tract and anterior spinothalamic tract ····· 262

图 524　皮质脊髓前束和侧束 Anterior corticospinal tract and lateral corticospinal tract ····· 263

图 525　牵张反射（模式图）Stretch reflex. Diagram ··· 263

图 526　屈曲反射（模式图）Flexion reflex. Diagram ··· 263

图 527　脑的底面 Basal surface of brain ·· 264

图 528　脑内侧面 Medial surface of brain ·· 264

图 529　脑干（腹面观）Brain stem. Ventral aspect ·· 265

图 530　脑干（背面观）Brain stem. Dorsal aspect ·· 265

图 531　脑干、小脑和第四脑室正中切面 Median section of brain stem,cerebellum
　　　　and the fourth ventricle ·· 266

图 532　小脑冠状切面 Coronal section of cerebellum ··· 266

图 533　第四脑室脉络组织 Tela choroidea of the fourth ventricle ····················· 266

图 534　脑神经核在脑干的投影（背面观）Projection of nuclei of cranial nerves in the
　　　　brain stem. Dorsal aspect ·· 267

图 535　脑神经核基本排列规律 Fundamental arrangement of nuclei of cranial nerves ····· 267

图 536　延髓横切面（经锥体交叉）Transverse section of medulla oblongata. Through the
　　　　decussation of pyramid ·· 268

图 537　延髓横切面（经内侧丘系交叉）Transverse section of medulla oblongata. Through the
　　　　decussation of medial lemniscus ·· 268

图 538　延髓横切面（经橄榄中部）Transverse section of medulla oblongata. Through the
　　　　middle portion of olive ·· 269

图 539　脑桥横切面（经面神经丘）Transverse section of pons. Through the facial colliculus ····· 269

图 540　脑桥横切面（经三叉神经根）Transverse section of pons. Through the root
　　　　of trigeminal nerve ·· 270

图 541　中脑横切面（经下丘）Transverse section of midbrain. Through the inferior colliculus ····· 270

图 542　中脑横切面（经上丘）Transverse section of midbrain. Through the superior colliculus ····· 271

图 543　脑干的动脉 Arteries of brain stem ··· 271

图 544　小脑（上面观）Cerebellum. Superior aspect ··· 272

图 545　小脑（下面观）Cerebellum. Inferior aspect ·· 272

图 546　小脑（前面观）Cerebellum. Anterior aspect ··· 272

图 547　小脑水平切面 Horizontal section of cerebellum ····································· 273

图 548　小脑脚（1）Peduncles of cerebellum（1）·· 273

图 549　小脑脚（2）Peduncles of cerebellum（2）·· 273

图 550　小脑齿状核和小脑脚 Dentate nucleus and peduncles of cerebellum ········· 274

图 551　间脑内侧面 Medial surface of diencephalon ··· 274

图 552　间脑的背面 Dorsal surface of diencephalon ··· 274

图 553　下丘脑的主要核团(矢状切面)Hypothalamic main nuclei. Sagittal section ·················· 275

图 554　下丘脑的纤维联系(矢状切面)Hypothalamic fiber connection. Sagittal section ·········· 275

图 555　脑外侧面(1)Lateral surface of brain(1) ·· 275

图 556　脑外侧面(2)Lateral surface of brain(2) ·· 276

图 557　岛叶 Insular lobe ·· 276

图 558　大脑半球内侧面 Medial surface of the cerebral hemisphere ····························· 277

图 559　端脑底面 Basal surface of telencephalon ··· 277

图 560　海马结构 Hippocampal formation ··· 278

图 561　人体各部在第Ⅰ躯体运动区的定位 Localization of different parts of human body
　　　　in primary somatomotor area ··· 278

图 562　人体各部在第Ⅰ躯体感觉区的定位 Localization of different parts of human body
　　　　in primary somesthetic area ··· 278

图 563　大脑皮质主要功能区(外侧面观)Main functional areas of cerebral cortex. Lateral aspect ········ 279

图 564　大脑皮质主要功能区(内侧面观)Main functional areas of cerebral cortex. Medial aspect ········ 279

图 565　基底核、背侧丘脑和内囊 Basal nuclei,dorsal thalamus and internal capsule ········ 280

图 566　基底核(内侧面观)Basal nuclei. Medial aspect ··· 280

图 567　基底核(外侧面观)Basal nuclei. Lateral aspect ··· 280

图 568　侧脑室(上面观)Lateral ventricle. Superior aspect ·· 281

图 569　海马旁回与海马结构的切面 Section through the parahippocampal gyrus and the
　　　　hippocampal formation ··· 281

图 570　脑室铸型(侧面观)Cast of ventricles of brain. Lateral aspect ·························· 282

图 571　脑室铸型(后面观)Cast of ventricles of brain. Posterior aspect ······················· 282

图 572　大脑半球内联络纤维 Association fibers in the cerebral hemisphere ···················· 283

图 573　穹隆和穹隆连合 Fornix and the commissure of fornix ····································· 283

图 574　扣带和胼胝体的辐射纤维 Fibers of cingulum and radiation of corpus callosum ········· 284

图 575　扣带 Cingulum ·· 284

图 576　锥体束 Pyramidal tract ·· 285

图 577　锥体交叉 Decussation of pyramid ·· 285

图 578　视束和视辐射 Optic tract and optic radiation ·· 286

图 579　内、外侧丘系 Medial and lateral lemniscus ·· 287

图 580　面神经在脑内的行路 Pathway of facial nerve in brain ····································· 287

图 581　内囊主要结构(模式图)Main structure of internal capsule. Diagram ················· 288

图 582　胼胝体(上面观)Corpus callosum. Superior aspect ··· 288

第十四章　周围神经系统 Peripheral Nervous System ·· **289**

图 583　脊神经 Spinal nerves ··· 289

图 584　颈丛的组成及颈襻 Formation of cervical plexus and ansa cervicalis ·················· 289

图 585　颈丛的皮支及分布 Distribution of cutaneous branches of cervical plexus ············ 290

图 586　膈神经 Phrenic nerve ·· 290

图 587　臂丛的组成 Formation of brachial plexus ··· 291

图 588　臂丛的主要分支 Main branches of brachial plexus ··· 291

图 589　上肢的神经 Nerves of upper limb ·· 292

图 590　臂部的神经(前面观)Nerves of arm. Anterior aspect ····································· 293

图 591 臂部的神经（后面观）Nerves of arm. Posterior aspect ·· 293

图 592 前臂的神经（前面观）Nerves of forearm. Anterior aspect ··· 294

图 593 前臂的神经（后面观）Nerves of forearm. Posterior aspect ······································· 294

图 594 手的神经（前面观1）Nerves of hand. Anterior aspect（1）··· 295

图 595 手的神经（前面观2）Nerves of hand. Anterior aspect（2）··· 295

图 596 手的神经（后面观）Nerves of hand. Posterior aspect ·· 296

图 597 肋间神经 Intercostal nerve ·· 296

图 598 胸神经前支的分布（前面观）Distribution of anterior branches of thoracic
nerve. Anterior aspect ·· 297

图 599 胸神经前支的分布（侧面观）Distribution of anterior branches of thoracic nerve.
Lateral aspect ·· 298

图 600 腹部肌的神经支配 Innervation of abdominal muscles ·· 299

图 601 背部皮神经的分布 Distribution of dorsal cutaneous nerves ·· 300

图 602 腰骶丛的组成 Formation of lumbar and sacral plexus ··· 301

图 603 腰骶丛 Lumbar and sacral plexus ·· 302

图 604 男性阴部神经 Male pudendal nerve ·· 303

图 605 女性会阴部的神经 Nerves of female perineum ··· 303

图 606 股部的神经（前面观）Nerves of thigh. Anterior aspect ·· 304

图 607 股部的神经（后面观1）Nerves of thigh. Posterior aspect（1）····································· 305

图 608 股部的神经（后面观2）Nerves of thigh. Posterior aspect（2）····································· 305

图 609 小腿的神经（前面观）Nerves of leg. Anterior aspect ·· 306

图 610 小腿的神经（后面观1）Nerves of leg. Posterior aspect（1）·· 306

图 611 小腿的神经（后面观2）Nerves of leg. Posterior aspect（2）·· 307

图 612 足背的神经 Dorsal nerves of foot ·· 307

图 613 足底的神经（1）Plantar nerves of foot（1）··· 308

图 614 足底的神经（2）Plantar nerves of foot（2）··· 308

图 615 脑神经（外侧面观1）Cranial nerves. Lateral aspect（1）··· 309

图 616 脑神经（外侧面观2）Cranial nerves. Lateral aspect（2）··· 310

图 617 眶腔内神经（外侧面观）Nerves in the orbital cavity. Lateral aspect ····························· 311

图 618 眶腔内神经（上面观）Nerves in the orbital cavity. Superior aspect ······························ 311

图 619 三叉神经 Trigeminal nerve ·· 312

图 620 下颌神经 Maxillary nerve ··· 312

图 621 上、下牙槽神经 Superior and inferior alveolar nerves ··· 313

图 622 眼外肌的神经与海绵窦 Cavernous sinus and nerves of extraocular muscles ···················· 313

图 623 面神经分支（1）Branches of facial nerve（1）··· 314

图 624 面神经分支（2）Branches of facial nerve（2）··· 315

图 625 鼓索、翼腭神经节与耳神经节 Chorda tympani, pterygopalatine ganglion and otic
ganglion ··· 316

图 626 舌咽神经和舌下神经 Glossopharyngeal and hypoglossal nerves ·································· 316

图 627 舌咽神经和迷走神经（后面观）Glossopharyngeal and vagus nerves. Posterior aspect ········ 317

图 628 舌咽神经的颈动脉窦支 Carotid sinus branch of glossopharyngeal nerve ······················· 318

图 629 喉部的神经（后面观）Nerves of the laryngeal cavity. Posterior aspect ························· 318

图 630 舌咽神经、迷走神经和副神经的分布 Distribution of glossopharyngeal, vagus and accessory nerves ································ 319

图 631 左侧喉返神经 Left recurrent laryngeal nerve ································ 320

图 632 右侧喉返神经 Right recurrent laryngeal nerve ································ 320

图 633 迷走神经的胃部分支(1)Gastric branches of vagus nerve(1)································ 321

图 634 迷走神经的胃部分支(2)Gastric branches of vagus nerve(2)································ 321

图 635 舌咽神经、迷走神经和副神经(后面观)Glossopharyngeal,vagus and accessory
nerves. Posterior aspect ································ 322

图 636 交感神经纤维走行(模式图)Course of sympathetic nerve. Diagram ································ 322

图 637 内脏运动神经(模式图)Diagram of viscera motor nerves ································ 323

图 638 交感干和交感干神经节 Sympathetic trunk and ganglia ································ 324

图 639 灰、白交通支 Grey and white communicating branches ································ 325

图 640 颈交感干和颈神经节 Cervical sympathetic trunk and cervical ganglia ································ 325

图 641 胸交感干和胸神经节 Thoracic sympathetic trunk and thoracic ganglia ································ 326

图 642 腰交感干和腰神经节 Lumbar sympathetic trunk and lumbar ganglia ································ 326

图 643 盆部内脏神经丛 Splanchnic plexus of pelvic part ································ 327

图 644 副交感神经的分布 Distribution of parasympathetic nerves ································ 327

图 645 心传入神经与皮肤传入神经中枢投射关系 Projectrelationship of the centers
between heart and skin afferent nerves ································ 328

图 646 肝胆牵涉性痛 Referred pain of liver and gallbladder ································ 328

第十五章 神经的传导通路 Nervous Pathways ································ **329**

图 647 躯干和四肢意识性本体感觉传导通路 Conscious proprioceptive pathway
of trunk and limbs ································ 329

图 648 躯干和四肢非意识性本体感觉传导通路 Unconscious proprioceptive
pathway of trunk and limbs ································ 329

图 649 痛温觉、粗略触觉和压觉传导通路 Pain,thermal,rude tactile and pressure
sensation pathways ································ 330

图 650 视觉传导通路 Visual pathway ································ 331

图 651 听觉传导通路 Auditory pathway ································ 332

图 652 平衡觉传导通路 Equilibratory sensation pathway ································ 332

图 653 皮质脊髓束与皮质核束 Corticospinal tract and corticonuclear tract ································ 333

图 654 皮质核束 Corticonuclear tract ································ 334

图 655 皮质-脑桥-小脑-皮质环路 Corticoponto-cerebellar-cortex circuit ································ 334

图 656 面神经瘫 Paralysis of the facial nerve ································ 335

图 657 舌下神经瘫 Paralysis of the hypoglossal nerve ································ 335

第十六章 脑和脊髓的被膜、血管及脑脊液循环 Meninges,Blood Vessels and Cerebrospinal Fluid
Circulation of Brain and Spinal Cord ································ **336**

图 658 脊髓的被膜 Coverings of spinal cord ································ 336

图 659 脑的被膜、蛛网膜粒和硬脑膜窦 Meninges of brain,arachnoid granulation and
sinuses of dura mater ································ 336

图 660 硬脑膜及硬脑膜窦 Cerebral dura mater and sinuses of dura mater ································ 337

图 661 海绵窦(冠状切面)Cavernous sinus. Coronal section ································ 337

图 662　脑动脉 Cerebral arteries ··· 338

图 663　脑底动脉 Arteries at the base of brain ··· 338

图 664　大脑外侧面的动脉 Arteries of lateral surface of cerebrum ····················· 339

图 665　大脑内侧面的动脉 Arteries of medial surface of cerebrum ···················· 339

图 666　大脑中动脉的皮质支和中央支 Central branches and cortical branches
　　　　of middle cerebral arteries ··· 340

图 667　大脑浅静脉(外侧面观)Superficial veins of cerebrum. Lateral aspect ········· 340

图 668　大脑的静脉(内侧面观)Veins of the cerebrum. Medial aspect ·················· 341

图 669　大脑大静脉及其属支 Great cerebral vein and its tributaries ···················· 341

图 670　脊髓动脉(前面观)Spinal arteries. Anterior aspect ·································· 342

图 671　脊髓动脉(后面观)Spinal arteries. Posterior aspect ································ 342

图 672　脊髓内部的血管分布 Distribution of vessels in spinal cord ····················· 343

图 673　脑脊液循环 Circulation of cerebrospinal fluid ·· 343

第十七章　内分泌系统 Endocrine System ··· **344**

图 674　垂体 Hypophysis ··· 344

图 675　松果体 Pineal body ·· 344

图 676　胸腺 Thymus ··· 344

图 677　甲状腺 Thyroid gland ·· 345

图 678　甲状旁腺 Parathyroid gland ··· 345

图 679　胰 Pancreas ·· 345

图 680　肾上腺 Suprarenal gland ·· 346

图 681　睾丸 Testis ·· 346

图 682　卵巢(后面观)Ovary. Posterior aspect ·· 346

第一章 绪论 Introduction

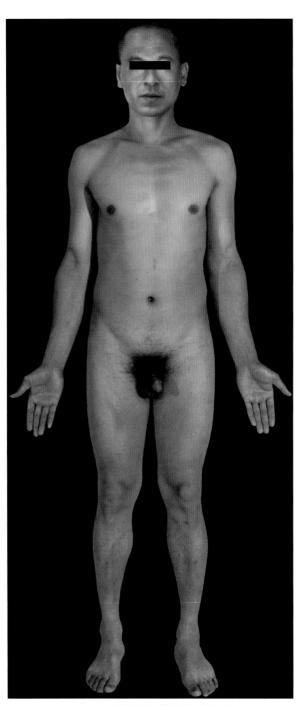

▲ 图 1 人体解剖学姿势（前面观）
Anatomical position. Anterior aspect

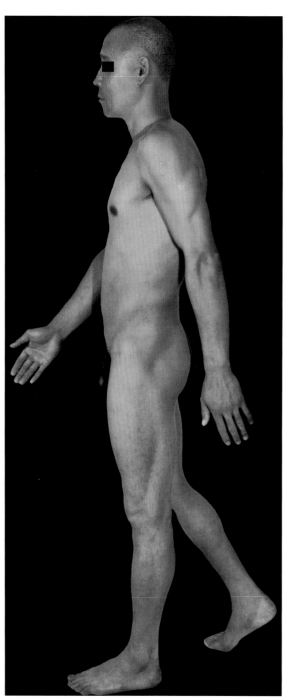

▲ 图 2 人体侧面观
Lateral aspect of human body

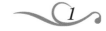

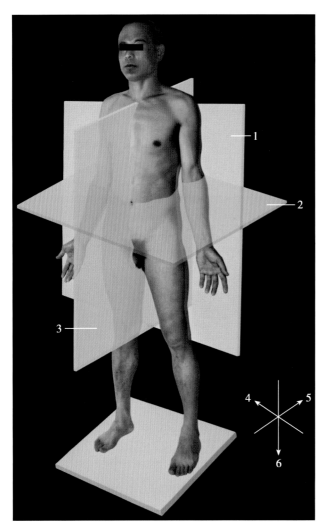

▲ 图3　人体的轴和面
Body axes and planes
1. 冠状面 coronal plane
2. 水平面 horizontal plane
3. 矢状面 sagittal plane
4. 冠状轴 frontal axis
5. 矢状轴 sagittal axis
6. 垂直轴 vertical axis

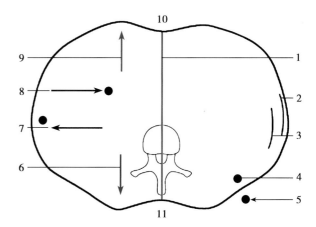

▲ 图4　人体的方向术语
Directional terms

1. 正中 center	7. 外侧 lateral
2. 浅 superficial	8. 内侧 medial
3. 深 deep	9. 前方 anterior
4. 内 internal	10. 腹侧 ventral
5. 外 external	11. 背侧 dorsal
6. 后方 posterior	

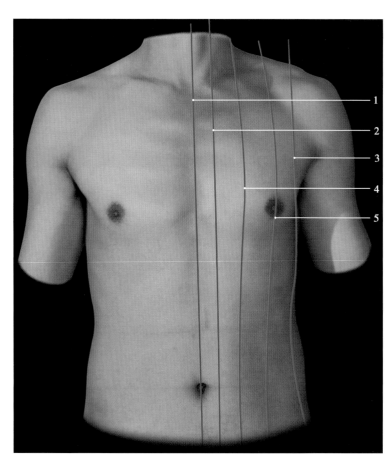

◀ 图 5

躯干的标志线（前面观）
Reference lines of trunk. Anterior aspect
1. 前正中线 anterior median line
2. 胸骨线 sternal line
3. 腋前线 anterior axillary line
4. 胸骨旁线 parasternal line
5. 锁骨中线 midclavicular line

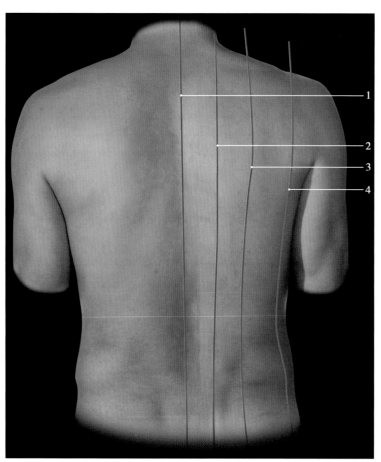

◀ 图 6

躯干的标志线（后面观）
Reference lines of trunk. Posterior aspect
1. 后正中线 posterior median line
2. 脊柱旁线 paravertebral line
3. 肩胛线 scapular line
4. 腋后线 posterior axillary line

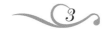

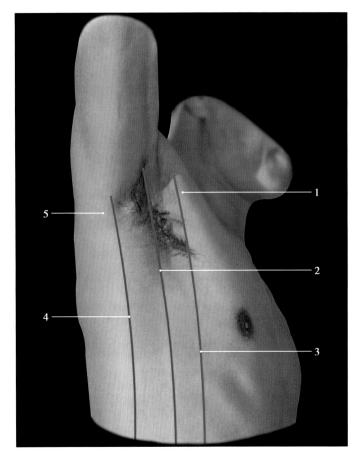

◀ 图 7

躯干的标志线（侧面观）
Reference lines of trunk. Lateral aspect
1. 腋前襞 anterior axillary fold
2. 腋中线 midaxillary line
3. 腋前线 anterior axillary line
4. 腋后线 posterior axillary line
5. 腋后襞 posterior axillary fold

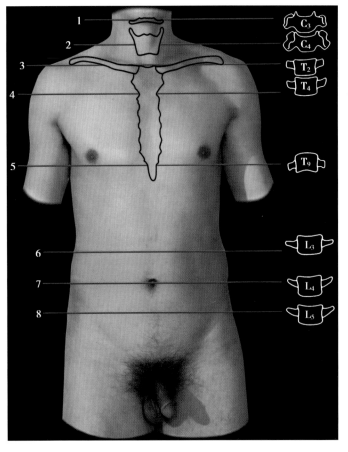

◀ 图 8

躯干的标志线（水平线）
Horizontal reference lines of trunk
1. 舌骨平面（平 C_3）level of hyoid bone. level of the 3rd cervical vertebra
2. 甲状软骨平面（平 C_4）level of thyroid cartilage. level of the 4th cervical vertebra
3. 颈静脉切迹平面（平 T_2）jugular notch plane. level of the 2nd thoracic vertebra
4. 胸骨角平面（平 T_4）sternal angle plane. level of the 4th thoracic vertebra
5. 剑胸结合平面（平 T_9）xiphisternal synchondrosis plane. level of the 9th thoracic vertebra
6. 肋下平面（平 L_3）subcostal plane. level of the 3rd lumbar vertebra
7. 脐平面（平 L_4）umbilical plane. level of the 4th lumbar vertebra
8. 棘间平面（平 L_5）interspinous plane. level of the 5th lumbar vertebra

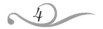

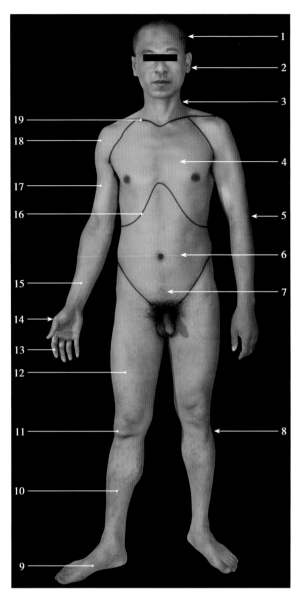

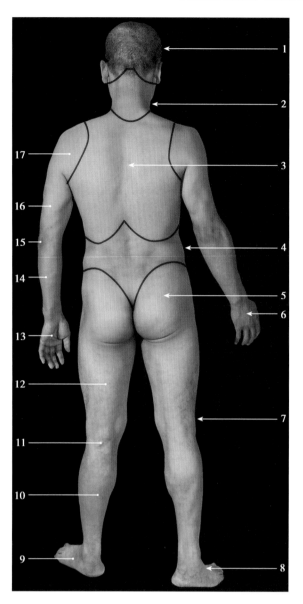

▲ 图9 人体的体表分区（前面观）
Body regions. Anterior aspect

1. 头 head
2. 面 face
3. 颈 neck
4. 胸 thorax
5. 上肢 upper limb
6. 腹 abdomen
7. 盆部 pelvis
8. 下肢 lower limb
9. 足 foot
10. 小腿 leg
11. 膝 knee
12. 股 thigh
13. 手指 finger
14. 手 hand
15. 前臂 forearm
16. 肋弓 costal arch
17. 臂 arm
18. 肩 shoulder
19. 锁骨 clavicle

▲ 图10 人体的体表分区（后面观）
Body regions. Posterior aspect

1. 头 head
2. 颈 neck
3. 背 back
4. 腰区 lumbar region
5. 臀区 gluteal region
6. 手背 back of hand
7. 下肢 lower limb
8. 足背 dorsum of foot
9. 足 foot
10. 小腿 leg
11. 腘窝 popliteal fossa
12. 股 thigh
13. 手掌 palm of hand
14. 前臂 forearm
15. 肘 elbow
16. 臂 arm
17. 肩后区 posterior shoulder region

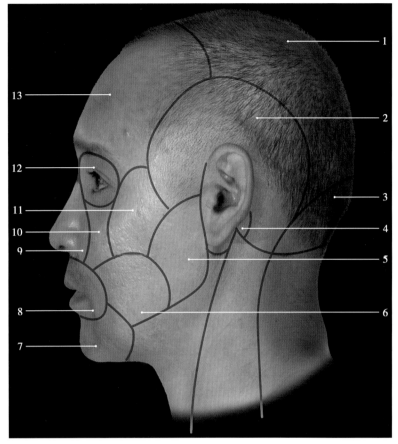

◀ 图 11

头面部的分区
Regions of head and face

1. 顶区 parietal region
2. 颞区 temporal region
3. 枕区 occipital region
4. 耳区 auricular region
5. 腮腺咬肌区 parotideomassetertic region
6. 颊区 buccal region
7. 颏区 mental region
8. 口区 oral region
9. 鼻区 nasal region
10. 眶下区 infraorbital region
11. 颧区 zygomatic region
12. 眶区 orbital region
13. 额区 frontal region

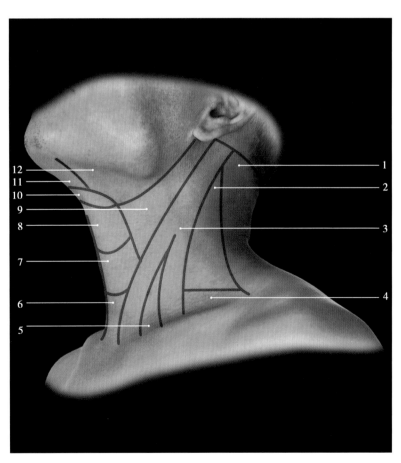

◀ 图 12

颈部的分区
Regions of neck

1. 颈后区 posterior region of neck
2. 枕三角 occipital triangle
3. 胸锁乳突肌区 sternocleidomastoid region
4. 锁骨上大窝 greater supraclavicular fossa
5. 锁骨上小窝 lesser supraclavicular fossa
6. 颈静脉窝 jugular fossa
7. 甲状腺区 thyroid region
8. 喉区 laryngeal region
9. 颈动脉三角 carotid triangle
10. 舌骨区 hyoid region
11. 颏下三角 submental triangle
12. 下颌下三角 submandibular triangle

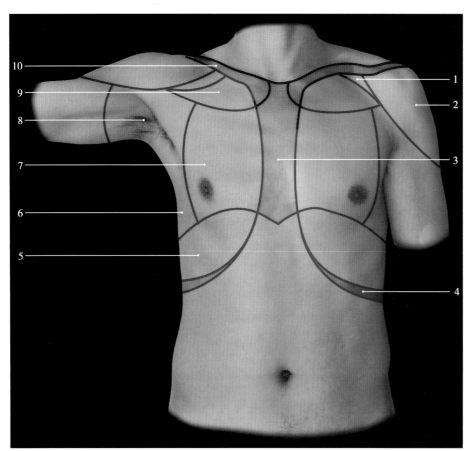

◀ 图 13
胸部的分区
Thoracic regions
1. 胸三角肌三角 deltopectoral triangle
2. 三角肌区 deltoid region
3. 胸骨区 sternal region
4. 肋骨弓 costal arch
5. 季肋区 hypochondriac region
6. 胸外侧区 lateral thoracic region
7. 乳房区 mammary region
8. 腋区 axillary region
9. 锁骨下区 infraclavicular region
10. 锁骨区 clavicular region

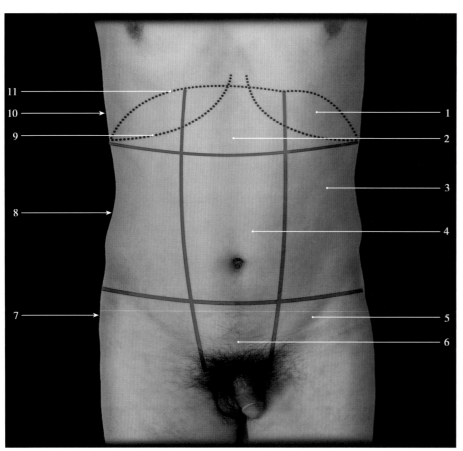

◀ 图 14
腹部的分区
Abdominal regions
1. 季肋区 hypochondriac region
2. 腹上区 epigastric region
3. 腹外侧区 lateral region of abdomen
4. 脐区 umbilical region
5. 腹股沟区 inguinal region
6. 耻区 pubic region
7. 下腹部 inferior abdomen
8. 中腹部 middle abdomen
9. 肋弓 costal arch
10. 上腹部 superior abdomen
11. 膈 diaphragm

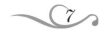

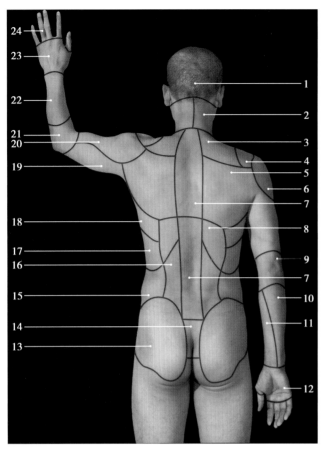

◀ 图15

背部和上肢的分区
Regions of back and upper limb
1. 枕区 occipital region
2. 颈后区 posterior region of neck
3. 肩胛上区 suprascapalar region
4. 肩峰区 acromial region
5. 肩胛区 scapular region
6. 三角肌区 deltoid region
7. 脊柱区 vertebral region
8. 肩胛下区 infrascapular region
9. 肘后区 posterior cubital region
10. 前臂后区 posterior antebrachial region
11. 前臂前区 anterior antebrachial region
12. 手掌 palm of hand
13. 臀区 gluteal region
14. 骶区 sacral region
15. 腹外侧区 lateral region of abdomen
16. 腰区 lumbar region
17. 季肋区 hypochondriac region
18. 胸外侧区 lateral thoracic region
19. 臂后区 posterior brachial region
20. 臂前区 anterior brachial region
21. 肘区 cubital area
22. 前臂后区 posterior antebrachial region
23. 手背 dorsum of hand
24. 手指 fingers

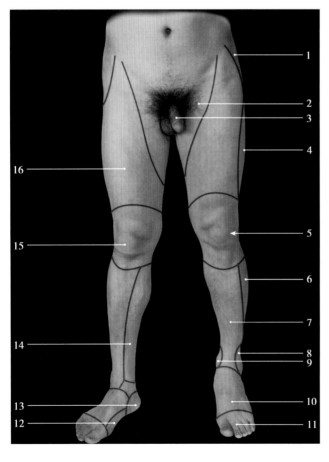

◀ 图16

下肢的分区(前面观)
Regions of lower limb. Anterior aspect
1. 臀区 gluteal region
2. 股内侧区 medial region of thigh
3. 外阴区 pudendal region
4. 股外侧区 lateral region of thigh
5. 膝 knee
6. 小腿后区 posterior crural region
7. 小腿前区 anterior crural region
8. 外踝 lateral malleolus
9. 内踝 medial malleolus
10. 足背 dorsum of foot
11. 足趾 toes
12. 足底 sole of foot
13. 跟区 calcaneal region
14. 小腿后区 posterior crural region
15. 髌骨 patella
16. 股前区 anterior region of thigh

第二章　骨学 Osteology

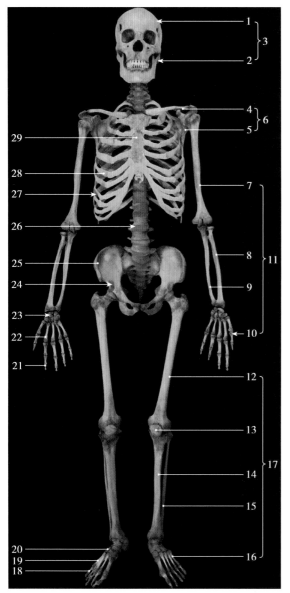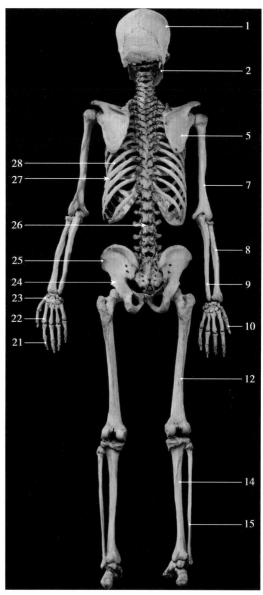

▲ 图 17　全身骨骼
Skeleton

1. 脑颅骨 cranial bone
2. 面颅骨 facial bone
3. 颅骨 skull
4. 锁骨 clavicle
5. 肩胛骨 scapula
6. 上肢带骨 shoulder girdle
7. 肱骨 humerus
8. 桡骨 radius
9. 尺骨 ulna
10. 手骨 bones of hand

11. 自由上肢骨 bones of free upper limb
12. 股骨 femur
13. 髌骨 patella
14. 胫骨 tibia
15. 腓骨 fibula
16. 足骨 bones of foot
17. 自由下肢骨 bones of free lower limb
18. 趾骨 phalanges of toes
19. 跖骨 metatarsal bones
20. 跗骨 tarsal bones

21. 指骨 phalanges of fingers
22. 掌骨 metacarpal bones
23. 腕骨 carpal bones
24. 骨盆 pelvis
25. 髋骨 hip bone
26. 脊柱 vertebral column
27. 胸廓 bones of free lower limb
28. 肋骨 costal bone
29. 胸骨 sternum

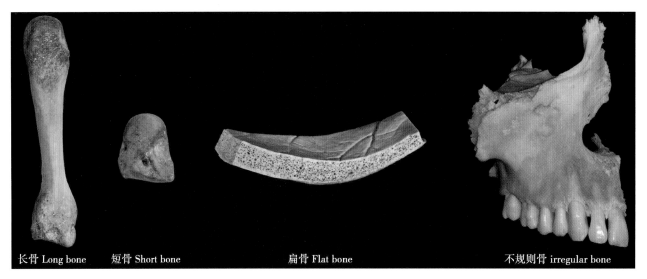

長骨 Long bone　　短骨 Short bone　　　　扁骨 Flat bone　　　　　　　不规则骨 irregular bone

▲ 图 18　骨的分类
Classification of bones

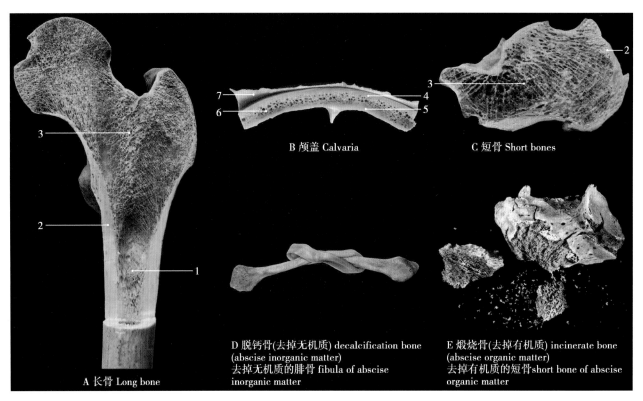

B 颅盖 Calvaria

C 短骨 Short bones

D 脱钙骨(去掉无机质) decalcification bone
(abscise inorganic matter)
去掉无机质的腓骨 fibula of abscise
inorganic matter

E 煅烧骨(去掉有机质) incinerate bone
(abscise organic matter)
去掉有机质的短骨 short bone of abscise
organic matter

A 长骨 Long bone

▲ 图 19　骨的内部构造
Interior of different bones

1. 髓腔 medullary cavity	5. 内板 inner plate
2. 骨密质 compact bone	6. 板障 diploë
3. 骨松质 spongy bone	7. 骨膜 periosteum
4. 外板 outer plate	

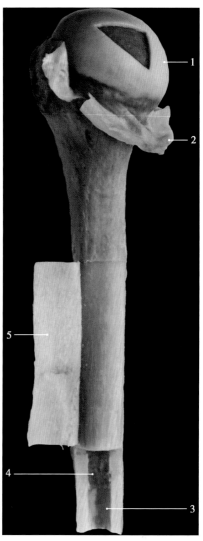

▲ 图 20　**长骨的构造**
Structure of long bone

1. 关节软骨 articular cartilage
2. 关节囊 articular capsule
3. 髓腔 medullary cavity
4. 骨髓 bone marrow
5. 骨膜 periosteum

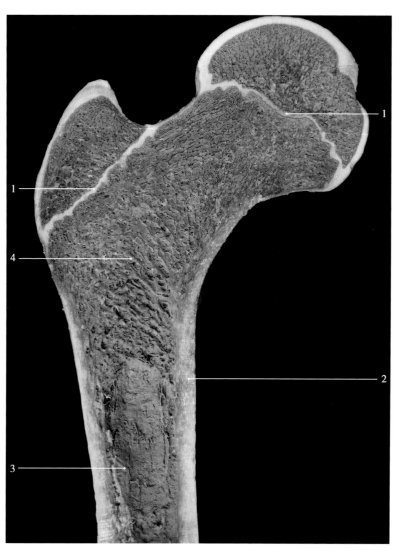

▲ 图 21　**骺软骨**
Epiphysial cartilage

1. 骺软骨 epiphysial cartilage
2. 骨密质 compact bone
3. 髓腔 medullary cavity
4. 骨松质 spongy bone

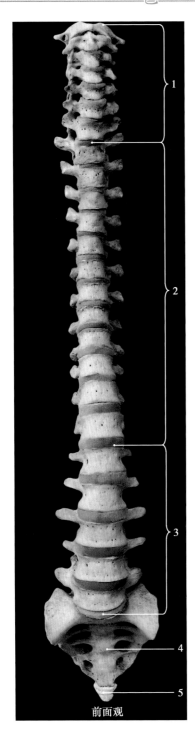

前面观

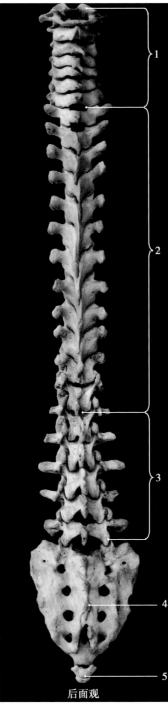

后面观

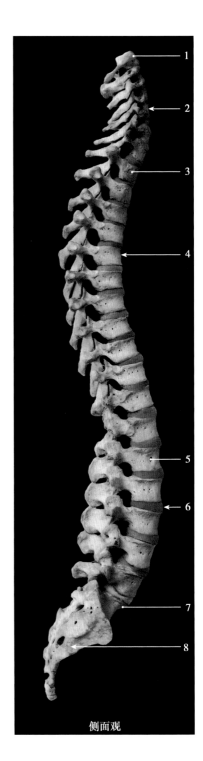

侧面观

▲ 图22 **脊柱**
Vertebral column

1. 颈椎 cervical vertebrae
2. 胸椎 thoracic vertebrae
3. 腰椎 lumbar vertebrae
4. 骶骨 sacrum
5. 尾骨 coccyx

1. 颈椎 cervical vertebrae
2. 胸椎 thoracic vertebrae
3. 腰椎 lumbar vertebrae
4. 骶骨 sacrum
5. 尾骨 coccyx

1. 寰椎 atlas
2. 颈曲 cervical curve
3. 第1胸椎 the 1st thoracic vertebra
4. 胸曲 thoracic curve
5. 第1腰椎 the 1st lumbar vertebra
6. 腰曲 lumbar curve
7. 岬 promontory
8. 骶曲 sacrum curve

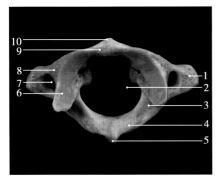

▲ 图23　寰椎（上面观）
Atlas. Superior aspect

1. 横突 transverse process
2. 椎孔 vertebral foramen
3. 椎动脉沟 groove for vertebral a.
4. 后弓 posterior arch
5. 后结节 posterior tubercle
6. 上关节面 superior articular surface
7. 横突孔 transverse foramen
8. 侧块 lateral mass
9. 前弓 anterior arch
10. 前结节 anterior tubercle

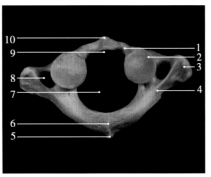

▲ 图24　寰椎（下面观）
Atlas. Inferior aspect

1. 前弓 anterior arch
2. 下关节面 inferior articular surface
3. 横突 transverse process
4. 侧块 lateral mass
5. 后结节 posterior tubercle
6. 后弓 posterior arch
7. 椎孔 vertebral foramen
8. 横突孔 transverse foramen
9. 齿突凹 dental fovea
10. 前结节 anterior tubercle

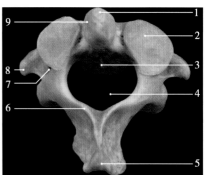

▲ 图25　枢椎（上面观）
Axis. Superior aspect

1. 齿突尖 apex of dens
2. 上关节面 superior articular surface
3. 椎体 vertebral body
4. 椎孔 vertebral foramen
5. 棘突 spinous process
6. 椎弓 vertebral arch
7. 横突孔 transverse foramen
8. 横突 transverse process
9. 齿突 dens

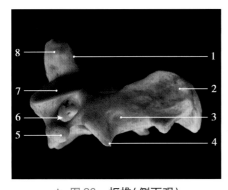

▲ 图26　枢椎（侧面观）
Axis. Lateral aspect

1. 后关节面 posterior articular facet
2. 棘突 spinous process
3. 椎弓 vertebral arch
4. 下关节突 inferior articular process
5. 横突 transverse process
6. 横突孔 transverse foramen
7. 上关节面 superior articular surface
8. 齿突 dens

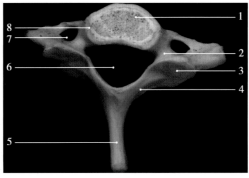

▲ 图27　颈椎（上面观）
Cervical vertebra. Superior aspect

1. 椎体 vertebral body
2. 椎弓根 pedicle of vertebral arch
3. 上关节突 superior articular process
4. 椎弓 vertebral arch
5. 棘突 spinous process
6. 椎孔 vertebral foramen
7. 横突孔 transverse foramen
8. 椎体钩 uncus of vertebral body

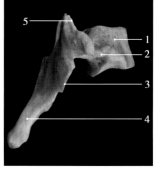

▲ 图28　颈椎（侧面观）
Cervical vertebra.
Lateral aspect

1. 椎体 vertebral body
2. 横突 transverse process
3. 下关节突 inferior articular process
4. 棘突 spinous process
5. 上关节突 superior articular process

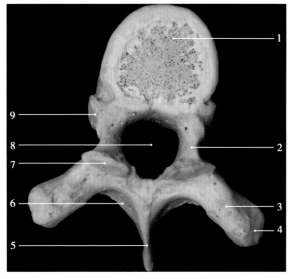

▲ 图 29　胸椎（上面观）
Thoracic vertebra. Superior aspect
1. 椎体 vertebral body
2. 椎弓根 pedicle of vertebral arch
3. 横突 transverse process
4. 横突肋凹 transverse costal fovea
5. 棘突 spinous process
6. 椎弓板 lamina of vertebral arch
7. 上关节突 superior articular process
8. 椎孔 vertebral foramen
9. 上肋凹 superior costal fovea

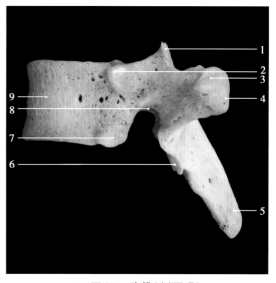

▲ 图 30　胸椎（侧面观）
Thoracic vertebra. Lateral aspect
1. 上关节突 superior articular process
2. 上肋凹 superior costal fovea
3. 横突肋凹 transverse costal fovea
4. 横突 transverse process
5. 棘突 spinous process
6. 下关节突 inferior articular process
7. 下肋凹 inferior costal fovea
8. 椎下切迹 inferior vertebral notch
9. 椎体 vertebral body

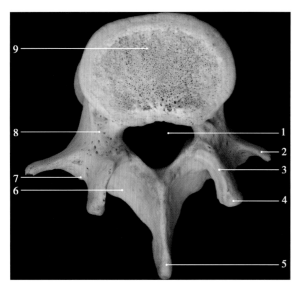

▲ 图 31　腰椎（上面观）
Lumbar vertebra. Superior aspect
1. 椎孔 vertebral foramen
2. 横突 transverse process
3. 上关节突 superior articular process
4. 乳突 mamillary process
5. 棘突 spinous process
6. 椎弓板 lamina of vertebral arch
7. 副突 accessory process
8. 椎弓根 pedicle of vertebral arch
9. 椎体 vertebral body

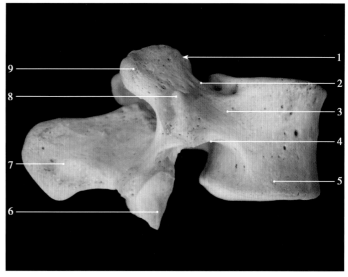

▲ 图 32　腰椎（侧面观）
Lumbar vertebra. Lateral aspect
1. 上关节突 superior articular process
2. 椎上切迹 superior vertebral notch
3. 椎弓根 pedicle of vertebral arch
4. 椎下切迹 inferior vertebral notch
5. 椎体 vertebral body
6. 下关节突 inferior articular process
7. 棘突 spinous process
8. 横突 transverse process
9. 乳突 mamillary process

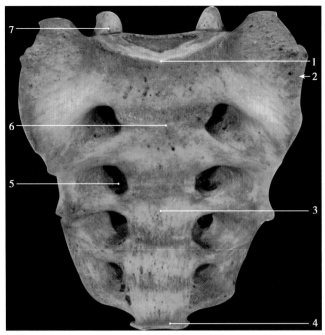

▲ 图 33　骶骨 (前面观)
Sacrum. Anterior aspect

1. 岬 promontory
2. 侧部 lateral part
3. 盆面 pelvic surface
4. 骶骨尖 apex of sacrum
5. 骶前孔 anterior sacral foramina
6. 横线 transverse line
7. 上关节突 superior articular process

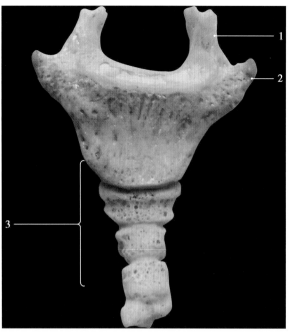

▲ 图 35　尾骨 (前面观)
Coccyx. Anterior aspect

1. 尾骨角 coccygeal cornu
2. 横突 transverse process
3. 尾骨 coccyx

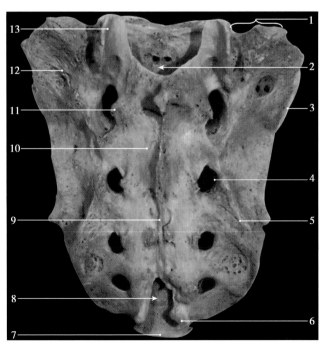

◀ 图 34

骶骨 (后面观)
Sacrum. Posterior aspect

1. 侧部 lateral part
2. 骶管 sacral canal
3. 耳状面 auricular surface
4. 骶后孔 posterior sacral foramina
5. 骶外侧嵴 lateral sacral crest
6. 骶角 sacral cornu
7. 骶骨尖 apex of sacrum
8. 骶管裂孔 sacral hiatus
9. 骶正中嵴 median sacral crest
10. 背侧面 dorsal surface
11. 骶中间嵴 median sacral crest
12. 骶粗隆 sacral tuberosity
13. 上关节突 superior articular
　　 process

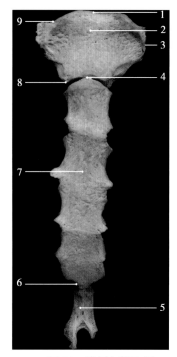

▲ 图36 胸骨(前面观)
Sternum. Anterior aspect
1. 颈静脉切迹 jugular notch
2. 胸骨柄 manubrium sterni
3. 第1肋切迹 1st costal notch
4. 胸骨角 sternal angle
5. 剑突 xiphoid process
6. 第7肋切迹 7th costal notch
7. 胸骨体 sternal body
8. 第2肋切迹 2nd costal notch
9. 锁切迹 clavicular notch

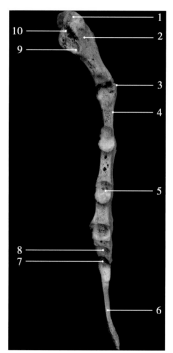

▲ 图37 胸骨(侧面观)
Sternum. Lateral aspect
1. 颈静脉切迹 jugular notch
2. 胸骨柄 manubrium sterni
3. 胸骨角 sternal angle
4. 胸骨体 sternal body
5. 第4肋切迹 4th costal notch
6. 剑突 xiphoid process
7. 第7肋切迹 7th costal notch
8. 第6肋切迹 6th costal notch
9. 第1肋切迹 1st costal notch
10. 锁切迹 clavicular notch

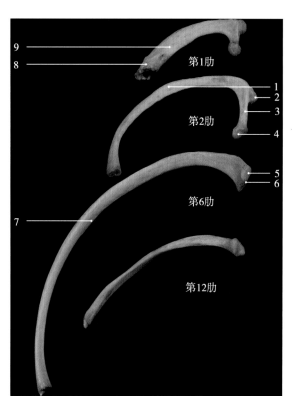

第1肋
第2肋
第6肋
第12肋

◀ 图38

肋骨
Costal bones
1. 前锯肌粗隆 tuberosity for serratus anterior
2. 肋结节 costal tubercle
3. 肋颈 costal neck
4. 肋头 costal head
5. 肋头关节面 articular facet of costal head
6. 肋头嵴 crest of costal head
7. 肋沟 costal groove
8. 锁骨下静脉沟 sulcus for subclavian v.
9. 锁骨下动脉沟 sulcus for subclavian a.

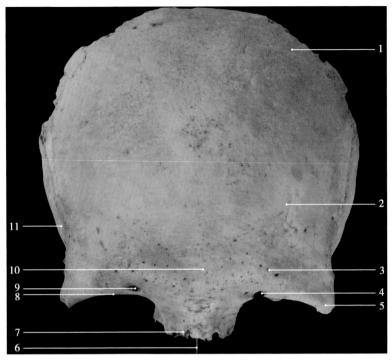

◀ 图 39

额骨（前面观）
Frontal bone. Anterior aspect
1. 额鳞 frontal squama
2. 额结节 frontal tuber
3. 眉弓 superciliary arch
4. 眶上切迹 supraorbital notch
5. 颧突 zygomatic process
6. 鼻棘 nasal spine
7. 鼻缘 nasal margin
8. 眶上缘 supraorbital margin
9. 眶上孔 supraorbital foramen
10. 眉间 glabella
11. 颞面 temporal surface

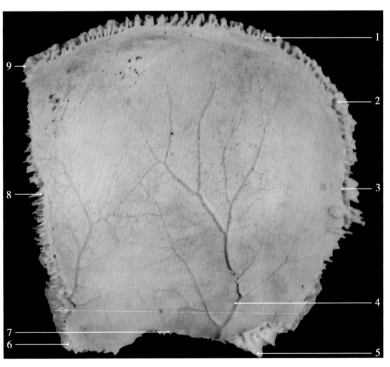

◀ 图 40

顶骨（内面观）
Parietal bone. Internal aspect
1. 矢状缘 sagittal border
2. 枕角 occipital angle
3. 枕缘 occipital border
4. 脑膜中动脉沟 sulcus for middle meningeal a.
5. 乳突角 mastoid angle
6. 蝶角 sphenoidal angle
7. 鳞缘 squamosal border
8. 额缘 frontal border
9. 额角 frontal angle

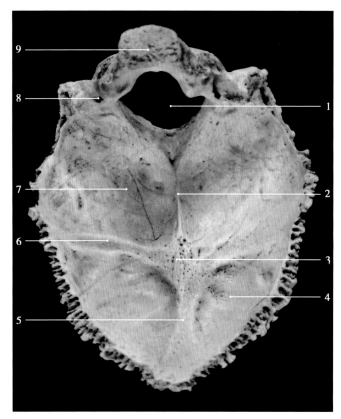

◀ 图 41

枕骨（内面观）
Occipital bone. Internal aspect
1. 枕骨大孔 foramen magnum of occipital bone
2. 枕内嵴 internal occipital crest
3. 枕内隆凸 internal occipital protuberance
4. 大脑窝 cerebral fossa
5. 上矢状窦沟 sulcus for superior sagittal sinus
6. 横窦沟 sulcus for transverse sinus
7. 小脑窝 cerebellar fossa
8. 髁管 condylar canal
9. 基底部 basilar part

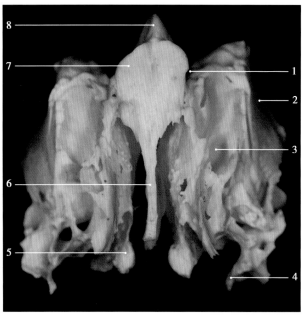

▲ 图 42　筛骨（前面观）
Ethmoid bone. Anterior aspect
1. 筛板 cribriform plate
2. 眶板 orbital plate
3. 筛窦及筛骨迷路 ethmoidal sinuses and
ethmoidal labyrinth
4. 钩突 uncinate process
5. 中鼻甲 middle concha
6. 垂直板 perpendicular plate
7. 鸡冠翼 ala of crista galli
8. 鸡冠 crista galli

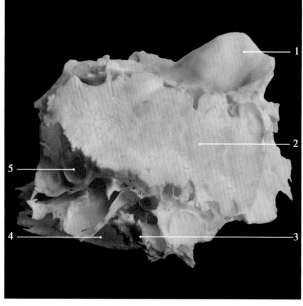

▲ 图 43　筛骨（侧面观）
Ethmoid bone. Lateral aspect
1. 鸡冠 crista galli
2. 眶板 orbital plate
3. 钩突 uncinate process
4. 中鼻甲 middle concha
5. 筛窦 ethmoidal sinuses

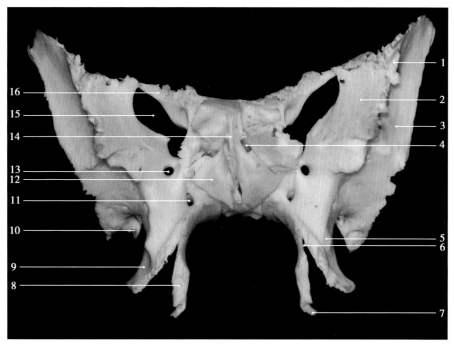

▲ 图44 **蝶骨（前面观）**
Sphenoid bone. Anterior aspect

1. 大翼 greater wing
2. 眶面 orbital surface
3. 颞面 temporal surface
4. 蝶窦口 aperture of sphenoidal sinus
5. 翼突 pterygoid process
6. 翼切迹 pterygoid fissure
7. 翼钩 pterygoid hamulus
8. 翼突内侧板 medial pterygoid plate
9. 翼突外侧板 lateral pterygoid plate
10. 蝶棘 spine of sphenoid bone
11. 翼管 pterygoid canal
12. 蝶骨体 sphenoid body
13. 圆孔 foramen rotundum
14. 蝶嵴 sphenoidal crest
15. 眶上裂 superior orbital fissure
16. 小翼 lesser wing

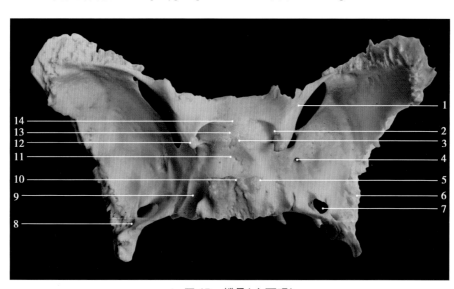

▲ 图45 **蝶骨（上面观）**
Sphenoid bone. Superior aspect

1. 小翼 lesser wing
2. 视神经管 optic canal
3. 鞍结节 tuberculum sellae
4. 圆孔 foramen rotundum
5. 后床突 posterior clinoid process
6. 鳞缘 squamosal margin
7. 卵圆孔 foramen ovale
8. 棘孔 foramen spinosum
9. 颈动脉沟 carotid sulcus
10. 鞍背 dorsum sellae
11. 垂体窝 hypophysial fossa
12. 前床突 anterior clinoid process
13. 交叉前沟 sulcus prechiasmaticus
14. 蝶轭 jugum sphenoidale

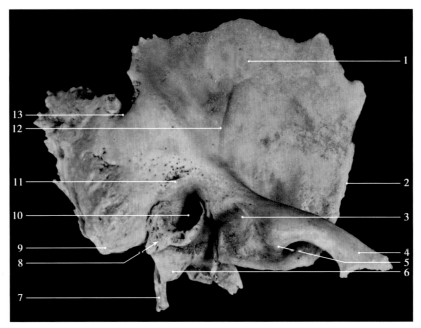

▲ 图46　颞骨(外面观)
Temporal bone. External aspect

1. 鳞部 squamous part
2. 蝶缘 sphenoidal margin
3. 下颌窝 mandibular fossa
4. 颧突 zygomatic process
5. 关节结节 articular tubercle
6. 茎突鞘 sheath of styloid process
7. 茎突 styloid process
8. 鼓部 tympanic part
9. 乳突 mastoid process
10. 外耳道 external acoustic meatus
11. 道上棘 suprameatal spine
12. 颞中动脉沟 sulcus for middle temporal a.
13. 顶切迹 parietal notch

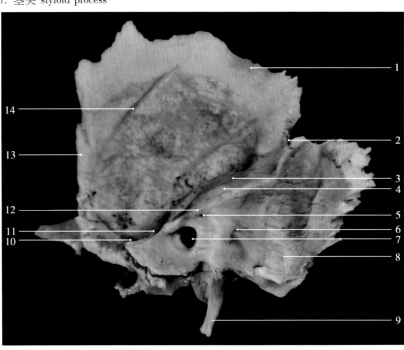

▲ 图47　颞骨(内面观)
Temporal bone. Internal aspect

1. 鳞部 squamous part
2. 顶切迹 parietal notch
3. 鼓室盖 tegmen tympani
4. 弓状隆起 arcuate eminence
5. 弓状下窝 subarcuate fossa
6. 前庭水管外口 external aperture of
   aqueduct of vestibule
7. 内耳门 internal acoustic pore
8. 乙状窦沟 sulcus for sigmoid sinus
9. 茎突 styloid process
10. 三叉神经压迹 trigeminal impression
11. 岩大神经沟 sulcus for greater petrosal n.
12. 岩上窦沟 sulcus for superior petrosal sinus
13. 蝶缘 sphenoidal margin
14. 脑膜中动脉沟 sulcus for middle meningeal a.

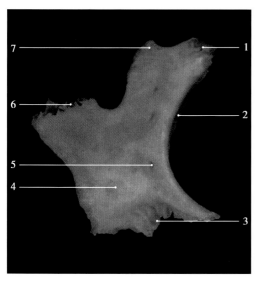

▲ 图 48 **颧骨**
Zygomatic bone

1. 额突 frontal process
2. 眶面 orbital surface
3. 上颌突 maxillary process
4. 外侧面 lateral surface
5. 颧面孔 zygomaticofacial foramen
6. 颞突 temporal process
7. 缘结节 marginal tubercle

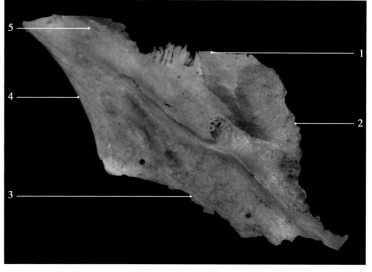

▲ 图 49 **犁骨**
Vomer

1. 上缘 superior border
2. 前缘 anterior border
3. 下缘 inferior border
4. 后缘 posterior border
5. 犁骨翼 ala of vomer

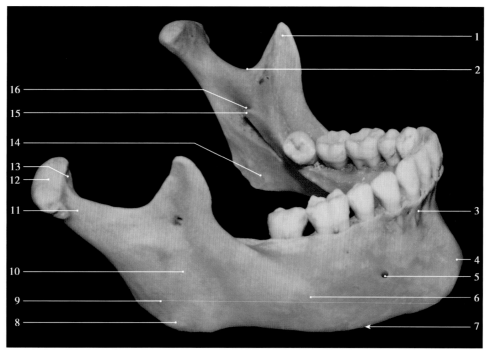

▲ 图 50 **下颌骨 (外侧面观)**
Mandible. Lateral aspect

1. 冠突 coronoid process
2. 下颌切迹 mandibular notch
3. 牙槽轭 juga alveolaria
4. 颏隆凸 mental protuberance
5. 颏孔 mental foramen
6. 下颌体 body of mandible
7. 下颌底 base of mandible
8. 下颌角 angle of mandible
9. 咬肌粗隆 masseteric tuberosity
10. 下颌支 ramus of mandible
11. 髁突 condylar process
12. 下颌头 head of mandible
13. 翼肌凹 pterygoid fovea
14. 翼肌粗隆 pterygoid tuberosity
15. 下颌小舌 mandibular lingula
16. 下颌孔 mandibular foramen

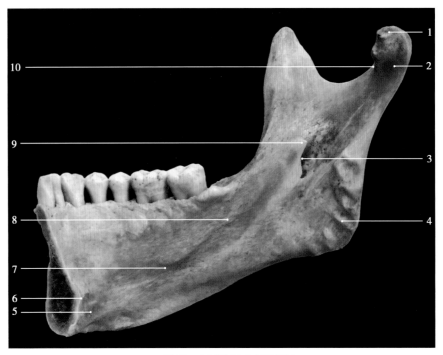

▲ 图51　下颌骨（内侧面观）
Mandible. Medial aspect

1. 下颌头 head of mandible
2. 翼肌凹 pterygoid fovea
3. 下颌孔 mandibular foramen
4. 翼肌粗隆 pterygoid tuberosity
5. 二腹肌窝 digastric fossa
6. 颏棘 mental spine
7. 下颌下腺凹 submandibular fovea
8. 下颌舌骨肌线 mylohyoid line
9. 下颌小舌 mandibular lingula
10. 下颌颈 neck of mandible

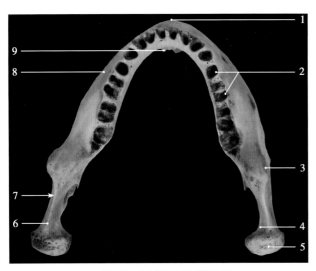

▲ 图52　下颌骨（牙槽面观）
Mandible. Dental alveoli aspect

1. 颏隆凸 mental protuberance
2. 牙槽 dental alveoli
3. 冠突 coronoid process
4. 翼肌凹 pterygoid fovea
5. 下颌头 head of mandible
6. 下颌颈 neck of mandible
7. 下颌切迹 mandibular notch
8. 下颌体 body of mandible
9. 颏棘 mental spine

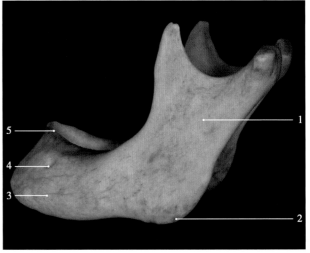

▲ 图53　下颌骨（老年）
Mandible. Aged

1. 下颌支 ramus of mandible
2. 下颌角 angle of mandible
3. 下颌体 body of mandible
4. 颏孔 mental foramen
5. 牙槽 dental alveoli

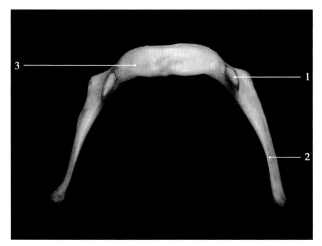

▲ 图54　舌骨(前面观)
Hyoid bone. Anterior aspect
1. 小角 lesser horn
2. 大角 greater horn
3. 舌骨体 body of hyoid bone

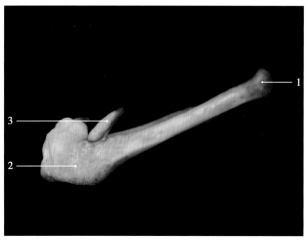

▲ 图55　舌骨(侧面观)
Hyoid bone. Lateral aspect
1. 大角 greater horn
2. 舌骨体 body of hyoid bone
3. 小角 lesser horn

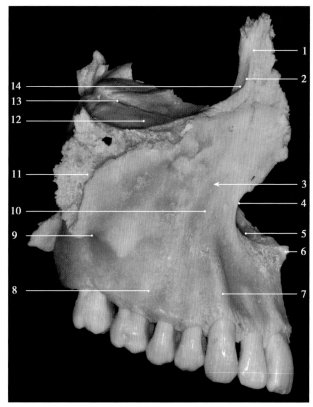

▲ 图56　上颌骨(外侧面观)
Maxilla. Lateral aspect

1. 额突 frontal process
2. 泪前嵴 anterior lacrimal crest
3. 前面 anterior surface
4. 鼻切迹 nasal notch
5. 腭突 palatine process
6. 鼻前棘 anterior nasal spine
7. 牙槽轭 juga alveolaria
8. 牙槽突 alveolar process
9. 颧下嵴 subzygomatic crest
10. 尖牙窝 canine fossa
11. 颧突 zygomatic process
12. 眶面 orbital surface
13. 眶下沟 infraorbital groove
14. 泪沟 lacrimal groove

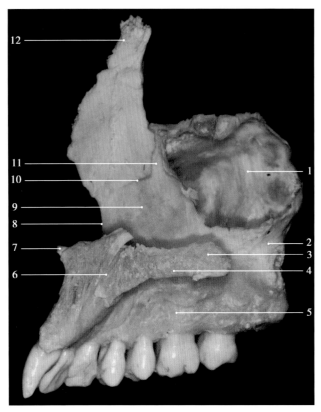

◀ 图57

上颌骨(内侧面观)
Maxilla. Medial aspect

1. 上颌窦 maxillary sinus
2. 腭大沟 greater palatine sulcus
3. 鼻嵴 nasal crest
4. 腭突 palatine process
5. 牙槽突 alveolar process
6. 切牙管 incisive canal
7. 鼻前棘 anterior nasal spine
8. 鼻切迹 nasal notch
9. 鼻面 nasal surface
10. 鼻甲嵴 conchal crest
11. 泪沟 lacrimal groove
12. 额突 frontal process

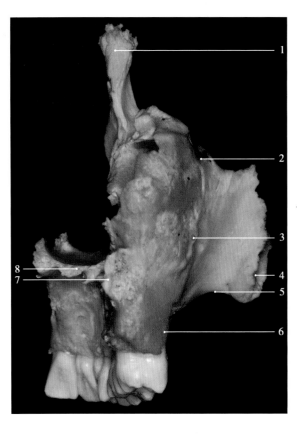

◀ 图58

上颌骨(后面观)
Maxilla. Posterior aspect

1. 额突 frontal process
2. 眶下沟 infraorbital groove
3. 牙槽孔 alveolar foramina
4. 颧突 zygomatic process
5. 颧下嵴 subzygomatic crest
6. 牙槽突 alveolar process
7. 腭大沟 greater palatine sulcus
8. 腭突 palatine process

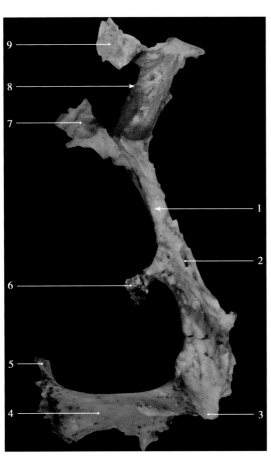

◀ 图 59

腭骨（后面观）
Palatine bone. Posterior aspect

1. 垂直板 perpendicular plate
2. 腭大沟 greater palatine sulcus
3. 锥突 pyramidal process
4. 水平板 horizontal plate
5. 鼻嵴 nasal crest
6. 鼻甲嵴 conchal crest
7. 蝶突 sphenoidal process
8. 蝶腭切迹 sphenopalatine notch
9. 眶突 orbital process

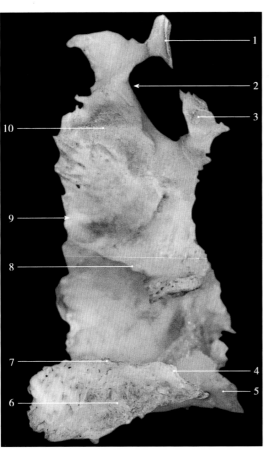

◀ 图 60

腭骨（内侧面观）
Palatine bone. Medial aspect

1. 眶突 orbital process
2. 蝶腭切迹 sphenopalatine notch
3. 蝶突 sphenoidal process
4. 鼻后棘 posterior nasal spine
5. 锥突 pyramidal process
6. 水平板 horizontal plate
7. 鼻嵴 nasal crest
8. 鼻甲嵴 conchal crest
9. 垂直板 perpendicular plate
10. 筛嵴 ethmoidal crest

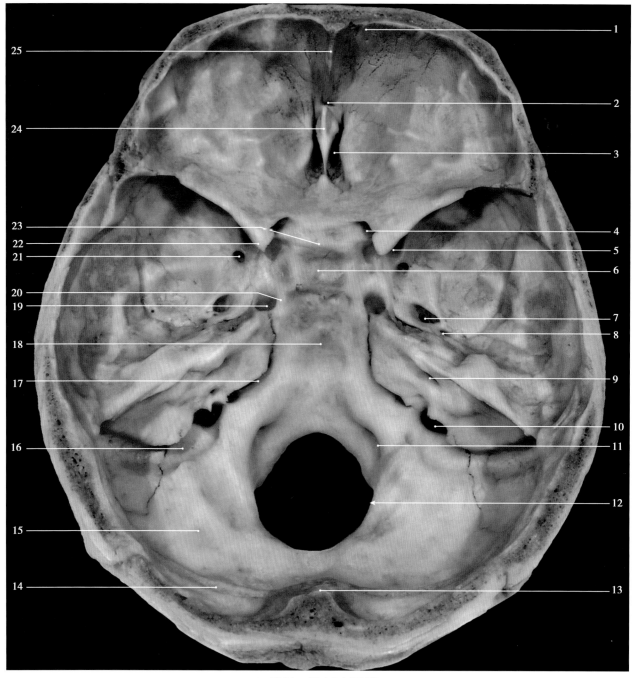

▲ 图61 颅底(内面观)
Internal surface of the base of skull

1. 额骨 frontal bone
2. 盲孔 foramen cecum
3. 筛板 cribriform plate
4. 视神经管 optic canal
5. 眶上裂 supraorbital fissure
6. 垂体窝 hypophysial fossa
7. 卵圆孔 foramen ovale
8. 棘孔 foramen spinosum
9. 内耳门 internal acoustic pore

10. 颈静脉孔 jugular foramen
11. 舌下神经管 hypoglossal canal
12. 枕骨大孔 foramen magnum of occipital bone
13. 枕内隆凸 internal occipital protuberance
14. 横窦沟 sulcus for transverse sinus
15. 小脑窝 cerebellar fossa
16. 乙状窦沟 sulcus for sigmoid sinus
17. 岩枕裂 petrooccipital fissure
18. 斜坡 clivus

19. 破裂孔 foramen lacerum
20. 后床突 posterior clinoid process
21. 圆孔 foramen rotundum
22. 前床突 anterior clinoid process
23. 鞍结节 tuberculum sellae
24. 鸡冠 crista galli
25. 额嵴 frontal crest

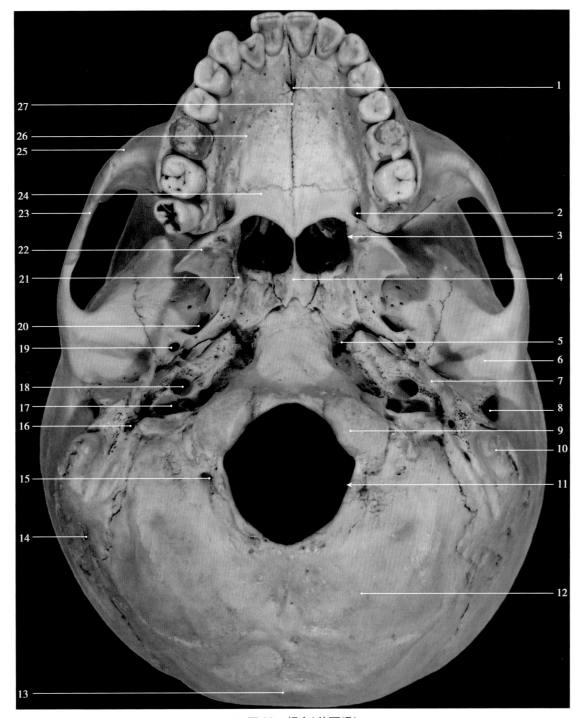

▲ 图 62　颅底（外面观）
External surface of the base of skull

1. 切牙孔 incisive foramina
2. 腭大孔 greater palatine foramen
3. 鼻后孔 posterior nasal apertures
4. 犁骨 vomer
5. 破裂孔 foramen lacerum
6. 下颌窝 mandibular fossa
7. 茎突 styloid process
8. 外耳门 external acoustic pore
9. 枕髁 occipital condyle

10. 乳突 mastoid process
11. 枕骨大孔 foramen magnum of occipital bone
12. 枕骨 occipital bone
13. 枕外隆凸 external occipital protuberance
14. 乳突孔 mastoid foramen
15. 髁管 condylar canal
16. 茎乳孔 stylomastoid foramen
17. 颈静脉窝 jugular fossa
18. 颈动脉管 carotid canal

19. 棘孔 foramen spinosum
20. 卵圆孔 foramen ovale
21. 翼突内侧板 medial pterygoid plate
22. 翼突外侧板 lateral pterygoid plate
23. 颧弓 zygomatic arch
24. 腭骨 palatine bone
25. 颧骨 zygomatic bone
26. 上颌骨 maxilla
27. 上颌间缝 intermaxillary suture

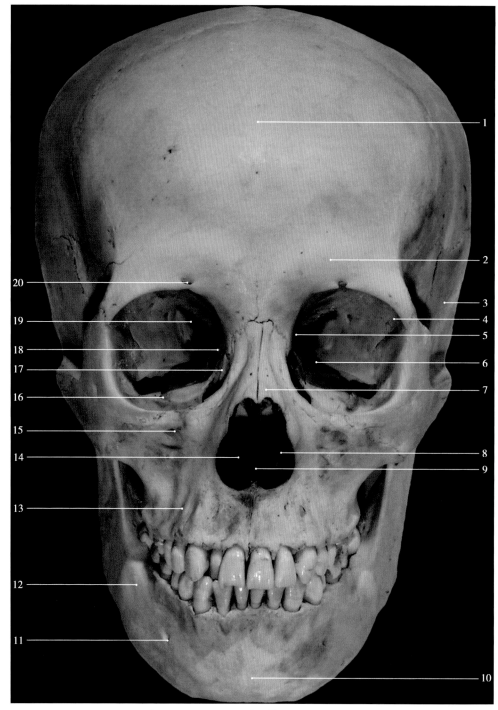

▲ 图63 颅(前面观)
Skull. Anterior aspect

1. 额骨 frontal bone
2. 眉弓 superciliary arch
3. 颞骨 temporal bone
4. 泪腺窝 fossa for lacrimal gland
5. 视神经管 optic canal
6. 眶下裂 inferior orbital fissure
7. 鼻骨 nasal bone

8. 下鼻甲 inferior nasal concha
9. 骨鼻中隔 bony septum of nose
10. 颏隆凸 mental protuberance
11. 颏孔 mental foramen
12. 下颌骨 mandible
13. 上颌骨 maxilla
14. 鼻腔 nasal cavity

15. 眶下孔 infraorbital foramen
16. 眶下沟 infraorbital groove
17. 泪骨 lacrimal bone
18. 筛骨 ethmoid bone
19. 眶上裂 superior orbital fissure
20. 眶上孔 supraorbital foramen

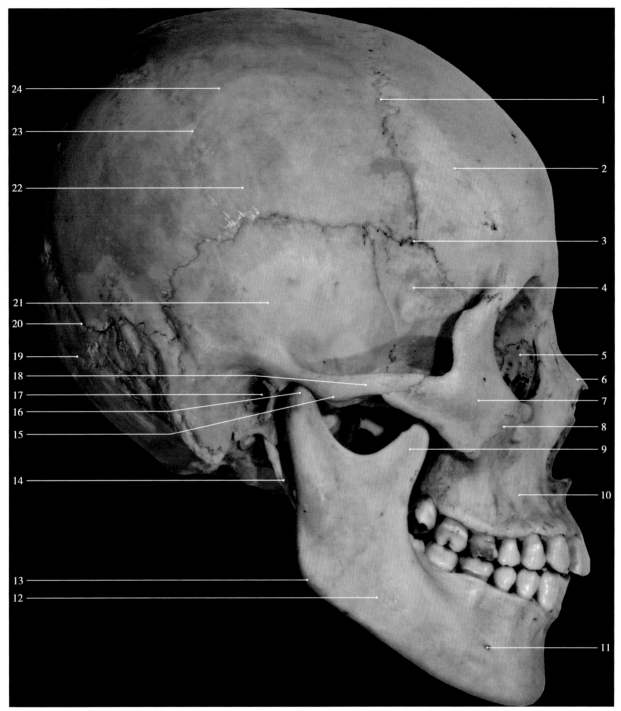

▲ 图64 颅(外侧面观)
Skull. Lateral aspect

1. 冠状缝 coronal suture
2. 额骨 frontal bone
3. 翼点 pterion
4. 蝶骨 sphenoid bone
5. 泪骨 lacrimal bone
6. 鼻骨 nasal bone
7. 颧骨 zygomatic bone
8. 颧上颌缝 zygomaticomaxillary suture

9. 冠突 coronoid process
10. 上颌骨 maxilla
11. 颏孔 mental foramen
12. 下颌骨 mandible
13. 下颌角 angle of mandible
14. 茎突 styloid process
15. 关节结节 articular tubercle
16. 下颌头 head of mandible

17. 外耳门 external acoustic pore
18. 颧弓 zygomatic arch
19. 枕骨 occipital bone
20. 人字缝 lambdoid suture
21. 颞骨 temporal bone
22. 下颞线 inferior temporal line
23. 顶骨 parietal bone
24. 上颞线 superior temporal line

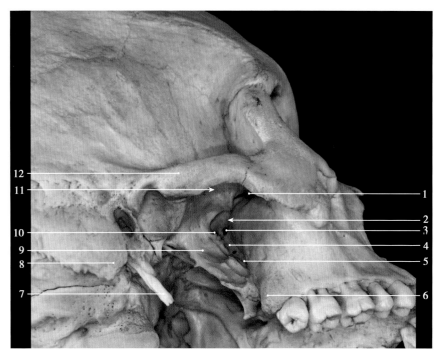

◀ 图65

翼腭窝
Pterygopalatine fossa
1. 眶下裂 inferior orbital fissure
2. 翼腭窝 pterygopalatine fossa
3. 蝶腭孔 sphenopalatine foramen
4. 腭骨垂直板 perpendicular plate of palatine bone
5. 翼腭管 pterygopalatine canal
6. 上颌结节 maxillary tuber
7. 茎突 styloid process
8. 乳突 mastoid process
9. 翼突外侧板 lateral pterygoid plate
10. 圆孔 foramen rotundum
11. 颞下窝 infratemporal fossa
12. 颧弓 zygomatic arch

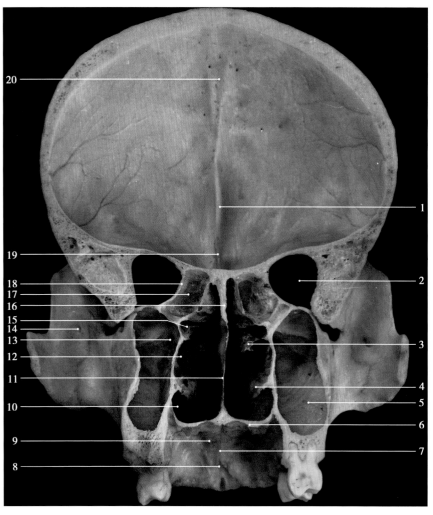

◀ 图66

颅冠状切面(经过第二磨牙)
Coronal section of skull through the second molar
1. 额嵴 frontal crest
2. 眶 orbit
3. 中鼻甲 middle nasal concha
4. 下鼻甲 inferior nasal concha
5. 上颌窦 maxillary sinus
6. 腭骨水平板 horizontal plate of palatine bone
7. 上颌间缝 intermaxillary suture
8. 切牙孔 incisive foramina
9. 上颌骨腭突 palatine process of maxilla
10. 下鼻道 inferior nasal meatus
11. 鼻中隔 nasal septum
12. 中鼻道 middle nasal meatus
13. 上颌窦裂孔 maxillary hiatus
14. 颧颞孔 zygomaticotemporal foramen
15. 上鼻道 superior nasal meatus
16. 筛骨垂直板 perpendicular plate of ethmoid bone
17. 筛小房 ethmoidal cellules
18. 筛骨眶板 orbital plate of ethmoid bone
19. 鸡冠 crista galli
20. 上矢状窦沟 sulcus for superior sagittal sinus

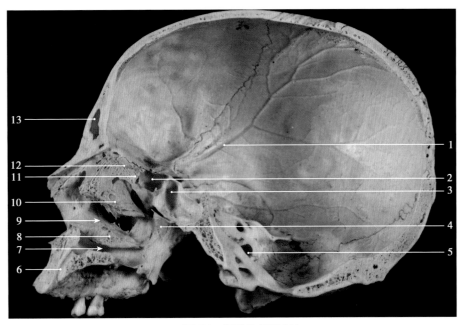

▲ 图 67　鼻腔外侧壁（1）
Lateral wall of nasal cavity（1）

1. 脑膜中动脉沟 sulcus for middle meningeal a.
2. 后筛窦 posterior ethmoidal sinuses
3. 蝶窦 sphenoidal sinus
4. 腭骨垂直板 perpendicular plate of palatine bone
5. 颈静脉孔 jugular foramen
6. 切牙管 incisive canal
7. 下鼻道 inferior nasal meatus
8. 下鼻甲 inferior nasal concha
9. 中鼻道 middle nasal meatus
10. 中鼻甲 middle nasal concha
11. 上鼻甲（切断）superior nasal concha
12. 筛板 cribriform plate
13. 额窦 frontal sinus

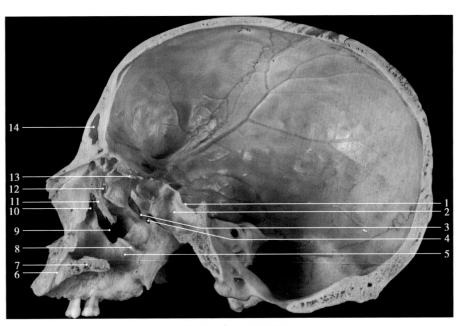

▲ 图 68　鼻腔外侧壁（2）
Lateral wall of nasal cavity（2）

1. 垂体窝 hypophysial fossa
2. 蝶窦 sphenoidal sinus
3. 后筛窦口 aperture of posterior ethmoidal sinuses
4. 蝶腭孔 sphenopalatine foramen
5. 腭骨垂直板 perpendicular plate of palatine bone
6. 切牙管 incisive canal
7. 上颌骨腭突 palatine process of maxilla
8. 鼻甲嵴 conchal crest
9. 上颌窦 maxillary sinus
10. 鼻泪管 nasolacrimal canal
11. 钩突 uncinate process
12. 中筛窦开口 aperture of middle ethmoidal sinuses
13. 筛板 cribriform plate
14. 额窦 frontal sinus

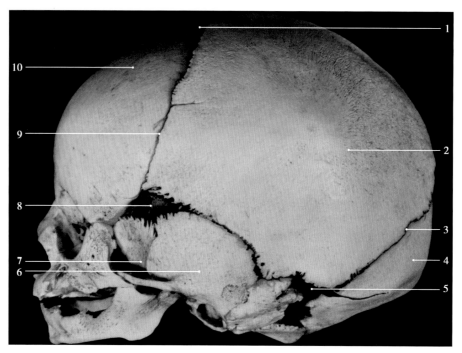

▲ 图 69　婴儿颅（侧面观）
Skull of infant. Lateral aspect

1. 前囟 anterior fontanelle　　6. 颞骨 temporal bone
2. 顶骨 parietal bone　　　　　7. 蝶骨 sphenoid bone
3. 人字缝 lambdoid suture　　8. 蝶囟 sphenoidal fontanelle
4. 枕骨 occipital bone　　　　9. 冠状缝 coronal suture
5. 乳突囟 mastoid fontanelle　10. 额骨 frontal bone

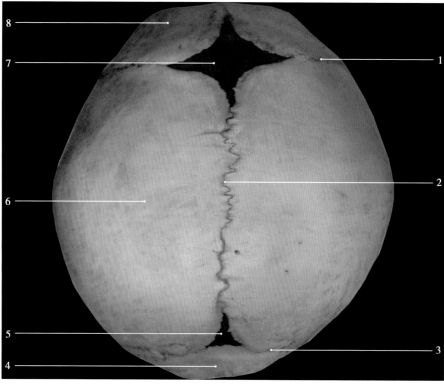

▲ 图 70　婴儿颅（上面观）
Skull of infant. Superior aspect

1. 冠状缝 coronal suture　　5. 后囟 posterior fontanelle
2. 矢状缝 sagittal suture　　6. 顶骨 parietal bone
3. 人字缝 lambdoid suture　7. 前囟 anterior fontanelle
4. 枕骨 occipital bone　　　8. 额骨 frontal bone

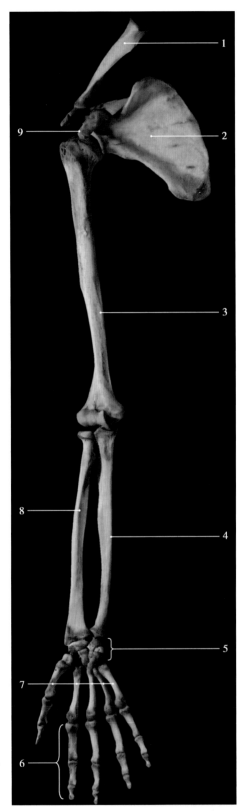

▲ 图71　**上肢骨**
Bones of upper limb

1. 锁骨 clavicle
2. 肩胛骨 scapular
3. 肱骨 humerus
4. 尺骨 ulna
5. 腕骨 carpal bones
6. 指骨 phalanges of fingers
7. 掌骨 metacarpal bones
8. 桡骨 radius
9. 喙突 coracoid process

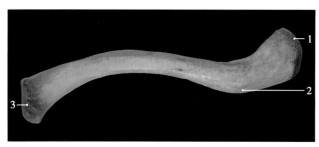

▲ 图72　锁骨（上面观）
Clavicle. Superior aspect

1. 肩峰端 acromial end
2. 锥状结节 conoid tubercle
3. 胸骨端 sternal end

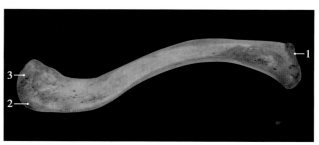

▲ 图73　锁骨（下面观）
Clavicle. Inferior aspect

1. 胸骨端 sternal end
2. 肩峰端 acromial end
3. 肩峰关节面 acromial articular facet

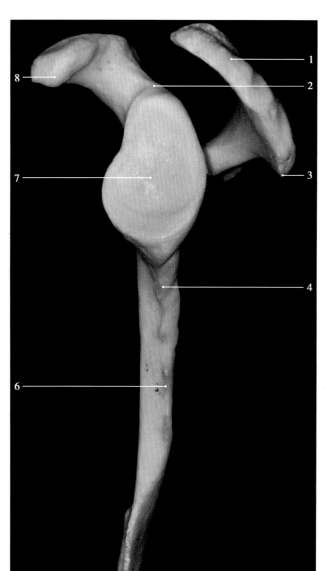

◀ 图74

肩胛骨（外侧面观）
Scapular. Lateral aspect

1. 肩峰 acromion
2. 盂上结节 supraglenoid tubercle
3. 肩峰角 acromial angle
4. 盂下结节 infraglenoid tubercle
5. 下角 inferior angle
6. 外侧缘 lateral border
7. 关节盂 glenoid cavity
8. 喙突 coracoid process

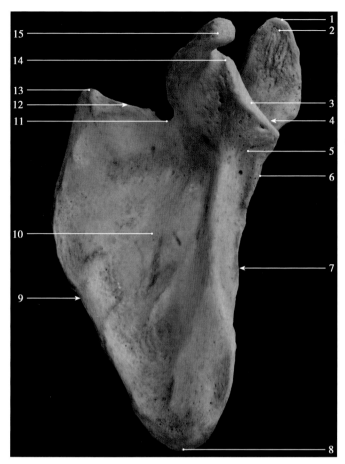

◀ 图 75

肩胛骨（前面观）
Scapular. Anterior aspect

1. 肩峰关节面 articular surface of acromion
2. 肩峰 acromion
3. 关节盂 glenoid cavity
4. 外侧角 lateral angle
5. 肩胛颈 neck of scapula
6. 盂下结节 infraglenoid tubercle
7. 外侧缘 lateral border
8. 下角 inferior angle
9. 内侧缘 medial border
10. 肩胛下窝 subscapular fossa
11. 肩胛切迹 notch of scapula
12. 上缘 superior border
13. 上角 superior angle
14. 盂上结节 supraglenoid tubercle
15. 喙突 coracoid process

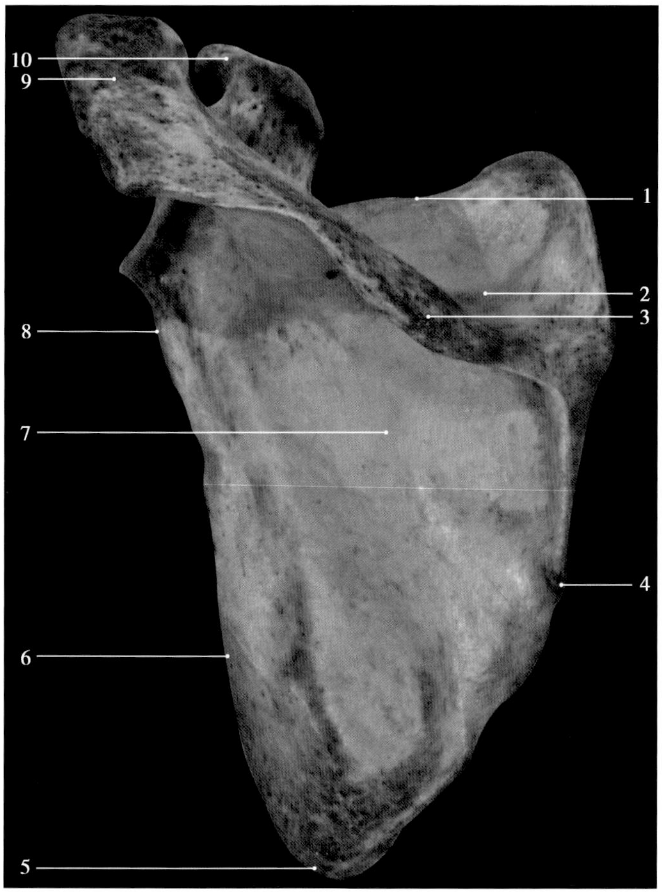

◀ 图 76

肩胛骨（后面观）
Scapular. Posterior aspect

1. 上缘 superior border
2. 冈上窝 supraspinous fossa
3. 肩胛冈 spine of scapula
4. 内侧缘 medial border
5. 下角 inferior angle
6. 外侧缘 lateral border
7. 冈下窝 infraspinous fossa
8. 盂下结节 infraglenoid tubercle
9. 肩峰 acromion
10. 喙突 coracoid process

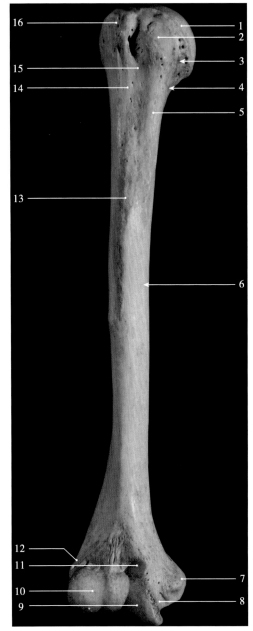

▲ 图77 肱骨（前面观）
Humerus. Anterior aspect

1. 肱骨头 head of humerus
2. 小结节 lesser tubercle
3. 解剖颈 anatomical neck
4. 外科颈 surgical neck
5. 小结节嵴 crest of lesser tubercle
6. 肱骨体 shaft of humerus
7. 内上髁 medial epicondyle
8. 尺神经沟 sulcus for ulnar n.
9. 肱骨滑车 trochlea of humerus
10. 肱骨小头 capitulum of humerus
11. 冠突窝 coronoid fossa
12. 外上髁 lateral epicondyle
13. 三角肌粗隆 deltoid tuberosity
14. 大结节嵴 crest of greater tubercle
15. 结节间沟 intertubercular sulcus
16. 大结节 greater tubercle

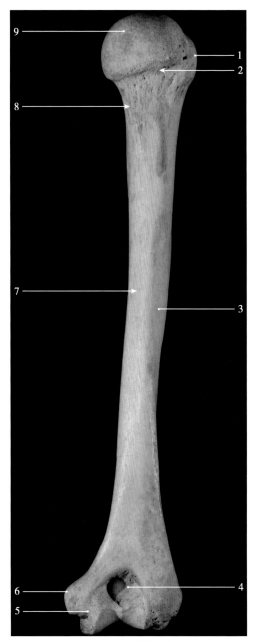

▲ 图78 肱骨（后面观）
Humerus. Posterior aspect

1. 大结节 greater tubercle
2. 解剖颈 anatomical neck
3. 桡神经沟 sulcus for radial n.
4. 鹰嘴窝 olecranon fossa
5. 尺神经沟 sulcus for ulnar n.
6. 内上髁 medial epicondyle
7. 肱骨体 shaft of humerus
8. 外科颈 surgical neck
9. 肱骨头 head of humerus

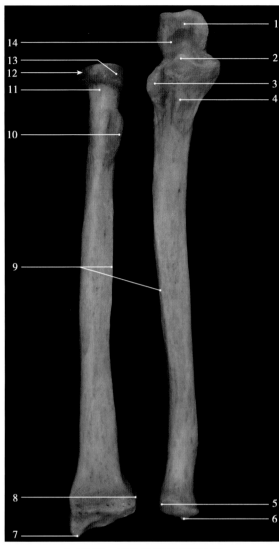
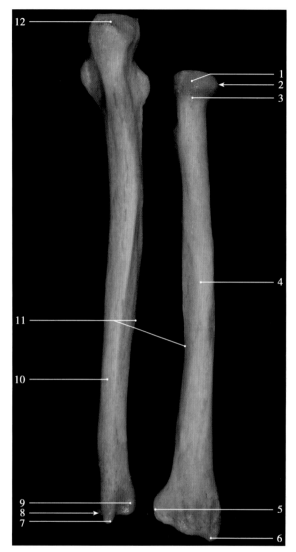

▲ 图79 桡骨和尺骨(前面观)
Radius and ulna. Anterior aspect

1. 鹰嘴 olecranon
2. 冠突 coronoid process
3. 桡切迹 radial notch
4. 尺骨粗隆 ulnar tuberosity
5. 尺骨环状关节面 articular circumference of ulna
6. 尺骨茎突 styloid process of ulna
7. 桡骨茎突 styloid process of radius
8. 尺切迹 ulnar notch
9. 骨间缘 interosseous border
10. 桡骨粗隆 radial tuberosity
11. 桡骨颈 neck of radius
12. 桡骨头 head of radius
13. 桡骨环状关节面 articular circumference of radius
14. 滑车切迹 trochlear notch

▲ 图80 桡骨和尺骨(后面观)
Radius and ulna. Posterior aspect

1. 桡骨环状关节面 articular circumference of radius
2. 桡骨头 head of radius
3. 桡骨颈 neck of radius
4. 后缘 posterior border
5. 尺切迹 ulnar notch
6. 桡骨茎突 styloid process of radius
7. 尺骨茎突 styloid process of ulna
8. 尺骨头 head of ulna
9. 尺骨环状关节面 articular circumference of ulna
10. 内侧面 medial surface
11. 骨间缘 interosseous border
12. 鹰嘴 olecranon

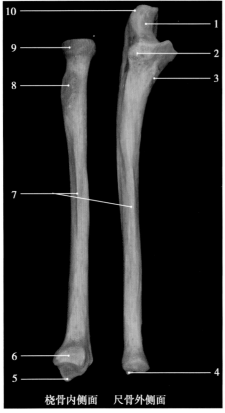

桡骨内侧面　尺骨外侧面

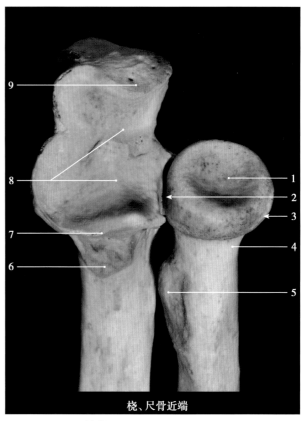

桡、尺骨近端

1. 滑车切迹 trochlear notch
2. 桡切迹 radial notch
3. 尺骨粗隆 ulnar tuberosity
4. 尺骨茎突 styloid process of ulna
5. 桡骨茎突 styloid process of radius
6. 尺切迹 ulnar notch
7. 骨间缘 interosseous border
8. 桡骨粗隆 radial tuberosity
9. 环状关节面 articular circumference
10. 鹰嘴 olecranon

1. 关节凹 articular fovea
2. 桡尺近侧关节 proximal radioulnar joint
3. 桡骨头 head of radius
4. 桡骨颈 neck of radius
5. 桡骨粗隆 radial tuberosity
6. 尺骨粗隆 ulnar tuberosity
7. 冠突 coronoid process
8. 滑车切迹 trochlear notch
9. 鹰嘴 olecranon

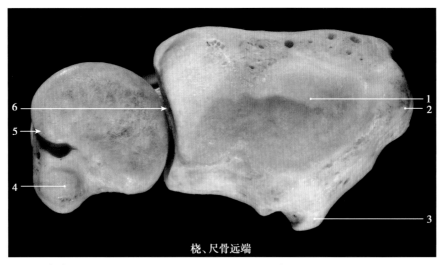

桡、尺骨远端

1. 腕关节面 carpal articular surface
2. 桡骨茎突 styloid process of radius
3. 背侧结节 dorsal tubercle
4. 尺骨茎突 styloid process of ulna
5. 尺骨头 head of radius
6. 桡尺远侧关节 distal radioulnar joint

▲ 图81　桡骨和尺骨
Radius and ulna

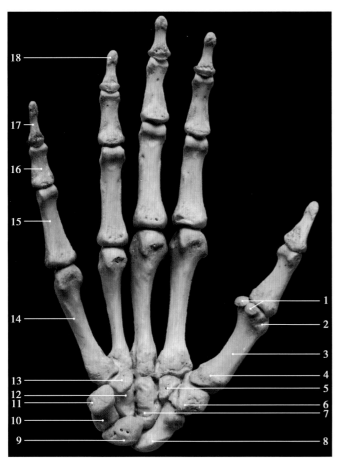

◀ 图 82

手骨(前面观)

Bones of hand. Anterior aspect

1. 籽骨 sesamoid bone
2. 掌骨头 head of metacarpal bone
3. 掌骨体 shaft of metacarpal bone
4. 掌骨底 base of metacarpal bone
5. 小多角骨 trapezoid bone
6. 大多角骨 trapezium bone
7. 头状骨 capitate bone
8. 手舟骨 scaphoid bone
9. 月骨 lunate bone
10. 三角骨 triquetral bone
11. 豌豆骨 pisiform bone
12. 钩骨 hamate bone
13. 钩骨钩 hamulus of hamate bone
14. 掌骨 metacarpal bone
15. 近节指骨 proximal phalanx
16. 中节指骨 middle phalanx
17. 远节指骨 distal phalanx
18. 远节指骨粗隆 tuberosity of distal phalanx

图 83 ▶

手骨(后面观)

Bones of hand. Posterior aspect

1. 远节指骨 distal phalanx
2. 中节指骨 middle phalanx
3. 近节指骨 proximal phalanx
4. 掌骨 metacarpal bone
5. 月骨 lunate bone
6. 第3掌骨茎突 styloid process of the 3rd metacarpal bone
7. 指骨底 base of phalanx
8. 指骨体 shaft of phalanx
9. 指骨滑车 trochlea of phalanx

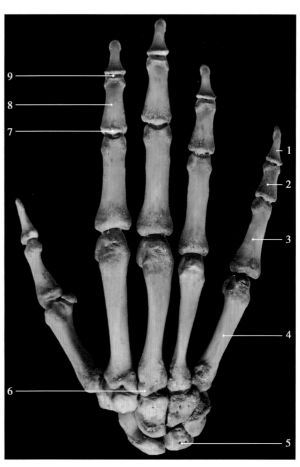

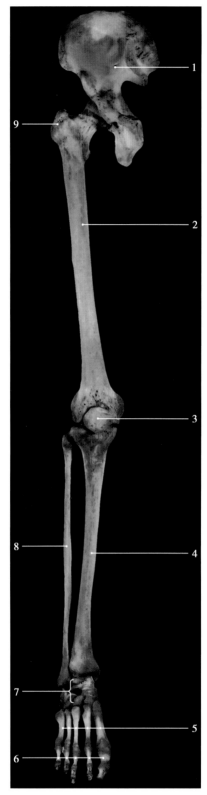

▲ 图84　下肢骨
Bones of lower limb

1. 髋骨 hip bone　　　　　6. 趾骨 phalanges of toes
2. 股骨 femur　　　　　　7. 跗骨 tarsal bones
3. 髌骨 patella　　　　　　8. 腓骨 fibula
4. 胫骨 tibia　　　　　　　9. 大转子 greater trochanter
5. 跖骨 metatarsal bone

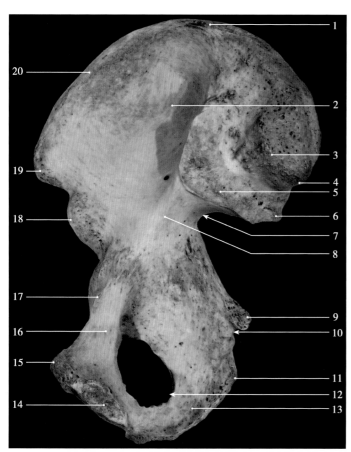

◀ 图 85

髋骨（内面观）
Hip bone. Internal aspect

1. 髂嵴 iliac crest
2. 髂窝 iliac fossa
3. 髂粗隆 iliac tuberosity
4. 髂后上棘 posterior superior iliac spine
5. 耳状面 auricular surface
6. 髂后下棘 posterior inferior iliac spine
7. 坐骨大切迹 greater sciatic notch
8. 弓状线 arcuate line
9. 坐骨棘 ischial spine
10. 坐骨小切迹 lesser sciatic notch
11. 坐骨结节 ischial tuberosity
12. 闭孔 obturator foramen
13. 坐骨支 ramus of ischium
14. 耻骨联合面 symphysial surface
15. 耻骨结节 pubic tuberosity
16. 耻骨上支 superior ramus of pubis
17. 耻骨梳 pecten pubis
18. 髂前下棘 anterior inferior iliac spine
19. 髂前上棘 anterior superior iliac spine
20. 内唇 inner lip

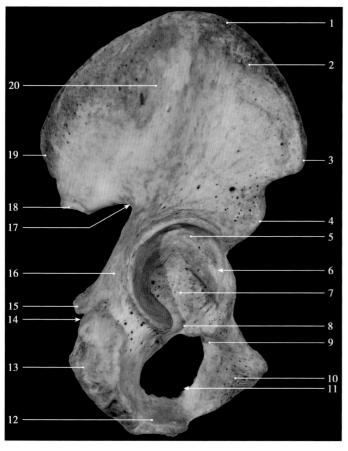

◀ 图 86

髋骨（外面观）
Hip bone. External aspect

1. 髂嵴 iliac crest
2. 髂结节 tubercle of iliac crest
3. 髂前上棘 anterior superior iliac spine
4. 髂前下棘 anterior inferior iliac spine
5. 月状面 lunate surface
6. 髋臼 acetabulum
7. 髋臼窝 acetabular fossa
8. 髋臼切迹 acetabular notch
9. 闭孔沟 obturator groove
10. 耻骨 pubis
11. 闭孔 obturator foramen
12. 坐骨支 ramus of ischium
13. 坐骨结节 ischial tuberosity
14. 坐骨小切迹 lesser sciatic notch
15. 坐骨棘 ischial spine
16. 坐骨体 body of ischium
17. 坐骨大切迹 greater sciatic notch
18. 髂后下棘 posterior inferior iliac spine
19. 髂后上棘 posterior superior iliac spine
20. 髂骨翼 ala of ilium

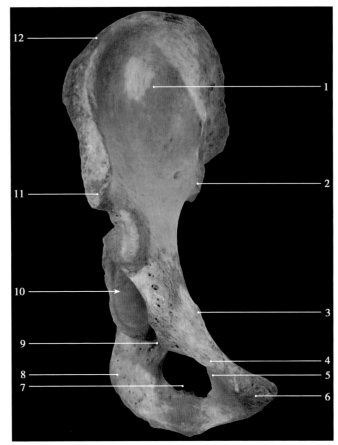

◀ 图87
髋骨（前面观）
Hip bone. Anterior aspect
1. 髂骨翼 ala of ilium
2. 髂后下棘 posterior inferior iliac spine
3. 髂耻隆起 iliopubic eminence
4. 耻骨上支 superior ramus of pubis
5. 闭孔沟 obturator groove
6. 耻骨 pubis
7. 闭孔 obturator foramen
8. 坐骨 ischium
9. 髋臼切迹 acetabular notch
10. 髋臼 acetabulum
11. 髂前上棘 anterior superior iliac spine
12. 髂嵴 iliac crest

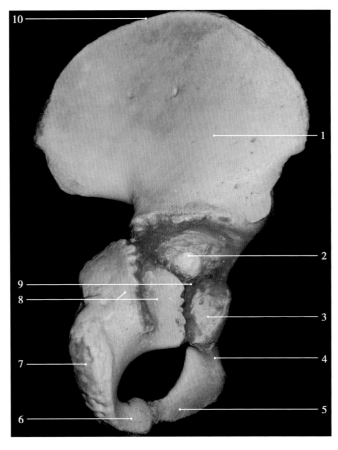

◀ 图88
幼儿髋骨
Hip bone of infant
1. 髂骨翼 ala of ilium
2. 髂骨体 body of ilium
3. 耻骨体 body of pubis
4. 耻骨上支 superior ramus of pubis
5. 耻骨下支 inferior ramus of pubis
6. 坐骨支 ramus of ischium
7. 坐骨结节 ischial tuberosity
8. 坐骨体 body of ischium
9. Y字软骨 "Y" cartilage
10. 髂嵴 iliac crest

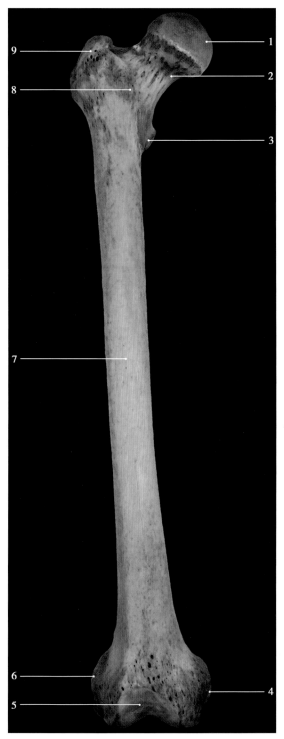

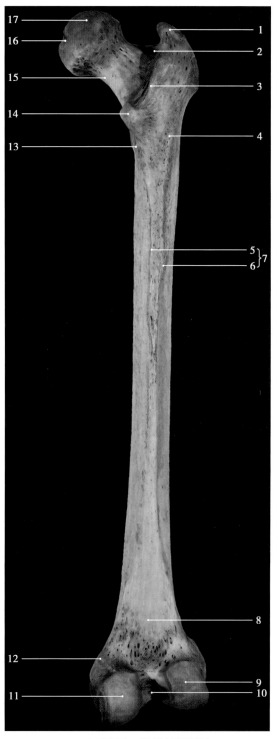

▲ 图89 股骨(前面观)
Femur. Anterior aspect

1. 股骨头 head of femur
2. 股骨颈 neck of femur
3. 小转子 lesser trochanter
4. 内上髁 medial epicondyle
5. 髌面 patellar surface
6. 外上髁 lateral epicondyle
7. 股骨体 shaft of femur
8. 转子间线 intertrochanteric line
9. 大转子 greater trochanter

▲ 图90 股骨(后面观)
Femur. Posterior aspect

1. 大转子 greater trochanter
2. 转子窝 trochanteric fossa
3. 转子间嵴 intertrochanteric crest
4. 臀肌粗隆 gluteal tuberosity
5. 内侧唇 medial lip
6. 外侧唇 lateral lip
7. 粗线 linea aspera
8. 腘面 popliteal surface
9. 外侧髁 lateral condyle

10. 髁间窝 intercondylar fossa
11. 内侧髁 medial condyle
12. 收肌结节 adductor tubercle
13. 耻骨肌线 pectineal line
14. 小转子 lesser trochanter
15. 股骨颈 neck of femur
16. 股骨头凹 fovea of femoral head
17. 股骨头 femoral head

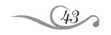

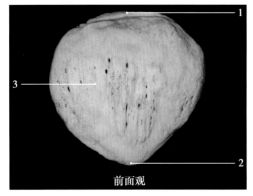

前面观

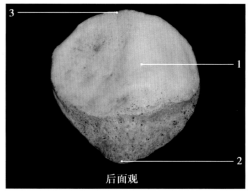

后面观

▲ 图91　髌骨
Patella

1. 髌底 base of patella
2. 髌尖 apex of patella
3. 前面 anterior surface

1. 关节面 articular surface
2. 髌尖 apex of patella
3. 髌底 base of patella

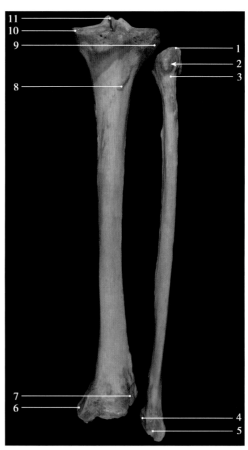

▲ 图 92　胫骨和腓骨（前面观）
Tibia and fibula. Anterior aspect

1. 髁间隆起 intercondylar eminence
2. 胫骨粗隆 tabial tuberosity
3. 外侧面 lateral surface
4. 前缘 anterior border
5. 内侧面 medial surface
6. 内踝 medial malleolus
7. 外踝关节面 articular facet of lateral malleolus
8. 外踝 lateral malleolus
9. 内侧面 medial surface
10. 前缘 anterior border
11. 骨间缘 interosseous border
12. 腓骨颈 neck of fibula
13. 腓骨头 fibular head
14. 腓骨头关节面 articular surface of fibular head
15. 外侧髁 lateral condyle

▲ 图 93　胫骨和腓骨（后面观）
Tibia and fibula. Posterior aspect

1. 腓骨头尖 apex of fibular head
2. 腓骨头 fibular head
3. 腓骨颈 neck of fibula
4. 外踝关节面 articular facet of lateral malleolus
5. 外踝窝 lateral malleolar fossa
6. 内踝 medial malleolus
7. 腓切迹 fibular notch
8. 比目鱼肌线 soleal line
9. 腓关节面 fibular articular facet
10. 内侧髁 medial condyle
11. 髁间隆起 intercondylar eminence

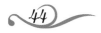

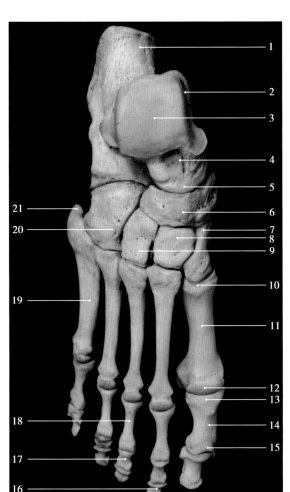

◀ 图 94

足骨 (上面观)

Bones of foot. Superior aspect

1. 跟骨 calcaneus
2. 距骨 talus
3. 距骨滑车 trochlea of talus
4. 距骨颈 neck of talus
5. 距骨头 head of talus
6. 足舟骨 navicular bone
7. 内侧楔骨 medial cuneiform bone
8. 中间楔骨 intermediate cuneiform bone
9. 外侧楔骨 lateral cuneiform bone
10. 跖骨底 base of metatarsal bone
11. 跖骨体 shaft of metatarsal bone
12. 跖骨头 head of metatarsal bone
13. 趾骨底 base of phalanx
14. 趾骨体 shaft of phalanx
15. 趾骨头 head of phalanx
16. 远节趾骨 distal phalanx
17. 中节趾骨 middle phalanx
18. 近节趾骨 proximal phalanx
19. 第 5 跖骨 5th metatarsal bone
20. 骰骨 cuboid bone
21. 第 5 跖骨粗隆 tuberosity of the 5th metatarsal bone

图 95 ▶

足骨 (下面观)

Bones of foot. Inferior aspect

1. 跟骨结节 calcaneal tuberosity
2. 跟骨 calcaneus
3. 骰骨 cuboid bone
4. 第 5 跖骨粗隆 tuberosity of the 5th metatarsal bone
5. 腓骨长肌腱沟 sulcus for tendon of peroneus longus
6. 第 5 跖骨 5th metatarsal bone
7. 近节趾骨 proximal phalanx
8. 中节趾骨 middle phalanx
9. 远节趾骨 distal phalanx
10. 远节趾骨粗隆 tuberosity of distal phalanx
11. 籽骨 sesamoid bone
12. 第 1 跖骨 1st metatarsal bone
13. 外侧楔骨 lateral cuneiform bone
14. 中间楔骨 intermediate cuneiform bone
15. 内侧楔骨 medial cuneiform bone
16. 足舟骨 navicular bone
17. 距骨 talus
18. 载距突 sustentaculum tali
19. 跗长屈肌腱沟 sulcus for tendon of flexor hallucis longus

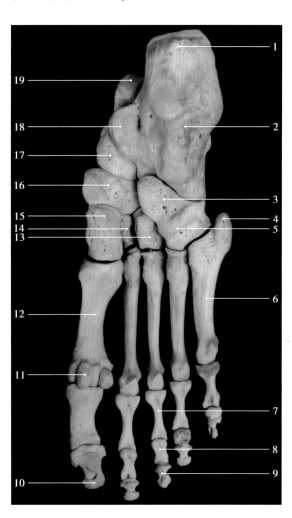

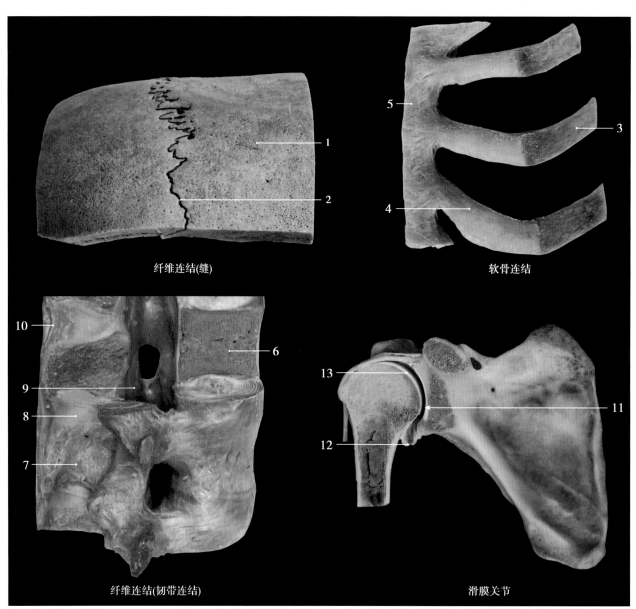

纤维连结(缝) 软骨连结

纤维连结(韧带连结) 滑膜关节

◀ 图96 骨连结分类
Joint classification

1. 顶骨 parietal bone
2. 冠状缝 coronal suture
3. 肋骨 costal bone
4. 肋软骨 costal cartilage
5. 胸骨 sternum
6. 椎体 vertebral body
7. 棘突 spinous process
8. 棘间韧带 interspinal lig.
9. 黄韧带 ligamenta flava
10. 棘上韧带 supraspinal lig.
11. 关节腔 articular cavity
12. 关节囊 articular capsule
13. 关节软骨 articular cartilage

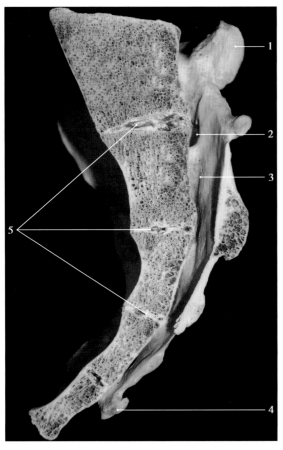

◀ 图 97

骨性结合
Synosteosis

1. 上关节突 superior articular process
2. 骶管侧壁内椎间孔 intervertebral foramina in the lateral wall of sacral canal
3. 骶管 sacral canal
4. 骶角 sacral cornu
5. 椎间盘遗迹 rudiment of intervertebral discs

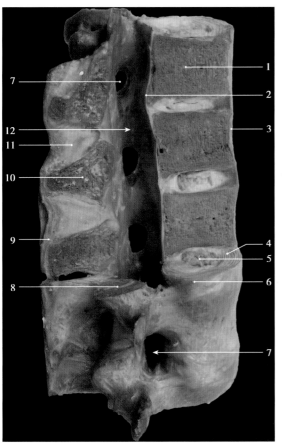

◀ 图 98

椎骨间连结
Joints between vertebrae

1. 椎体 vertebral body
2. 后纵韧带 posterior longitudinal lig.
3. 前纵韧带 anterior longitudinal lig.
4. 纤维环 anulus fibrosus
5. 髓核 nucleus pulposus
6. 椎间盘 intervertebral disc
7. 椎间孔 intervertebral foramen
8. 关节突关节 zygapophyseal joint
9. 棘上韧带 supraspinal lig.
10. 棘突 spinous process
11. 棘间韧带 interspinal lig.
12. 椎管 vertebral canal

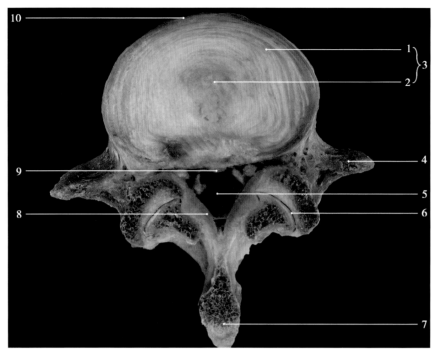

▲ 图 99　椎间盘和关节突关节
Intervertebral disc and zygapophyseal joint

1. 纤维环 anulus fibrosus
2. 髓核 nucleus pulposus
3. 椎间盘 intervertebral disc
4. 横突 transverse process
5. 椎孔 vertebral foramen
6. 关节突关节 zygapophysial joint
7. 棘突 spinous process
8. 黄韧带 ligamenta flava
9. 后纵韧带 posterior longitudinal lig.
10. 前纵韧带 anterior longitudinal lig.

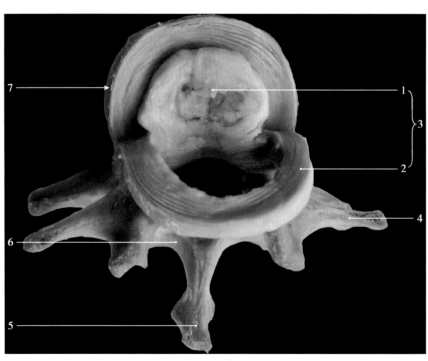

▲ 图 100　椎间盘
Intervertebral disc

1. 髓核 nucleus pulposus
2. 纤维环 anulus fibrosus
3. 椎间盘 intervertebral disc
4. 横突 transverse process
5. 棘突 spinous process
6. 椎弓板 lamina of vertebral arch
7. 椎体 vertebral body

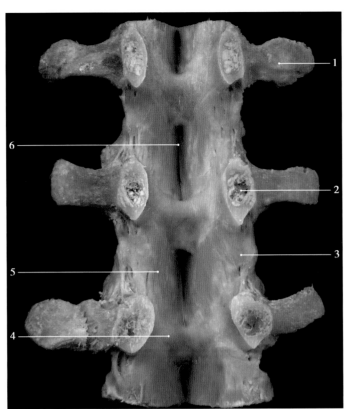

◀ 图 101

黄韧带

Ligamenta flava

1. 横突 transverse process
2. 椎弓根 pedicle of vertebral arch
3. 黄韧带与关节突关节囊混合部 the part that ligamenta flava mixed with articular capsule of zygapophysial joint
4. 椎弓板 lamina of vertebral arch
5. 黄韧带 ligamenta flava
6. 黄韧带间隙 space between ligamenta flava

图 102 ▶

项韧带

Ligamentum nuchae

1. 环椎 atlas
2. 枢椎 axis
3. 隆椎 vertebra prominens
4. 棘上韧带 supraspinal lig.
5. 棘间韧带 interspinal lig.
6. 项韧带 ligamentum nuchae
7. 枕外隆凸 external occipital protuberance

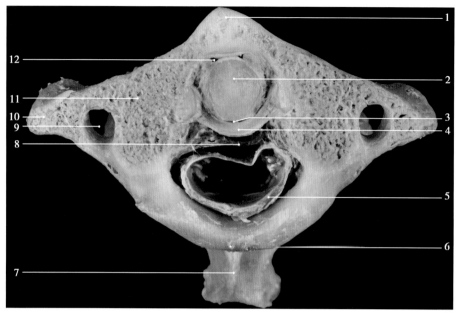

▲ 图103　寰枢关节（水平切面）
Atlantoaxial joint. Horizontal section

1. 寰椎前结节 anterior tubercle of atlas
2. 齿突 dens
3. 寰齿后关节 posterior atlantodens joint
4. 寰椎横韧带 transverse ligament of atlas
5. 硬脊膜 spinal dura mater
6. 寰椎后结节 posterior tubercle of atlas
7. 枢椎棘突 spinous process of axis
8. 覆膜 tectorial membrane
9. 横突孔 transverse foramen
10. 横突 transverse process
11. 寰椎侧块 lateral mass of atlas
12. 寰齿前关节 anterior atlantodens join

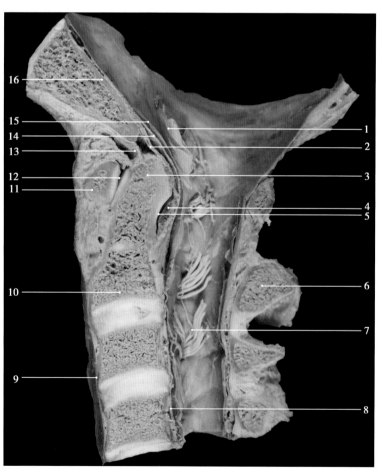

◄ 图104
寰枕寰枢关节（矢状切面）
Atlantooccipital joint and atlantoaxial joint. Sagittal section

1. 蛛网膜 arachnoid mater
2. 纵束 longitudinal brands
3. 齿突 dens
4. 寰椎横韧带 transverse ligament of atlas
5. 寰齿后关节 posterior atlantodens joint
6. 棘突 spinous process
7. 脊神经根丝 rootlets of spinal n.
8. 后纵韧带 posterior longitudinal lig.
9. 前纵韧带 anterior longitudinal lig.
10. 枢椎 axis
11. 寰椎前弓 anterior arch of atlas
12. 寰齿前关节 anterior atlantodens joint
13. 齿突尖韧带 apical ligament of dens
14. 覆膜 tectorial membrane
15. 硬脊膜 spinal dura mater
16. 斜坡 clivus

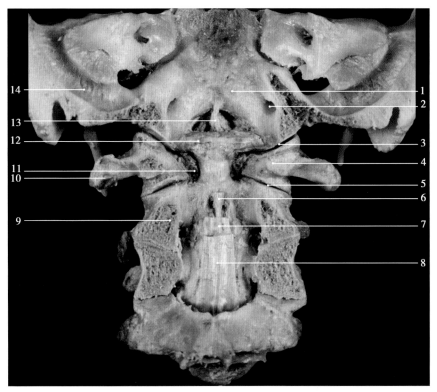

▲ 图 105　**寰枕、寰枢关节（后面观）**
Atlantooccipital joint and atlantoaxial joint. Posterior aspect

1. 斜坡 clivus of occipital bone
2. 舌下神经管 hypoglossal canal
3. 寰枕关节 atlantooccipital joint
4. 寰椎 atlas
5. 寰枢外侧关节 lateral atlantoaxial joint
6. 纵束（下部）longitudinal bands
7. 覆膜 tectorial membrane
8. 后纵韧带 posterior longitudinal lig.
9. 枢椎 axis
10. 寰椎横突 transverse process of atlas
11. 寰椎横韧带 transverse ligament of atlas
12. 翼状韧带 alar lig.
13. 纵束（上部）longitudinal bands
14. 乙状窦沟 sulcus for sigmoid sinus

图 106 ▶

肋椎关节（上面观）
Costovertebral joint.
Superior aspect

1. 肋头关节 joint of costal head
2. 肋头 costal head
3. 肋横突关节 costotransverse joint
4. 肋 rib
5. 棘突 spinous process
6. 肋横突外侧韧带 lateral costotransverse lig.
7. 横突 transverse processes
8. 上关节突 superior articular process
9. 肋头辐状韧带 radiate ligament of costal head
10. 椎体 vertebral body

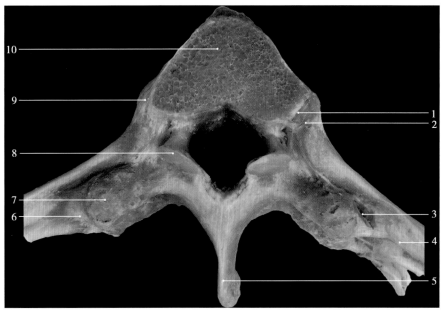

51

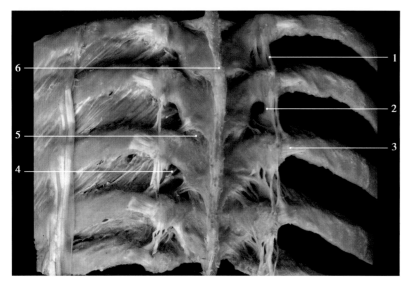

◀ 图 107

肋椎关节（后面观）
Costovertebral joint. Posterior aspect
1. 横突间韧带 intertransverse lig.
2. 肋横突上韧带 superior costotransverse lig.
3. 肋横突外侧韧带 lateral costotransverse lig.
4. 胸神经后支 posterior branch of thoracic n.
5. 黄韧带 ligamenta flava
6. 棘上韧带 supraspinal lig.

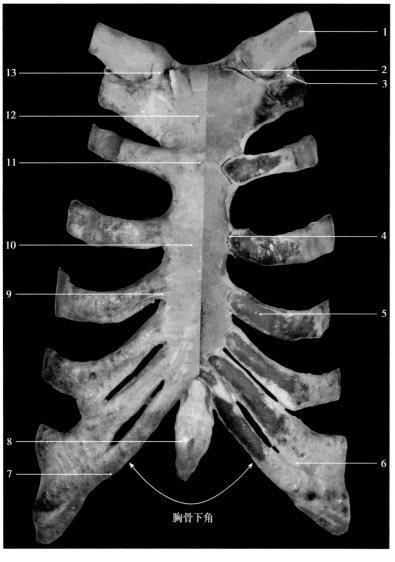

胸骨下角

◀ 图 108

胸肋关节和胸锁关节
Sternocostal joint and sternoclavicular joint
1. 锁骨 clavicle
2. 关节盘 articular disc
3. 肋锁韧带 costoclavicular lig.
4. 胸肋关节腔 sternocostal joint cavity
5. 肋软骨 costal cartilage
6. 软骨间连接 interchondral joints
7. 肋弓 costal arch
8. 剑突 xiphoid process
9. 胸肋辐状韧带 radiate sternocostal lig.
10. 胸骨体 body of sternum
11. 胸骨角 sternal angle
12. 胸骨柄 manubrium sterni
13. 胸锁韧带 sternoclavicular lig.

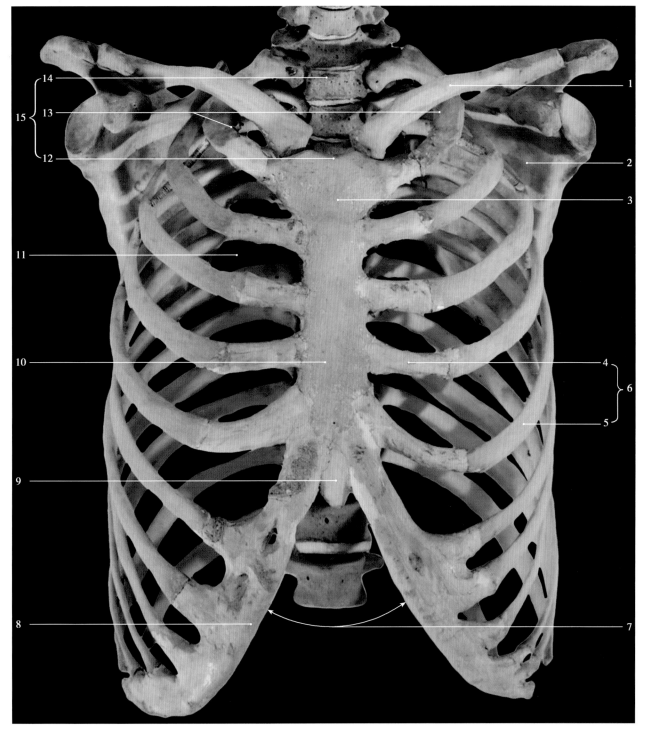

▲ 图 109 胸廓(前面观)
Thorax. Anterior aspect

1. 锁骨 clavicle
2. 肩胛骨 scapula
3. 胸骨柄 manubrium sterni
4. 肋软骨 costal cartilage
5. 肋骨 costal bone
6. 肋 rib
7. 胸骨下角 infrasternal angle
8. 肋弓 costal arch
9. 剑突 xiphoid process
10. 胸骨体 body of sternum
11. 肋间隙 intercostal space
12. 胸骨柄上缘 superior border of manubrium sterni
13. 第 1 肋 1st costal bone
14. 第 1 胸椎椎体 Vertebral body of the 1st thoracic vertebra
15. 胸廓上口 superior aperture of thorax

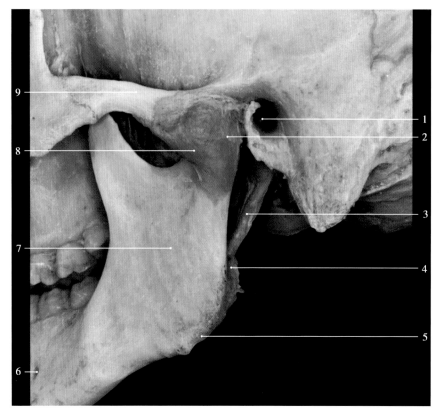

◀ 图 110

颞下颌关节(外侧面观)
Temporomandibular joint.
Lateral aspect
1. 外耳道 external acoustic meatus
2. 关节囊 articular capsule
3. 茎突 styloid process
4. 茎突下颌韧带 stylomandibular lig.
5. 下颌角 angle of mandible
6. 颏孔 mental foramen
7. 下颌支 ramus of mandible.
8. 外侧韧带 lateral lig.
9. 颧弓 zygomatic arch

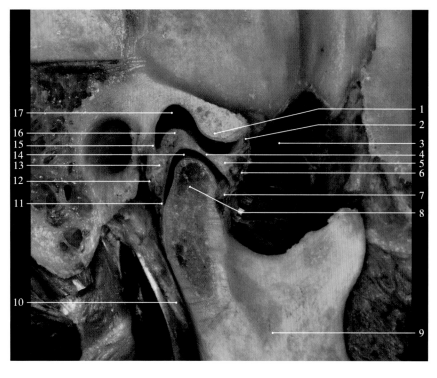

◀ 图 111

颞下颌关节(矢状切面)
Temporomandibular joint.
Sagittal section
1. 关节结节 articular tubercle
2. 颞前附着 attachment anterior to temporal bone
3. 翼外肌 lateral pterygoid
4. 中间带 intermediate zone
5. 前带 prozone
6. 关节囊前壁 anterior wall of articular capsule
7. 下颌前附着 attachment anterior to mandible
8. 下颌头 head of mandible
9. 下颌支 ramus of mandible
10. 茎突 styloid process
11. 下颌后附着 attachment posterion to mandible
12. 关节囊后壁 posterior wall of articular capsule
13. 双极区 bilaminar zone
14. 下关节腔 inferior articular cavity
15. 颞后附着 attachment posterior to temporal bone
16. 后带 posterior band
17. 上关节腔 superior articular cavity

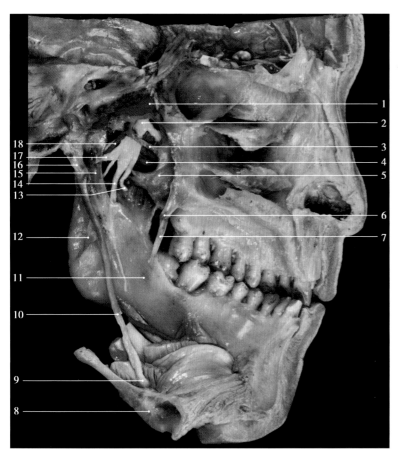

◄ 图 112
颞下颌关节（内侧面观）
Temporomandibular joint. Medial aspect
1. 颈内动脉 internal carotid a.
2. 下颌神经 mandibular n.
3. 翼棘韧带 pterygospinous lig.
4. 翼外肌 lateral pterygoid
5. 翼突外侧板 lateral pterygoid plate
6. 翼钩 pterygoid hamulus
7. 翼下颌韧带 pterygomandibular lig.
8. 舌骨 hyoid bone
9. 舌骨小角 lesser horn of hyoid bone
10. 茎突舌骨韧带 stylohyoid lig.
11. 下颌骨 mandible
12. 茎突下颌韧带 stylomandibular lig.
13. 舌神经 lingual n.
14. 下牙槽神经 inferior alveolar n.
15. 蝶下颌韧带 sphenomandibular lig.
16. 茎突 styloid process
17. 耳颞神经 auriculotemporal n.
18. 脑膜中动脉 middle meningeal a.

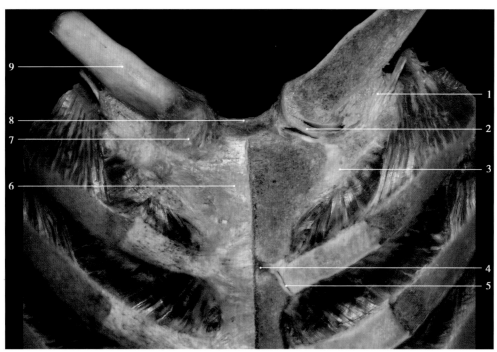

▲ 图 113 **胸锁关节**
Sternoclavicular joint

1. 肋锁韧带 costoclavicular lig.
2. 关节盘 articular disc
3. 第 1 肋胸结合 sternocostal synchondrosis of the first rib
4. 柄胸联合 manubriosternal symphysis
5. 胸肋关节 sternocostal joint
6. 胸骨柄 manubrium sterni
7. 胸锁前韧带 anterior sternoclavicular lig.
8. 锁间韧带 interclavicular lig.
9. 锁骨 clavicle

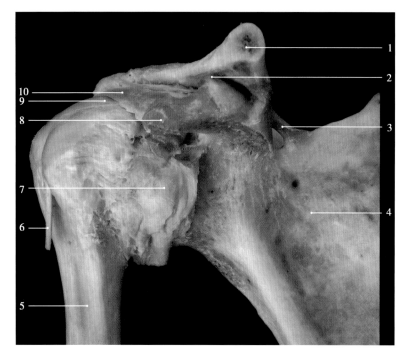

◀ 图 114

肩关节（前面观 1）
Shoulder joint. Anterior aspect（1）
1. 锁骨 clavicle
2. 斜方韧带 trapezoid lig.
3. 肩胛上横韧带 superior transverse scapular lig.
4. 肩胛骨 scapula
5. 肱骨 humerus
6. 肱二头肌长头腱 long head tendon of biceps brachii
7. 关节囊 articular capsule
8. 喙突 coracoid process
9. 喙肱韧带 coracohumeral lig.
10. 喙肩韧带 coracoacromial lig.

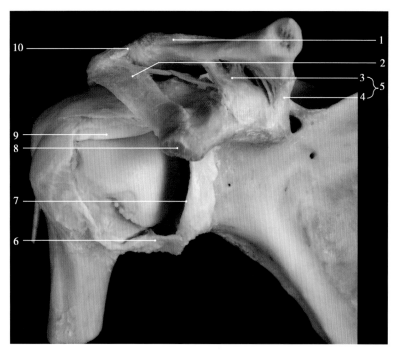

◀ 图 115

肩关节（前面观 2）
Shoulder joint. Anterior aspect（2）
1. 肩峰 acromion
2. 喙肩韧带 coracoacromial lig.
3. 斜方韧带 trapezoid lig.
4. 锥状韧带 conoid lig.
5. 喙锁韧带 coracoclavicular lig.
6. 关节囊 articular capsule
7. 盂唇 glenoid labrum
8. 喙突 coracoid process
9. 肱二头肌长头腱 long head tendon of biceps brachii
10. 肩锁韧带 acromioclavicular lig.

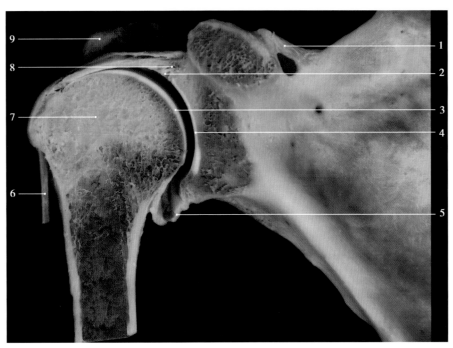

▲ 图 116 肩关节 (冠状切面)
Shoulder joint. Coronal section

1. 肩胛上横韧带 superior transverse scapular lig.
2. 盂唇 glenoid labrum
3. 关节软骨 articular cartilage
4. 关节盂 glenoid cavity
5. 关节囊 articular capsule
6. 肱二头肌长头腱 long head tendon of biceps brachii
7. 肱骨头 head of humerus
8. 盂上结节 supraglenoid tubercle
9. 肩峰 acromion

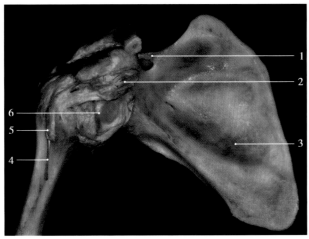

▲ 图 117 肩关节腔 (前面观)
Cavity of shoulder joint. Anterior aspect

1. 肩胛上横韧带 superior transverse scapular lig.
2. 肩胛下肌腱下囊 subtendinous bursa of subscapularis
3. 肩胛骨 scapula
4. 肱二头肌长头腱 long head tendon of biceps brachii
5. 结节间滑膜鞘 intertubercular vagina synovialis
6. 关节囊滑膜层 synovial layer of articular capsule

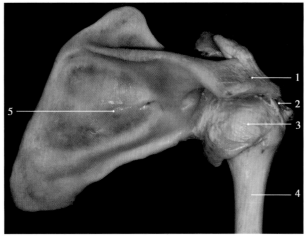

▲ 图 118 肩关节腔 (后面观)
Cavity of shoulder joint. Posterior aspect

1. 肩峰 acromion
2. 肩峰下滑液囊 synovial sac below acromion
3. 滑膜层 synovial layer
4. 肱骨 humerus
5. 肩胛骨 scapula

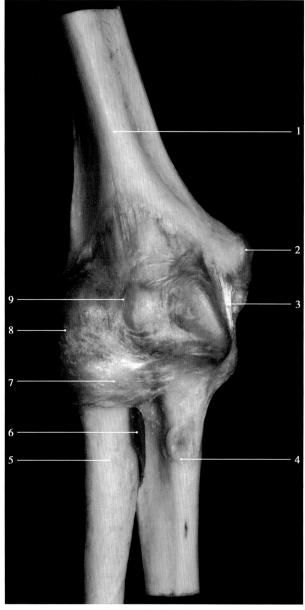

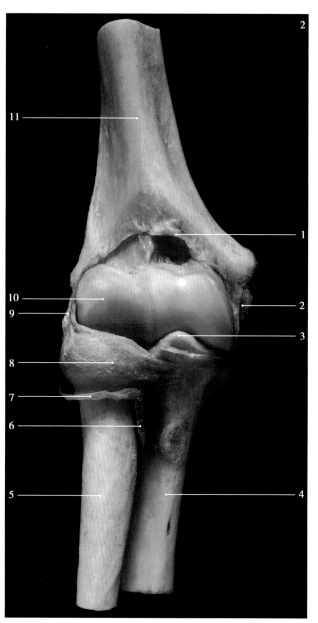

▲ 图 119　肘关节（前面观 1 ）
Elbow joint. Anterior aspect (1)

1. 肱骨 humerus
2. 内上髁 medial epicondyle
3. 尺侧副韧带 ulnar collateral lig.
4. 尺骨 ulna
5. 桡骨 radius
6. 肱二头肌腱 tendon of biceps brachii
7. 桡骨环状韧带 annular ligament of radius
8. 桡侧副韧带 radial collateral lig.
9. 关节囊 articular capsule

▲ 图 120　肘关节（前面观 2 ）
Elbow joint. Anterior aspect (2)

1. 关节囊 articular capsule
2. 尺侧副韧带 ulnar collateral lig.
3. 冠突 coronoid process
4. 尺骨 ulna
5. 桡骨 radius
6. 肱二头肌腱 tendon of biceps brachii
7. 滑膜层 synovial layer
8. 桡骨环状韧带 annular ligament of radius
9. 桡侧副韧带 radial collateral lig.
10. 肱骨小头 capitulum of humerus
11. 肱骨 humerus

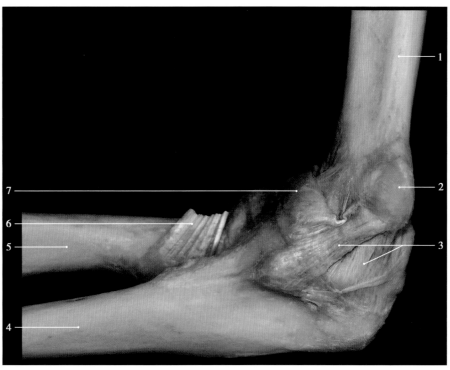

▲ 图 121　肘关节 (内侧面观)
Elbow joint. Medial aspect

1. 肱骨 humerus
2. 内上髁 medial epicondyle
3. 尺侧副韧带 ulnar collateral lig.
4. 尺骨 ulna
5. 桡骨 radius
6. 肱二头肌腱 tendon of biceps brachii
7. 关节囊 articular capsule

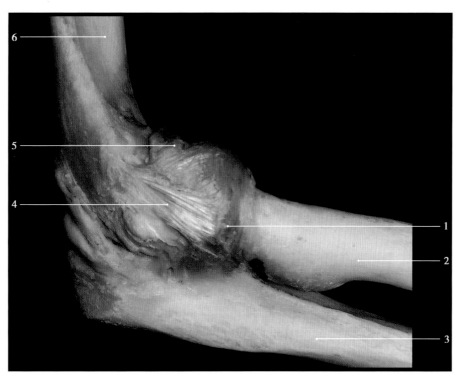

▲ 图 122　肘关节 (外侧面观)
Elbow joint. Lateral aspect

1. 桡骨环状韧带 annular lig. of radius
2. 桡骨 radius
3. 尺骨 ulna
4. 桡侧副韧带 radial collateral lig.
5. 关节囊 articular capsule
6. 肱骨 humerus

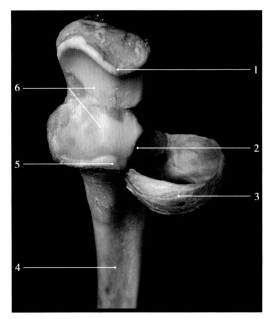

◀ 图 123

桡骨环状韧带
Annular ligament of radius

1. 鹰嘴 olecranon
2. 桡切迹 radial notch
3. 桡骨环状韧带 annular ligament of radius
4. 尺骨 ulna
5. 冠突 coronoid process
6. 滑车切迹 trochlear notch

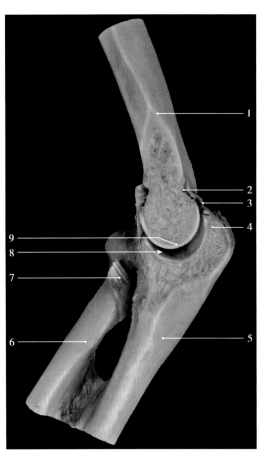

▲ 图 124 **肘关节（矢状切面）**
Elbow joint. Sagittal section

1. 肱骨 humerus
2. 冠突窝 coronoid fossa
3. 关节囊 articular capsule
4. 鹰嘴 olecranon
5. 尺骨 ulna
6. 桡骨 radius
7. 肱二头肌腱 tendon of biceps brachii
8. 关节腔 articular cavity
9. 肱骨滑车 trochlea of humerus

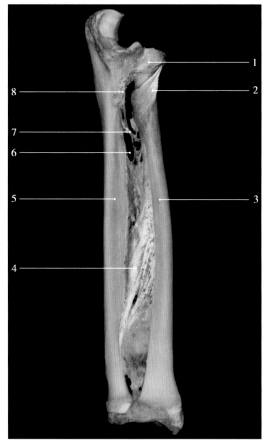

▲ 图 125 **前臂骨间膜**
Interosseous membrane of forearm

1. 桡骨环状韧带 annular ligament of radius
2. 肱二头肌腱 tendon of biceps brachii
3. 桡骨 radius
4. 前臂骨间膜 interosseous membrane of forearm
5. 尺骨 ulna
6. 血管裂孔 hiatus of blood vessel
7. 斜索 oblique cord
8. 肱肌腱 tendon of brachialis

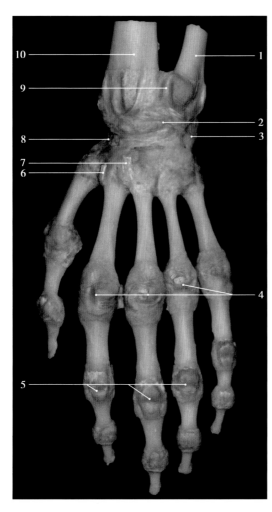

◀ 图 126

手关节（背面观）
Joints of hand. Dorsal aspect
1. 尺骨 ulna
2. 桡腕背侧韧带 dorsal radiocarpal lig.
3. 腕尺侧副韧带 ulnar carpal collateral lig
4. 掌指关节 metacarpophalangeal joint
5. 指骨间关节 interphalangeal joints of hand
6. 桡侧腕长伸肌腱 tendon of extensor carpi radialis longas
7. 桡侧腕短伸肌腱 tendon of extensor carpi radialis brevis
8. 腕桡侧副韧带 radial carpal collateral lig.
9. 桡尺远侧关节 distal radioulnar joint
10. 桡骨 radius

图 127 ▶

手关节（掌面观）
Joints of hand. Palmar aspect
1. 桡骨 radius
2. 腕桡侧副韧带 radial carpal collateral lig.
3. 掌骨掌侧韧带 palmar metacarpal lig.
4. 掌指关节 metacarpophalangeal joints
5. 掌骨深横韧带 deep transverse metacarpal lig.
6. 指骨间远侧关节 distal interphalangeal joints of hand
7. 指骨间近侧关节 proximal interphalangeal joints of hand
8. 掌侧韧带 palmar lig.
9. 钩骨 hamate bone
10. 豆钩韧带 pisohamate lig.
11. 豆掌韧带 pisometacarpal lig.
12. 豌豆骨 pisiform bone
13. 腕尺侧副韧带 ulnar carpal collateral lig
14. 尺骨 ulna

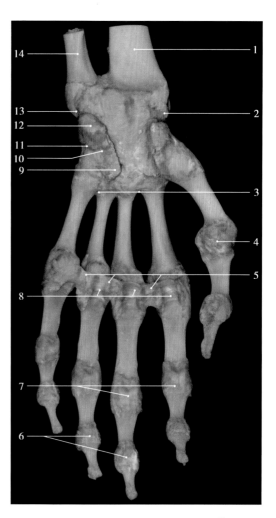

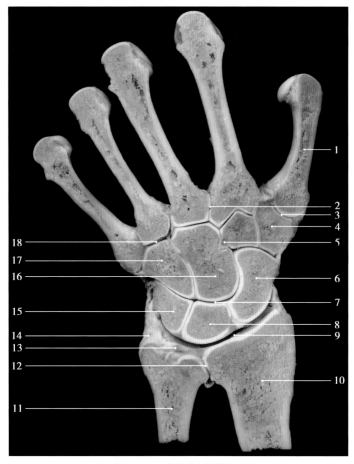

▲ 图 128　**手关节（冠状切面）**
Joints of hand. Coronal section

1. 第 1 掌骨 1st metacarpal bone
2. 掌骨间关节 intermetacarpal joint
3. 拇指腕掌关节 carpometacarpal joint of thumb
4. 大多角骨 trapezium bone
5. 腕骨间骨间韧带 interosseous intercarpal lig.
6. 手舟骨 scaphoid bone
7. 腕骨间关节 intercarpal joint
8. 月骨 lunate bone
9. 桡腕关节 radiocarpal joint

10. 桡骨 radius
11. 尺骨 ulna
12. 桡尺远侧关节 distal radioulnar joint
13. 关节盘 articular disc
14. 腕尺侧副韧带 ulnar carpal collateral lig.
15. 三角骨 triquetral bone
16. 头状骨 capitate bone
17. 钩骨 hamate bone
18. 腕掌关节 carpometacarpal joint

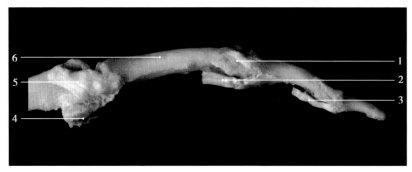

▲ 图 129　**指骨间关节（侧面观）**
Interphalangeal joints of hand. Lateral aspect

1. 指骨间关节侧副韧带 collateral ligaments of interphalangeal joint
2. 指浅屈肌腱 tendon of flexor digitorum superficialis
3. 指深屈肌腱 tendon of flexor digitorum profundus
4. 掌侧韧带 palmar lig.
5. 掌指关节侧副韧带 collateral ligament of metacarpophalangeal joint
6. 近节指骨 proximal phalanx

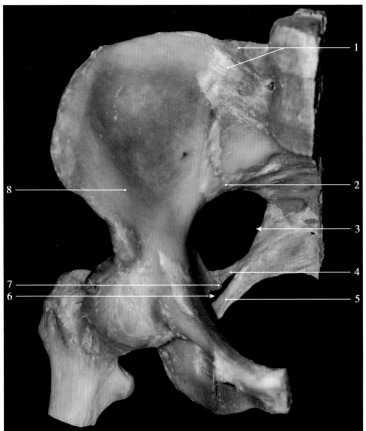

◀ 图 130
骨盆的韧带（前面观）
Ligaments of pelvis. Anterior aspect
1. 髂腰韧带 iliolumbar lig.
2. 骶髂前韧带 anterior sacroiliac lig.
3. 坐骨大孔 greater sciatic foramen
4. 骶棘韧带 sacrospinous lig.
5. 骶结节韧带 sacrotuberous lig.
6. 坐骨小孔 lesser sciatic foramen
7. 坐骨棘 ischial spine
8. 髂骨 ilium

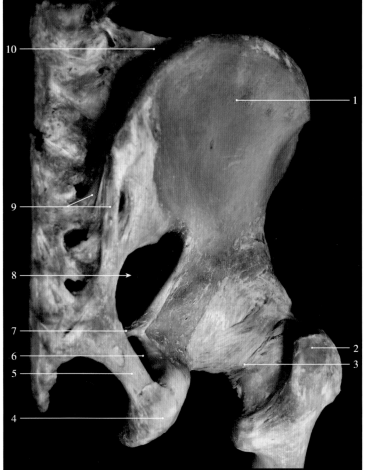

◀ 图 131
骨盆的韧带（后面观）
Ligaments of pelvis. Posterior aspect
1. 髂骨 ilium
2. 大转子 greater trochanter
3. 关节囊 articular capsule
4. 坐骨结节 ischial tuberosity
5. 骶结节韧带 sacrotuberous lig.
6. 坐骨小孔 lesser sciatic foramen
7. 骶棘韧带 sacrospinous lig.
8. 坐骨大孔 greater sciatic foramen
9. 骶髂后韧带 posterior sacroiliac lig.
10. 髂腰韧带 iliolumbar lig.

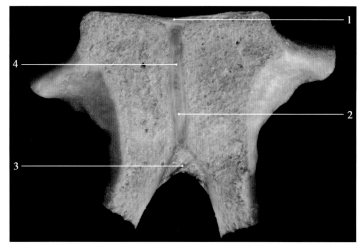

▲ 图 132 　耻骨联合(冠状切面)
Pubic symphysis. Coronal section

1. 耻骨上韧带 superior pubic lig.　　3. 耻骨弓状韧带 arcuate pubic lig.
2. 耻骨间盘 interpubic disc　　　　4. 耻骨联合腔 symphysial cavity

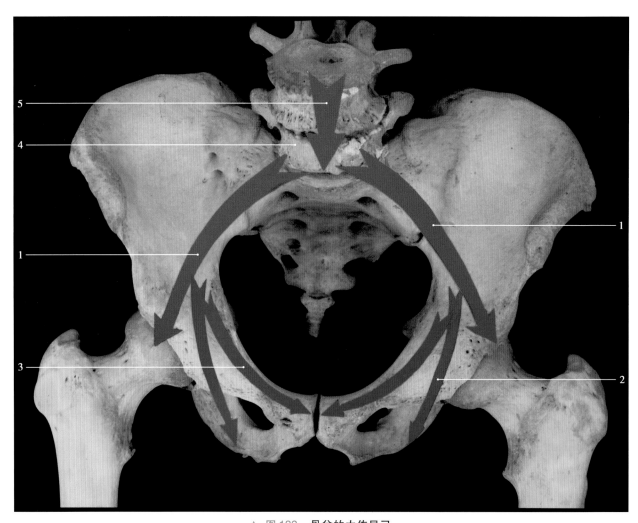

▲ 图 133 　骨盆的力传导弓
Arcus of mechanotransduction of pelvis

1. 股骶弓 femorosacral arch　　　4. 第 5 腰椎 5th lumbar vertebra
2. 坐骶弓 ischiosacral arch　　　　5. 重力 gravity
3. 右约束弓 right constraint arch

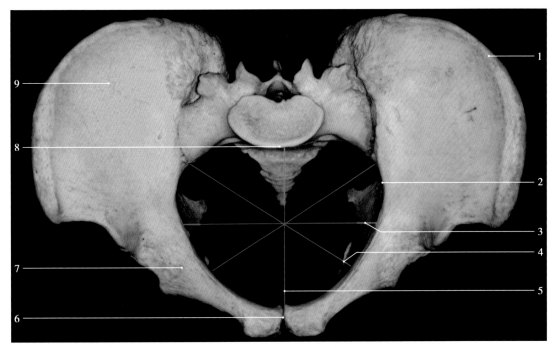

▲ 图 134　**骨盆径线（上面观）**
Diameter of pelvis. Superior aspect

1. 髂嵴 iliac crest
2. 弓状线 arcuate line
3. 横径 transverse diameter
4. 斜径 oblique diameter
5. 入口前后径 anteroposterior diameter of pelvic inlet
6. 耻骨联合 pubic symphysis
7. 髂耻隆起 iliopubic eminence
8. 岬 promontory
9. 髂骨翼 iliac ala

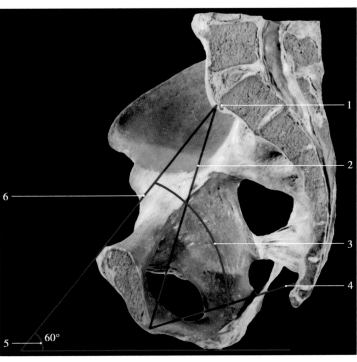

▲ 图 135　**骨盆径线（侧面观）**
Diameter of pelvis. Lateral aspect

1. 岬 promontory
2. 对角径 diameter diagonalis
3. 骨盆轴 pelvic axis
4. 出口前后径 anteroposterior diameter of pelvic outlet
5. 骨盆倾斜度 inclination of pelvis
6. 入口前后径 anteroposterior diameter of pelvic inlet

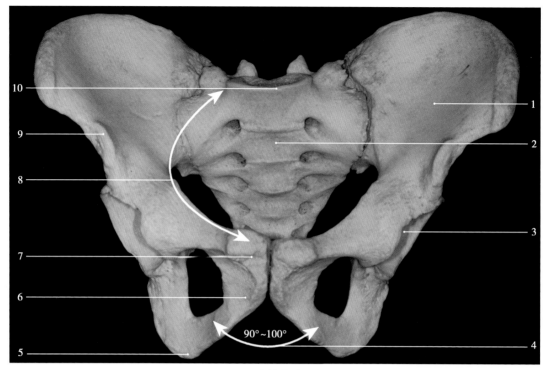

▲ 图136 女性骨盆（前面观）
Pelvis of female. Anterior aspect

1. 髂骨 ilium
2. 骶骨 sacrum
3. 髋臼 acetabulum
4. 耻骨下角 subpudic angle
5. 坐骨结节 ischial tuberosity
6. 耻骨下支 inferior ramus of pubis
7. 耻骨 pubis
8. 界线 terminal line
9. 髂前下棘 anterior inferior iliac spine
10. 岬 promontory

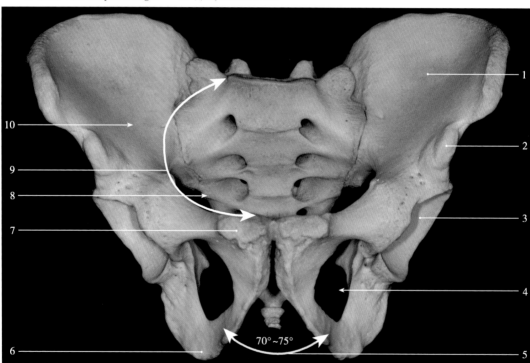

▲ 图137 男性骨盆（前面观）
Pelvis of male. Anterior aspect

1. 髂骨 ilium
2. 髂前下棘 anterior inferior iliac spine
3. 髋臼 acetabulum
4. 闭孔 obturator foramen
5. 耻骨下角 subpubic angle
6. 坐骨 ischium
7. 耻骨 pubis
8. 小骨盆 lesser pelvis
9. 界线 terminal line
10. 大骨盆 greater pelvis

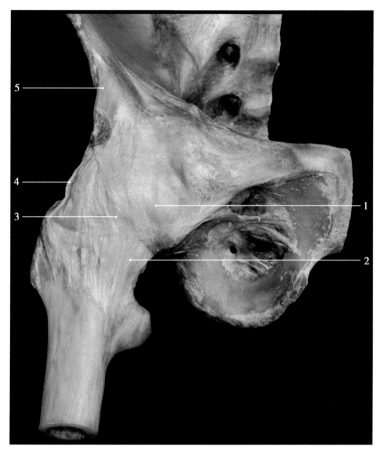

◀ 图 138

髋关节（前面观）
Hip joint . Anterior aspect

1. 关节囊 articular capsule
2. 耻股韧带 pubofemoral lig.
3. 髂股韧带下束 inferior bundle of iliofemoral lig.
4. 髂股韧带上束 superior bundle of iliofemoral lig.
5. 股直肌直头 straight head of rectus femoris

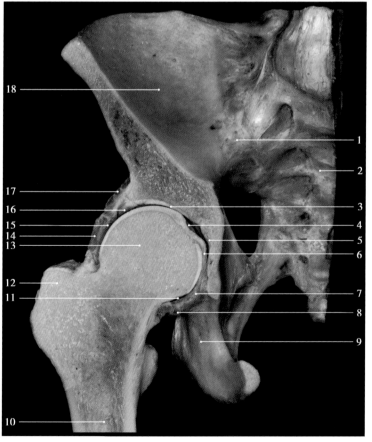

◀ 图 139

髋关节冠状切面
Coronal section through hip joint

1. 骶髂关节 sacroiliac joint
2. 骶骨 sacrum
3. 关节软骨 articular cartilage
4. 股骨头凹 fovea of femoral head
5. 哈佛森腺 Haversian gland
6. 股骨头韧带 ligament of head of femur
7. 髋臼横韧带 transverse acetabular lig.
8. 关节囊纤维膜 fibrous membrane of articular capsule
9. 坐骨 ischium
10. 股骨 femur
11. 关节腔 articular cavity
12. 大转子 greater trochanter
13. 股骨头 femoral head
14. 轮匝带 zona orbicularis
15. 滑膜 synovium
16. 髋臼唇 acetabular labrum
17. 股直肌反折头 reflected head of rectus femoris
18. 髂骨 ilium

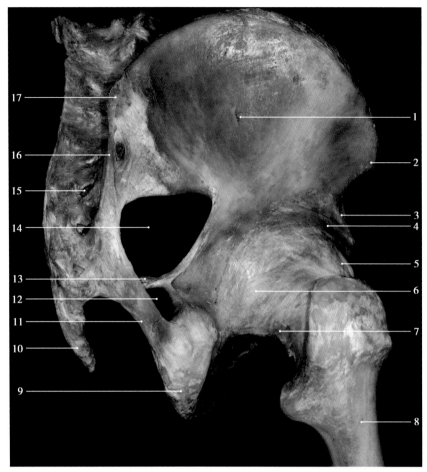

◀ 图 140

髋关节(后面观1)
Hip joint. Posterior aspect(1)
1. 髂骨 ilium
2. 髂前上棘 anterior superior iliac spine
3. 股直肌直头 straight head of rectus femoris
4. 股直肌反折头 reflected head of rectus femoris
5. 髂股韧带 iliofemoral lig.
6. 坐股韧带 ischiofemoral lig.
7. 关节囊 articular capsule
8. 股骨 femur
9. 坐骨结节 ischial tuberosity
10. 尾骨 coccyx
11. 骶结节韧带 sacrotuberous lig.
12. 坐骨小孔 lesser sciatic foramen
13. 骶棘韧带 sacrospinous lig.
14. 坐骨大孔 greater sciatic foramen
15. 骶后孔 posterior sacral foramina
16. 骶髂后韧带 posterior sacroiliac lig.
17. 髂后上棘 posterior superior iliac spine

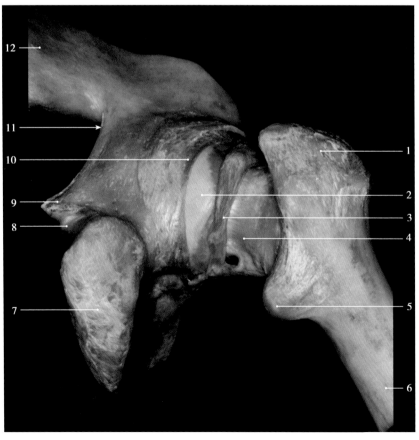

◀ 图 141

髋关节(后面观2)
Hip joint. Posterior aspect(2)
1. 大转子 greater trochanter
2. 股骨头 femoral head
3. 轮匝带 zona orbicularis
4. 股骨颈 neck of femur
5. 小转子 lesser trochanter
6. 股骨 femur
7. 坐骨结节 ischial tuberosity
8. 坐骨小切迹 lesser sciatic notch
9. 坐骨棘 ischial spine
10. 髋臼唇 acetabular labrum
11. 坐骨大切迹 greater sciatic notch
12. 髂骨 ilium

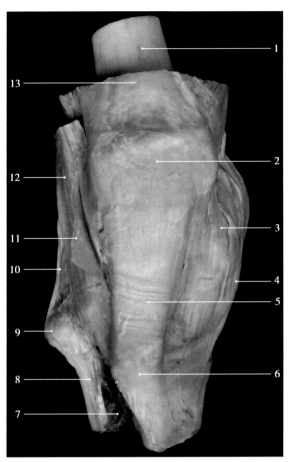

◀ 图 142

膝关节（前面观）
Knee joint. Anterior aspect

1. 股骨 femur
2. 髌骨 patella
3. 髌内侧支持带 medial patellar retinaculum
4. 胫侧副韧带 tibial collateral lig.
5. 髌韧带 patellar lig.
6. 胫骨粗隆 tuberosity of tibia
7. 骨间膜 interosseous membrane
8. 腓骨 fibula
9. 腓骨头 fibular head
10. 腓侧副韧带 fibular collateral lig.
11. 髌外侧支持带 lateral patellar retinaculum
12. 髂胫束 iliotibial tract
13. 股四头肌腱 tendon of quadriceps femoris

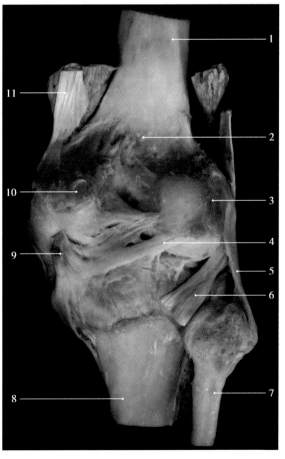

◀ 图 143

膝关节（后面观）
Knee joint. Posterior aspect

1. 股骨 femur
2. 腘平面 popliteal surface
3. 腓肠肌外侧头 lateral head of gastrocnemius
4. 腘斜韧带 oblique popliteal lig.
5. 腓侧副韧带 fibular collateral lig.
6. 腘肌腱 tendon of popliteus
7. 腓骨 fibula
8. 胫骨 tibia
9. 半膜肌腱 tendon of semimembranosus
10. 腓肠肌内侧头 medial head of gastrocnemius
11. 大收肌腱 tendon of adductor magnus

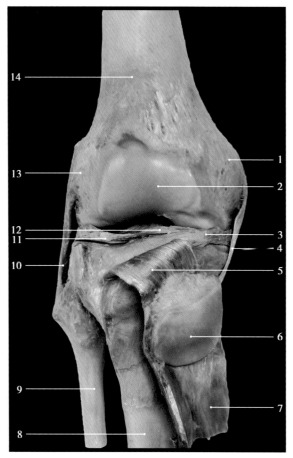

◀ 图 144

膝关节（囊切开前面观）
Opened knee joint. Anterior aspect

1. 内上髁 medial epicondyle
2. 髌面 patellar surface
3. 内侧半月板 medial meniscus
4. 胫侧副韧带 tibial collateral lig.
5. 髌韧带 patellar lig.
6. 髌关节面 patellar articular surface
7. 股四头肌腱 tendon of quadriceps femoris
8. 胫骨 tibia
9. 腓骨 fibula
10. 腓侧副韧带 fibular collateral lig.
11. 外侧半月板 lateral meniscus
12. 膝横韧带 transverse ligament of knee
13. 外上髁 lateral epicondyle
14. 股骨 femur

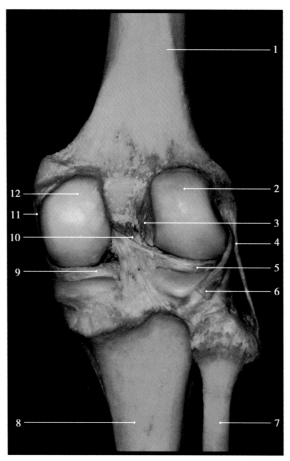

◀ 图 145

膝关节（囊切开后面观）
Opened knee joint. Posterior aspect

1. 股骨 femur
2. 外侧髁 lateral condyle
3. 前交叉韧带 anterior cruciate lig.
4. 腓侧副韧带 fibular collateral lig.
5. 外侧半月板 lateral meniscus
6. 腘肌腱 tendon of popliteus
7. 腓骨 fibula
8. 胫骨 tibia
9. 内侧半月板 medial meniscus
10. 后交叉韧带 posterior cruciate lig
11. 胫侧副韧带 tibial collateral lig.
12. 内侧髁 medial condyle

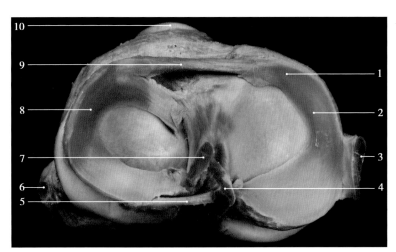

◀ 图 146

膝关节半月板(上面观)
Menici of knee joint. Superior aspect

1. 内侧半月板前角 anterior angle of medial meniscus
2. 内侧半月板 medial meniscus
3. 胫侧副韧带 tibial collateral lig.
4. 后交叉韧带 posterior cruciate lig.
5. 板股后韧带 posterior meniscofemoral lig.
6. 腓侧副韧带 fibular collateral lig.
7. 前交叉韧带 anterior cruciate lig.
8. 外侧半月板 lateral meniscus
9. 膝横韧带 transverse ligament of knee
10. 胫骨粗隆 tuberosity of tibia

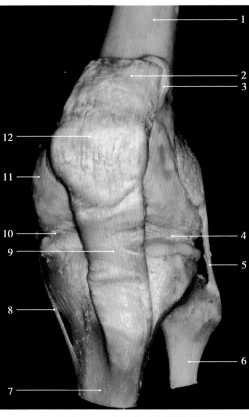

▲ 图 147　膝关节腔(前面观)
Cavity of knee joint. Anterior aspect

1. 股骨 femur
2. 股四头肌腱 tendon of quadriceps femoris
3. 髌上囊 suprapatellar bursa
4. 外侧半月板 lateral meniscus
5. 腓侧副韧带 fibular collateral lig.
6. 腓骨 fibula
7. 胫骨 tibia
8. 胫侧副韧带 tibial collateral lig.
9. 髌韧带 patellar lig.
10. 内侧半月板 medial meniscus
11. 关节囊 articular capsule
12. 髌骨 patella

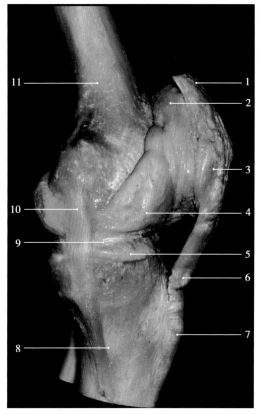

▲ 图 148　膝关节腔(内侧面观)
Cavity of knee joint. Medial aspect

1. 股四头肌腱 tendon of quadriceps femoris
2. 髌上囊 suprapatellar bursa
3. 髌骨 patella
4. 上部(内髁部)upper part of medial condyle
5. 下部(内髁部)lower part of medial condyle
6. 髌韧带 patellar lig.
7. 胫骨粗隆 tuberosity of tibia
8. 胫骨 tibia
9. 内侧半月板 medial meniscus
10. 胫侧副韧带 tibial collateral lig.
11. 股骨 femur

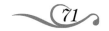

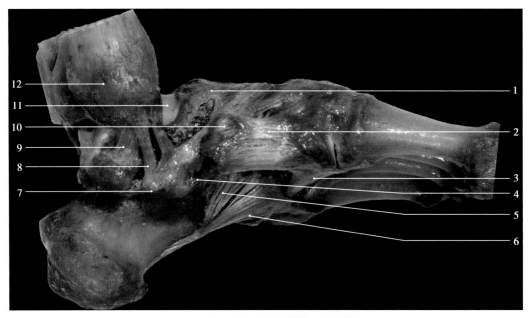

▲ 图149　足的关节韧带 (内侧面观)
Joints and ligaments of foot. Medial aspect

1. 距舟韧带 talonavicular lig.
2. 楔舟背侧韧带 dorsal cuneonavicular lig.
3. 腓骨长肌腱 tendon of peroneus longus
4. 跟舟足底韧带 plantar calcaneonavicular lig.
5. 跟骰足底韧带 plantar calcaneocuboid lig.
6. 跖长韧带 long plantar lig.
7. 载距突 sustentaculum tali
8. 胫跟部 tibiocalcaneal part
9. 胫距后部 posterior tibiotalar part
10. 足舟骨 navicular bone
11. 距骨颈 neck of talus
12. 内踝 medial malleolus

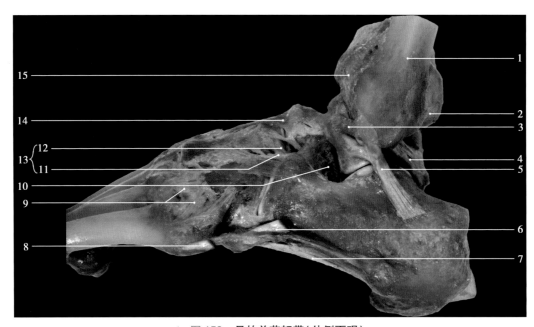

▲ 图150　足的关节韧带 (外侧面观)
Joints and ligaments of foot. Lateral aspect

1. 腓骨 fibula
2. 胫腓后韧带 posterior tibiofibular lig.
3. 距腓前韧带 anterior talofibular lig.
4. 距腓后韧带 posterior talofibular lig
5. 跟腓韧带 calcaneofibular lig.
6. 腓骨长肌腱 tendon of peroneus longus
7. 跖长韧带 long plantar lig.
8. 腓骨短肌腱 tendon of peroneus brevis
9. 跗跖背侧韧带 dorsal tarsometatarsal lig.
10. 距跟骨间韧带 interosseous talocalcaneal lig.
11. 跟骰韧带 calcaneocuboid lig
12. 跟舟韧带 calcaneonavicular lig
13. 分歧韧带 bifurcated lig.
14. 距舟韧带 talonavicular lig.
15. 胫腓前韧带 anterior tibiofibular lig.

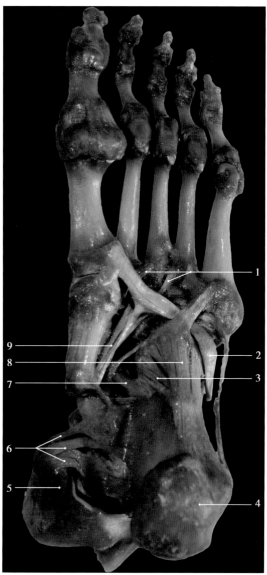

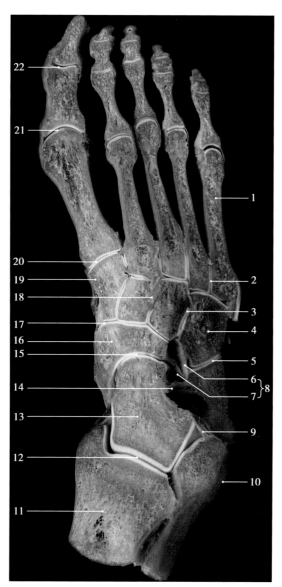

▲ 图 151 足的关节韧带（足底面观）
Joints and ligaments of foot. Plantar aspect

1. 跗跖足底韧带 plantar tarsometatarsal lig.
2. 腓骨长肌腱 tendon of peroneus longus
3. 跟骰足底韧带 plantar calcaneocuboid lig.
4. 跟结节 tuberosity of calcaneus
5. 内踝 medial malleolus
6. 内侧韧带 medial lig.
7. 跟舟足底韧带 plantar calcaneonavicular lig.
8. 跖长韧带 long plantar lig.
9. 胫骨后肌腱 tendon of tibialis posterior

▲ 图 152 足的关节（水平切面）
Joints of foot. Horizontal section

1. 跖骨 metatarsal bone
2. 跖骨间关节 intermetatarsal joint
3. 楔骰关节 cuneocuboid joint
4. 骰骨 cuboid bone
5. 跟骰关节 calcaneocuboid joint
6. 跟骰韧带 calcaneocuboid lig.
7. 跟舟韧带 calcaneonavicular lig.
8. 分歧韧带 bifurcated lig.
9. 距腓前韧带 anterior talofibular lig.
10. 外踝 lateral malleolus
11. 胫骨 tibia
12. 踝关节 ankle joint
13. 距骨 talus
14. 距跟骨间韧带 interosseous talocalcaneal lig.
15. 距舟关节 talonavicular joint
16. 足舟骨 navicular bone
17. 楔舟关节 cuneonavicular joint
18. 楔间骨间韧带 interosseous intercuneiform lig.
19. 内侧楔骨 medial cuneiform bone
20. 跗跖关节 tarsometatarsal joint
21. 跖趾关节 metatarsophalangeal joint
22. 趾骨间关节 interphalangeal joints of foot

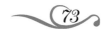

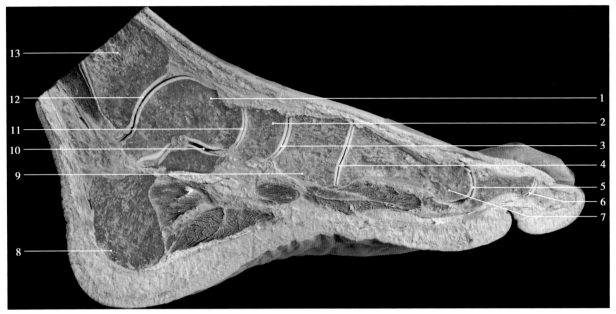

▲ 图 153　足的关节 (矢状切面)
Joints of foot. Sagittal section

1. 距骨 talus
2. 足舟骨 navicular bone
3. 楔舟关节 cuneonavicular joint
4. 跗跖关节 tarsometatarsal joint
5. 跖趾关节 metatarsophalangeal joint
6. 趾骨间关节 interphalangeal joint of foot
7. 跖骨 metatarsal bone
8. 跟骨 calcaneus
9. 内侧楔骨 medial cuneiform bone
10. 距跟关节 (距下关节) talocalcaneal joint
11. 距舟关节 talonavicular joint
12. 距小腿关节 talocrural joint
13. 胫骨 tibia

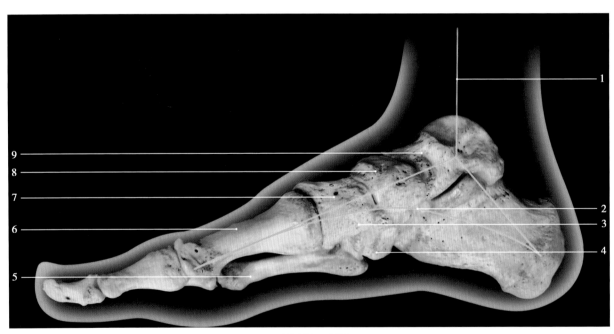

▲ 图 154　足弓
Arch of foot

1. 重力线 weight line
2. 内侧纵弓 medial longitudinal arch
3. 横弓 transverse arch
4. 骰骨 cuboid bone
5. 第 5 跖骨 5th metatarsal bone
6. 第 1 跖骨 1st metatarsal bone
7. 内侧楔骨 medial cuneiform bone
8. 足舟骨 navicular bone
9. 距骨 talus

第四章 肌学 Myology

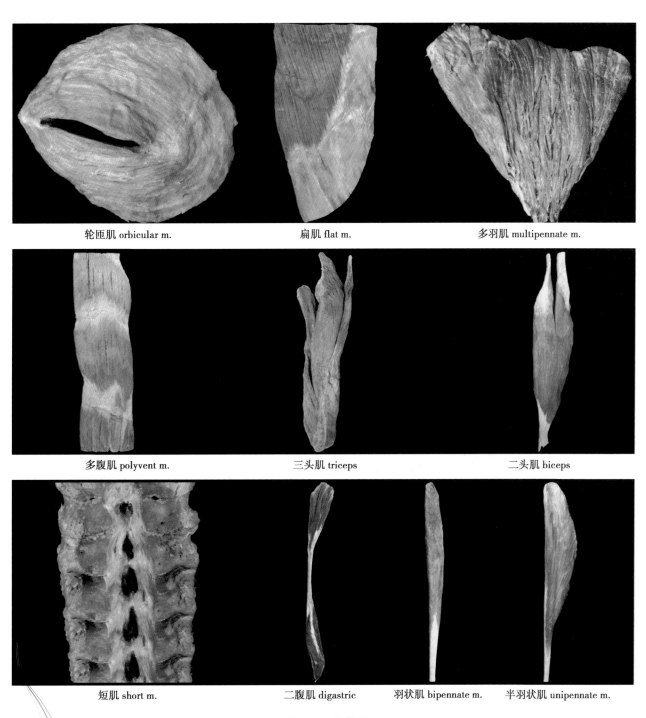

轮匝肌 orbicular m.　　　　扁肌 flat m.　　　　多羽肌 multipennate m.

多腹肌 polyvent m.　　　　三头肌 triceps　　　　二头肌 biceps

短肌 short m.　　　　二腹肌 digastric　　　羽状肌 bipennate m.　　半羽状肌 unipennate m.

▲ 图 155　肌的形态
Various shapes of muscles

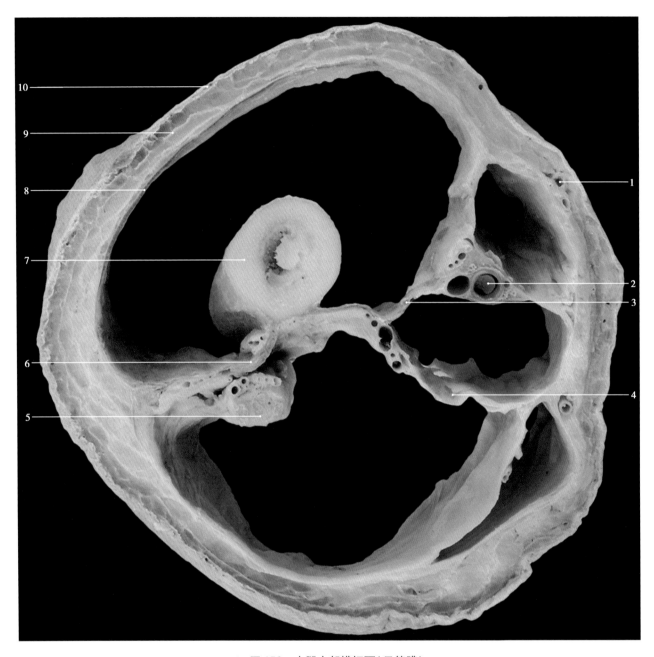

▲ 图156 大腿中部横切面 (示筋膜)
Transverse section through middle of thigh. Showing fasciae

1. 大隐静脉 greater saphenous v.
2. 股动脉 femoral a.
3. 股内侧肌间隔 medial femoral intermuscular septum
4. 股后肌间隔 posterior femoral intermuscular septum
5. 坐骨神经 sciatic n.
6. 股外侧肌间隔 external femoral intermuscular septum
7. 股骨 femur
8. 深筋膜 deep fascia
9. 浅筋膜 superficial fascia
10. 皮肤 skin

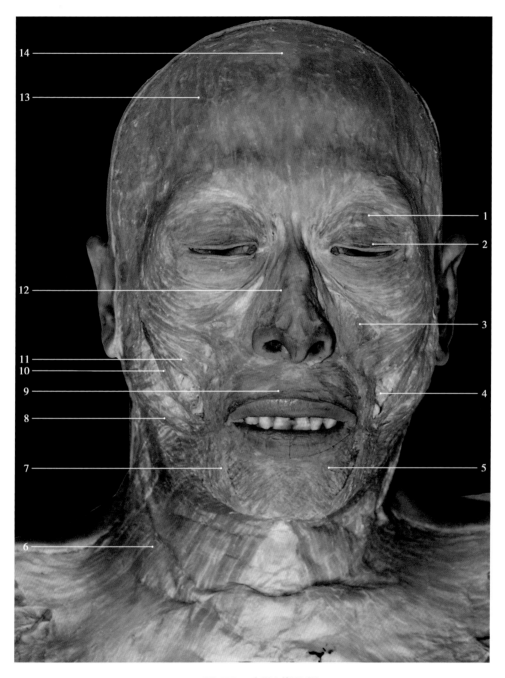

▲ 图157 头肌(前面观)
Muscles of head. Anterior aspect

1. 眶部(眼轮匝肌) orbital part(orbicularis oculi)
2. 睑部(眼轮匝肌) palpebral part (orbicularis oculi)
3. 提上唇肌 levator labii superioris
4. 颊脂肪垫 buccal fat pad
5. 降下唇肌 depressor labii inferioris
6. 颈阔肌 platysma m.
7. 降口角肌 depressor anguli oris

8. 笑肌 risorius
9. 口轮匝肌 orbicularis oris
10. 颧大肌 zygomaticus major
11. 颧小肌 zygomaticus minor
12. 鼻肌 nasalis
13. 枕额肌额腹 frontal belly of occipitofrontalis
14. 帽状腱膜 galea aponeurotica

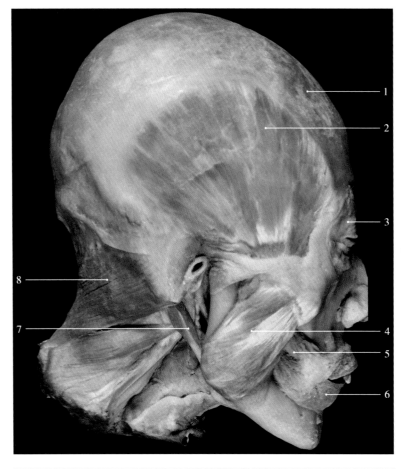

◀ 图 158

头肌(侧面观 1)
Muscles of head. Lateral aspect(1)
1. 额骨 frontal bone
2. 颞肌 temporalis
3. 眶隔 orbital septum
4. 咬肌 masseter
5. 颊肌 buccinator
6. 口轮匝肌 orbicularis oris
7. 二腹肌后腹 posterior belly of digastric
8. 头夹肌 splenius capitis

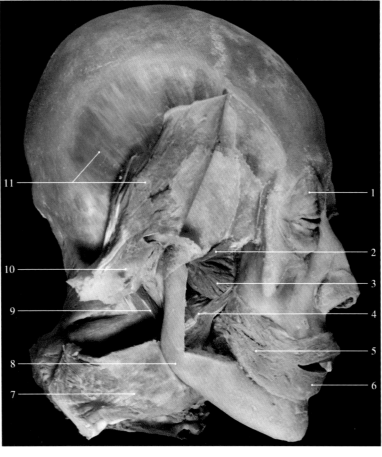

◀ 图 159

头肌(侧面观 2)
Muscles of head. Lateral aspect(2)
1. 眶隔 orbital septum
2. 翼外肌上头 superior head of lateral pterygoid
3. 翼外肌下头 inferior head of lateral pterygoid
4. 翼内肌 medial pterygoid
5. 颊肌 buccinator
6. 口轮匝肌 orbicularis oris
7. 咬肌 masseter
8. 下颌角 angle of mandible
9. 二腹肌后腹 posterior belly of digastric
10. 冠突(切断) coronoid process
11. 颞肌 temporalis

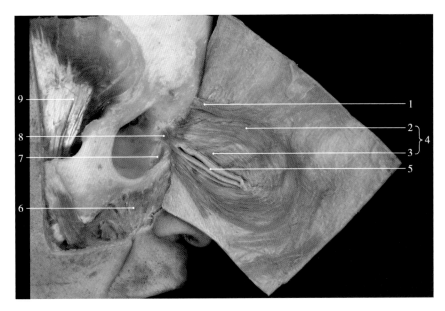

▲ 图160　眼轮匝肌泪部与泪囊的关系
Relationship of lacrimal part of orbicularis oculi and lacrimal sac

1. 皱眉肌 corrugator supercilii
2. 眶部 orbital part
3. 睑部 palpebral part
4. 眼轮匝肌 orbicularis oculi
5. 睑裂 palpebral fissure
6. 提上唇肌 levator labii superioris
7. 泪囊 lacrimal sac
8. 眼轮匝肌泪囊部 lacrimal part of orbicularis oculi
9. 颞肌 temporalis

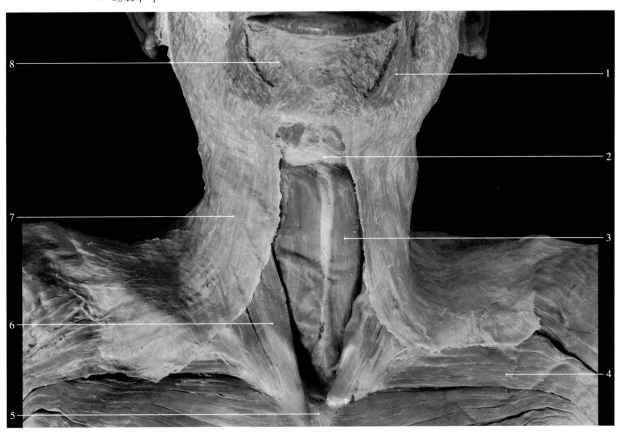

▲ 图161　颈阔肌
Platysma

1. 降口角肌 depressor anguli oris
2. 舌骨 hyoid bone
3. 胸骨舌骨肌 sternohyoid
4. 胸大肌 pectoralis major
5. 颈静脉切迹 jugular notch
6. 胸锁乳突肌 sternocleidomastoid
7. 颈阔肌 platysma
8. 降下唇肌 depressor labii inferioris

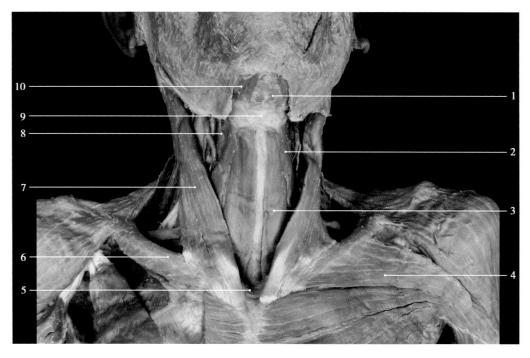

▲ 图162 颈肌（前面观1）
Muscles of neck. Anterior aspect（1）

1. 下颌舌骨肌 mylohyoideus
2. 肩胛舌骨肌 omohyoid
3. 胸骨舌骨肌 sternohyoid
4. 胸大肌 pectoralis major
5. 锁间韧带 interclavicular lig.

6. 锁骨 clavicle
7. 胸锁乳突肌 sternocleidomastoid
8. 甲状舌骨肌 thyrohyoid
9. 舌骨 hyoid bone
10. 二腹肌前腹 anterior belly of digastric

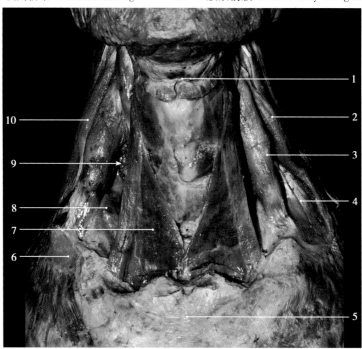

▲ 图163 颈肌（前面观2）
Muscles of neck. Anterior aspect（2）

1. 舌骨 hyoid bone
2. 中斜角肌 scalenus medius
3. 前斜角肌 scalenus anterior
4. 小斜角肌 scalenus minimus
5. 胸骨柄 manubrium sterni

6. 第1肋 1st rib
7. 胸骨甲状肌 sternothyroid
8. 胸膜 pleura
9. 斜角肌间隙 scalenus space
10. 后斜角肌 scalenus posterior

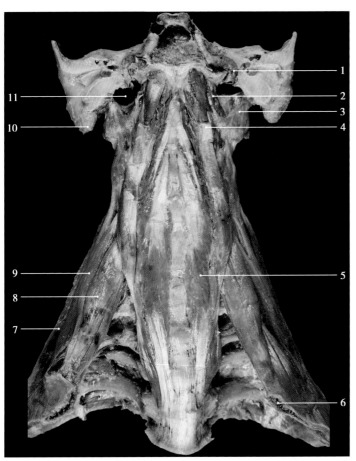

◀ 图 164

颈肌（前面观 3）

Muscles of neck. Anterior aspect（3）

1. 颈内动脉 internal carotid a.
2. 头前直肌 rectus capitis anterior
3. 头外侧直肌 rectus capitis lateralis
4. 头长肌 longus capitis
5. 颈长肌 longus colli
6. 第 1 肋骨 1st rib
7. 后斜角肌 scalenus posterior
8. 前斜角肌 scalenus anterior
9. 中斜角肌 scalenus medius
10. 乳突 mastoid process
11. 颈静脉孔 jugular foramen

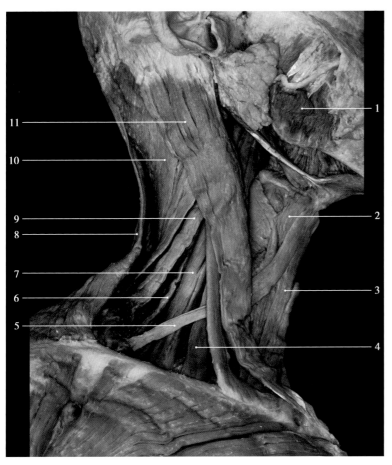

◀ 图 165

颈肌（侧面观）

Muscles of neck. Lateral aspect

1. 咬肌 masseter
2. 甲状舌骨肌 thyrohyoid
3. 胸骨舌骨肌 sternohyoid
4. 前斜角肌 scalenus anterior
5. 肩胛舌骨肌 omohyoid
6. 后斜角肌 scalenus posterior
7. 中斜角肌 scalenus medius
8. 斜方肌 trapezius
9. 肩胛提肌 levator scapulae
10. 头夹肌 splenius capitis
11. 胸锁乳突肌 sternocleidomastoid

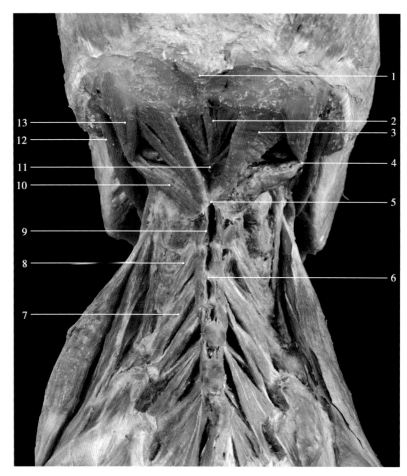

◀ 图 166

椎枕肌

Vertebrooccipital muscles

1. 枕外隆凸 external occipital protuberance
2. 头后小直肌 rectus capitis posterior minor
3. 头后大直肌 rectus capitis posterior major
4. 寰椎横突 transverse process of atlas
5. 枢椎棘突 spinous process of axis
6. 棘突 spinous process
7. 多裂肌 multifidi
8. 颈回旋肌 rotatores cervicis
9. 颈棘间肌 interspinales cervicis
10. 头下斜肌 obliquus capitis inferior
11. 寰椎后结节 posterior tubercle of atlas
12. 二腹肌后腹 posterior belly of digastric
13. 头上斜肌 obliquus capitis superior

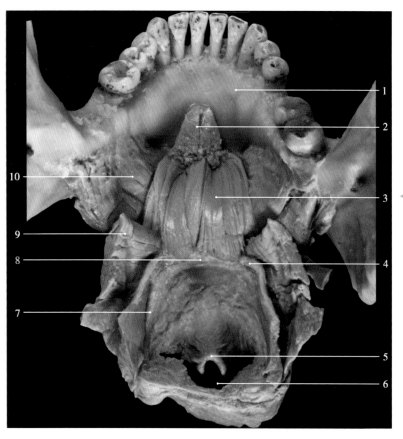

◀ 图 167

口底肌

Muscles of base of oral cavity

1. 下颌骨 mandible
2. 颏舌肌 genioglossus
3. 颏舌骨肌 geniohyoid
4. 舌骨小角 lesser horn of hyoid bone
5. 会厌 epiglottis
6. 咽腔 pharynx cavity
7. 舌骨大角 greater horn of hyoid bone
8. 舌骨 hyoid bone
9. 舌骨舌肌 hyoglossus
10. 下颌舌骨肌 mylohyoid

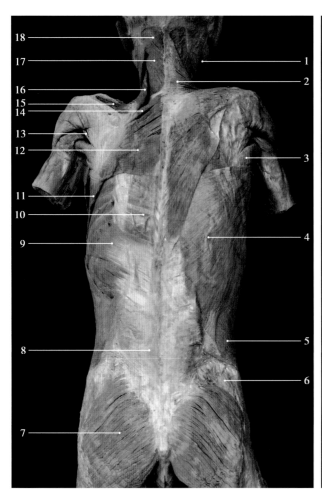

▲ 图 168　背肌（1）
Muscles of back（1）

1. 胸锁乳突肌 sternocleidomastoid
2. 斜方肌 trapezius
3. 大圆肌 teres major
4. 背阔肌 latissimus dorsi
5. 腹外斜肌 obliquus externus abdominis
6. 臀中肌筋膜 fascia of gluteus medius
7. 臀大肌 gluteus maximus
8. 胸腰筋膜 thoracolumbar fascia
9. 下后锯肌 serratus posterior inferior
10. 竖脊肌 erector spinae
11. 前锯肌 serratus anterior
12. 大菱形肌 rhomboideus major
13. 小圆肌 teres minor
14. 小菱形肌 rhomboideus minor
15. 冈上肌 supraspinatus
16. 肩胛提肌 levator scapulae
17. 头夹肌 splenius capitis
18. 头半棘肌 semispinalis capitis

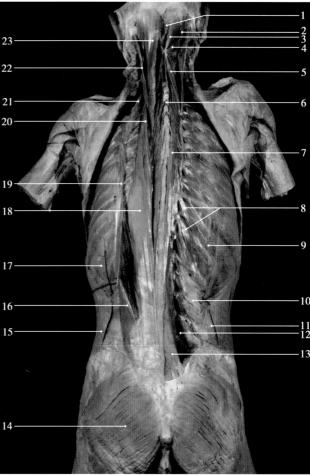

▲ 图 169　背肌（2）
Muscles of back（2）

1. 头后小直肌 rectus capitis posterior minor
2. 头上斜肌 obliquus capitis superior
3. 头后大直肌 rectus capitis posterior major
4. 头下斜肌 obliquus capitis inferior
5. 颈半棘肌 semispinalis cervicis
6. 棘间肌 interspinales
7. 棘肌 spinalis
8. 肋提肌 levatores costarum
9. 肋间外肌 intercostales externi
10. 胸腰筋膜深层 deep layer of thoracolumbar fascia
11. 腹内斜肌 obliquus internus abdominis
12. 横突间肌 intertransversarii
13. 多裂肌 multifidi
14. 臀大肌 gluteus maximus
15. 腹外斜肌 obliquus externus abdominis
16. 腰髂肋肌 iliocostalis lumborum
17. 下后锯肌 serratus posterior inferior
18. 胸最长肌 longissimus thoracis
19. 胸髂肋肌 iliocostalis thoracis
20. 颈最长肌 longissimus cervicis
21. 颈髂肋肌 iliocostalis cervicis
22. 头最长肌 longissimus capitis
23. 头半棘肌 semispinalis capitis

83

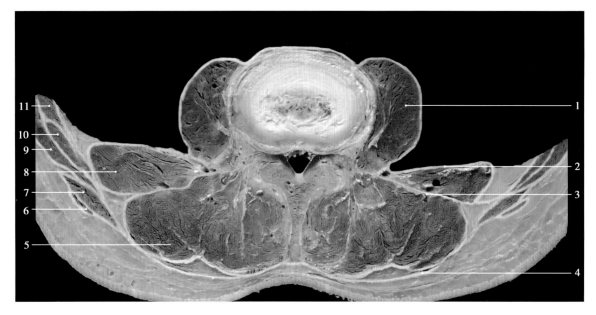

▲ 图170　胸腰筋膜
Thoracolumbar fascia

1. 腰大肌 psoas major
2. 胸腰筋膜深层 deep layer of thoracolumbar fascia
3. 胸腰筋膜中层 middle layer of thoracolumbar fascia
4. 胸腰筋膜浅层 superficial layer of thoracolumbar fascia
5. 竖脊肌 erector spinae
6. 背阔肌 latissimus dorsi

7. 下后锯肌 serratus posterior inferior
8. 腰方肌 quadratus lumborum
9. 腹外斜肌 obliquus externus abdominis
10. 腹内斜肌 obliquus internus abdominis
11. 腹横肌 transverses abdominis

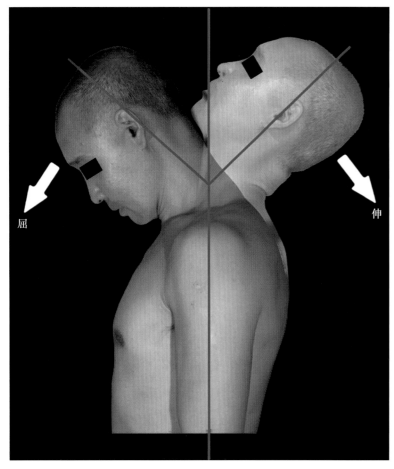

▲ 图171　颈部的屈和伸
Flexion and extension of neck

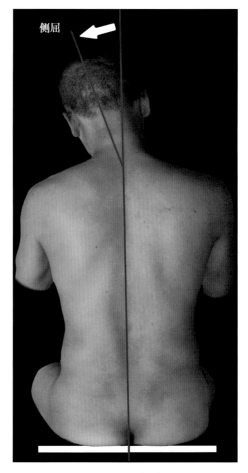

▲ 图172　颈部的侧屈
Lateral flection of neck

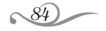

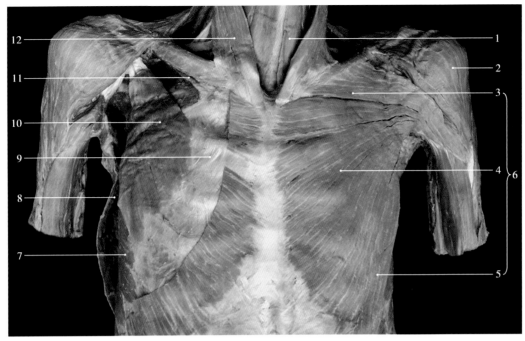

▲ 图 173 胸肌
Muscles of thorax

1. 胸骨舌骨肌 sternohyoideus
2. 三角肌 deltoid
3. 胸大肌锁骨部 clavicular part of pectoralis major
4. 胸大肌胸骨部 sternal part of pectoralis major
5. 胸大肌腹部 abdominal part of pectoralis major
6. 胸大肌 pectoralis major
7. 前锯肌 serratus anterior
8. 背阔肌 latissimus dorsi
9. 肋间内肌 intercostales interni
10. 胸小肌 pectoralis minor
11. 锁骨下肌 subclavius
12. 胸锁乳突肌 sternocleidomastoid

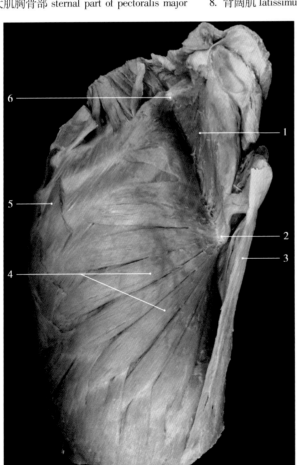

◀ 图 174

前锯肌
Serratus anterior

1. 肩胛下肌 subscapularis
2. 肩胛骨下角 inferior angle of scapula
3. 背阔肌 latissimus dorsi
4. 前锯肌 serratus anterior
5. 胸小肌（切断）pectoralis minor
6. 肩胛骨上角 superior angle of scapula

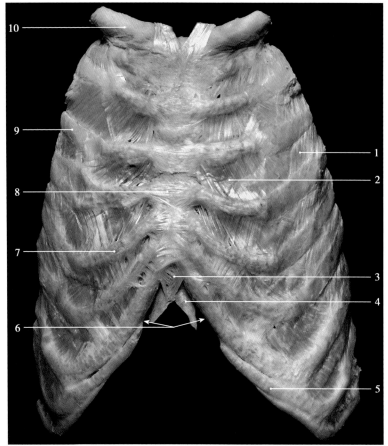

◀ 图 175

肋间肌(前面观)
Intercostales. Anterior aspect
1. 肋间外肌 intercostales externi
2. 肋间内肌 intercostales interni
3. 肋剑突韧带 costoxiphoid lig.
4. 剑突 xiphoid process
5. 肋弓 costal arch
6. 胸骨下角 infrasternal angle
7. 肋软骨 costal cartilage
8. 胸骨 sternum
9. 肋骨 costal bone
10. 锁骨 clavicle

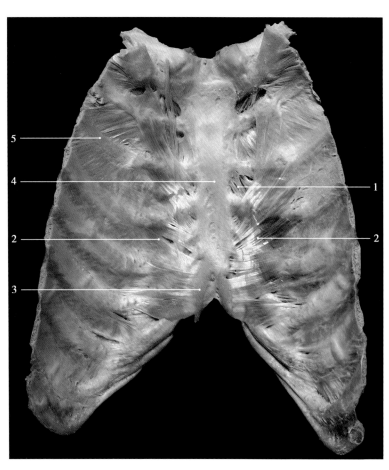

◀ 图 176

胸横肌(后面观)
Transverses thoracis. Posterior aspect
1. 肋间内肌 intercostales interni
2. 胸横肌 transverses thoracis
3. 剑突 xiphoid process
4. 胸骨 sternum
5. 肋骨 costal bone

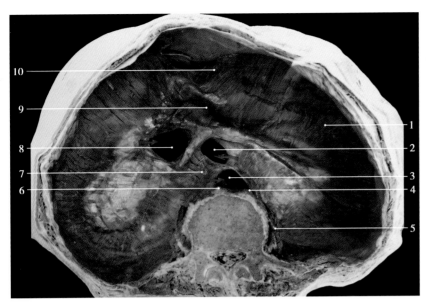

◀ 图 177

膈（下面观）
Diaphragm. Inferior aspect
1. 肋部 costal part
2. 食管裂孔 esophageal hiatus
3. 主动脉裂孔 aortic hiatus
4. 左脚 left crus
5. 腰大肌 psoas major
6. 右脚 right crus
7. 腰部 lumbar part
8. 腔静脉孔 vena caval foramen
9. 中心腱 central tendon
10. 胸骨部 sternal part

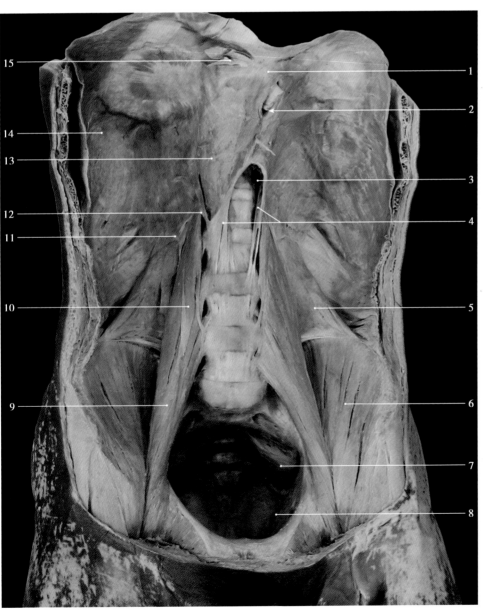

◀ 图 178

腹后壁肌
Muscles of posterior abdominal wall
1. 膈中心腱 central tendon of diaphragm
2. 食管裂孔 esophageal hiatus
3. 主动脉裂孔 aortic hiatus
4. 膈脚 crus of diaphragm
5. 腰方肌 quadratus lumborum
6. 髂肌 iliacus
7. 梨状肌 piriformis
8. 盆底肌 pelvic floor muscles
9. 腰大肌 psoas major
10. 腰小肌 psoas minor
11. 外侧弓状韧带 lateral arcuate lig.
12. 内侧弓状韧带 medial arcuate lig.
13. 膈（腰部）diaphragm (lumbar part)
14. 膈（肋部）diaphragm (costal part)
15. 腔静脉孔 vena caval foramen

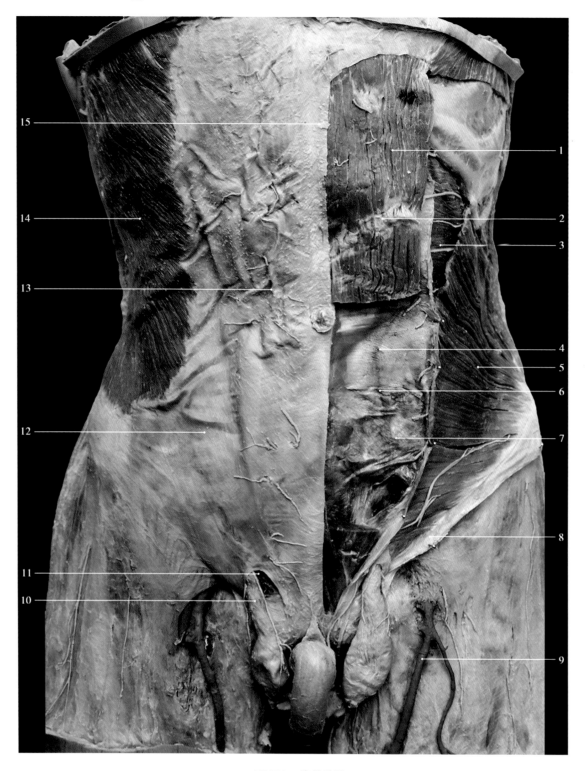

▲ 图 179　腹前壁肌
Muscles of anterior abdominal wall

1. 腹直肌 rectus abdominis
2. 腱划 tendinous intersections
3. 腹横肌 transverse abdominis
4. 腹直肌鞘后层 posterior layer of sheath of rectus abdominis
5. 腹内斜肌 obliquus internus abdominis
6. 弓状线 arcuate line
7. 腹横筋膜 transverse fascia
8. 腹股沟韧带 inguinal lig.

9. 大隐静脉 great saphenous v.
10. 精索 spermatic cord
11. 腹股沟管浅环 superficial inguinal ring
12. 腹外斜肌腱膜 aponeurosis of obliquus externus abdominis
13. 腹直肌鞘前层 anterior layer of sheath of rectus abdominis
14. 腹外斜肌 obliquus externus abdominis
15. 白线 linea alba

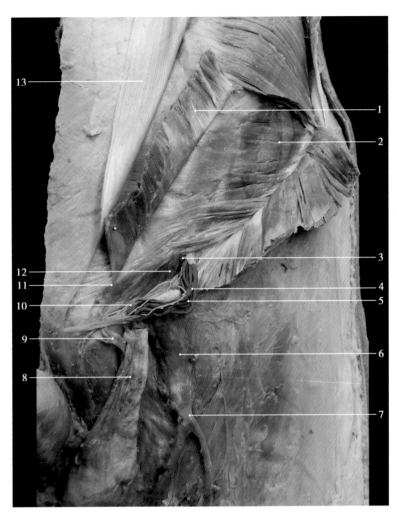

◀ 图 180

腹股沟区
Inguinal region

1. 腹内斜肌 obliquus internus abdominis
2. 腹横肌 transverse abdominis
3. 腹股沟管深环 deep inguinal ring
4. 蔓状静脉丛 pampiniform plexus
5. 睾丸动脉 testicular a.
6. 股鞘 femoral sheath
7. 大隐静脉 great saphenous v.
8. 精索 spermatic cord
9. 提睾肌（耻骨头）cremaster
10. 输精管 deferent duct
11. 腹股沟镰 inguinal falx
12. 腹壁下动脉 inferior epigastric a.
13. 腹外斜肌腱膜 aponeurosis of obliquus externus abdominis

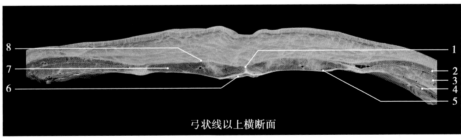

弓状线以上横断面

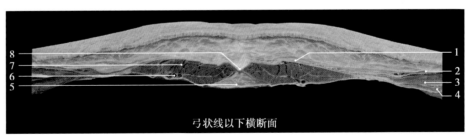

弓状线以下横断面

▲ 图 181 **腹壁的横断面**
Transverse sections of abdominal wall

1. 白线 linea alba
2. 腹外斜肌 obliquus externus abdominis
3. 腹内斜肌 obliquus internus abdominis
4. 腹横肌 transverse abdominis
5. 腹直肌鞘后层 posterior layer of sheath of rectus abdominis
6. 腹横筋膜 transverse fascia
7. 腹直肌 rectus abdominis
8. 腹直肌鞘前层 anterior layer of sheath of rectus abdominis

1. 腹直肌鞘前层 anterior layer of sheath of rectus abdominis
2. 腹外斜肌腱膜 aponeurosis of obliquus externus abdominis
3. 腹内斜肌 obliquus internus abdominis
4. 腹横肌 transverse abdominis
5. 腹横筋膜 transverse fascia
6. 腹壁下动脉 inferior epigastric a.
7. 腹直肌 rectus abdominis
8. 白线 linea alba

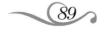

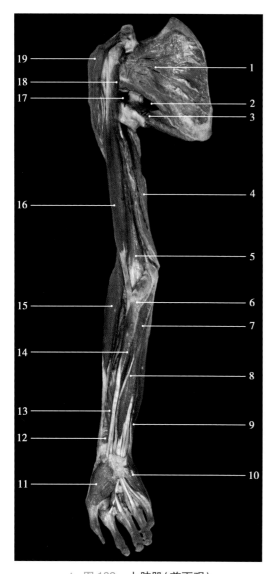

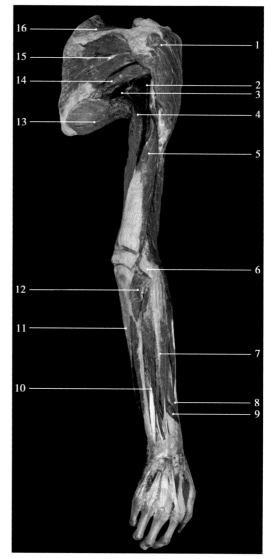

▲ 图 182　上肢肌（前面观）
Muscles of upper limb. Anterior aspect
1. 肩胛下肌 subscapularis
2. 三边孔 trilateral foramen
3. 大圆肌 teres major
4. 肱三头肌 triceps brachii
5. 肱肌 brachialis
6. 肱二头肌腱膜 bicipital aponeurosis
7. 掌长肌 palmaris longus
8. 指浅屈肌 flexor digitorum superiicialis
9. 尺侧腕屈肌 flexor carpi ulnaris
10. 小鱼际 hypothenar
11. 鱼际 thenar
12. 旋前方肌 pronator quadratus
13. 拇长屈肌 flexor pollicis longus
14. 桡侧腕屈肌 flexor carpi radialis
15. 肱桡肌 brachioradialis
16. 肱二头肌 biceps brachii
17. 四边孔 quadrilateral foramen
18. 喙肱肌 coracobrachialis
19. 三角肌 deltoid

▲ 图 183　上肢肌（后面观）
Muscles of upper limb. Posterior aspect
1. 三角肌 deltoid
2. 四边孔 quadrilateral foramen
3. 三边孔 trilateral foramen
4. 肱三头肌长头 long head of triceps brachii
5. 肱三头肌外侧头 lateral head of biceps brachii
6. 外上髁 lateral epicondyle
7. 指伸肌 extensor digitorum
8. 拇长展肌 abductor pollicis longus
9. 拇短伸肌 extensor pollicis brevis
10. 尺侧腕伸肌 extensor carpi ulnaris
11. 尺侧腕屈肌 flexor carpi ulnaris
12. 肘肌 anconeus
13. 大圆肌 teres major
14. 小圆肌 teres minor
15. 冈下肌 infraspinatus
16. 冈上肌 supraspinatus

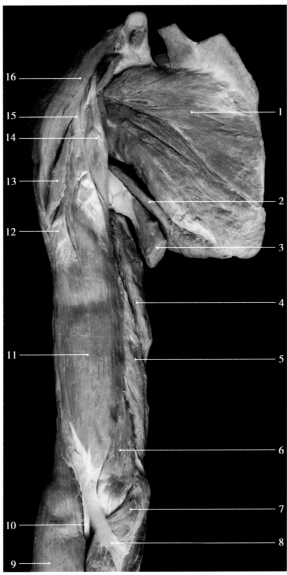

▲ 图 184　肩、臂部肌（前面观 1）
Muscles of shoulder and upper arm.
Anterior aspect（1）

1. 肩胛下肌 subscapularis
2. 大圆肌 teres major
3. 背阔肌 latissimus dorsi
4. 肱三头肌长头 long head of triceps brachii
5. 肱三头肌内侧头 medial head of biceps brachii
6. 肱肌 brachialis
7. 旋前圆肌 pronator teres
8. 肱二头肌腱膜 bicipital aponeurosis
9. 肱桡肌 brachioradialis
10. 肱二头肌腱 tendon of biceps brachii
11. 肱二头肌 biceps brachii
12. 肱二头肌长头 long head of biceps brachii
13. 胸大肌 pectoralis major
14. 喙肱肌 coracobrachialis
15. 肱二头肌短头 short head of biceps brachii
16. 三角肌 deltoid

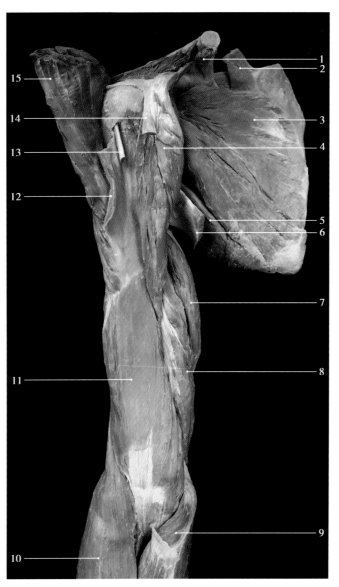

▲ 图 185　肩、臂部肌（前面观 2）
Muscles of shoulder and upper arm.
Anterior aspect（2）

1. 锁骨下肌 subclavius
2. 肩胛舌骨肌 omohyoid
3. 肩胛下肌 subscapularis
4. 喙肱肌 coracobrachialis
5. 大圆肌 teres major
6. 背阔肌 latissimus dorsi
7. 肱三头肌长头 long head of triceps brachii
8. 肱三头肌内侧头 medial head of biceps brachii
9. 旋前圆肌 pronator teres
10. 肱桡肌 brachioradialis
11. 肱肌 brachialis
12. 胸大肌 pectoralis major
13. 肱二头肌长头 long head of biceps brachii
14. 肱二头肌短头 short head of biceps brachii
15. 三角肌 deltoid

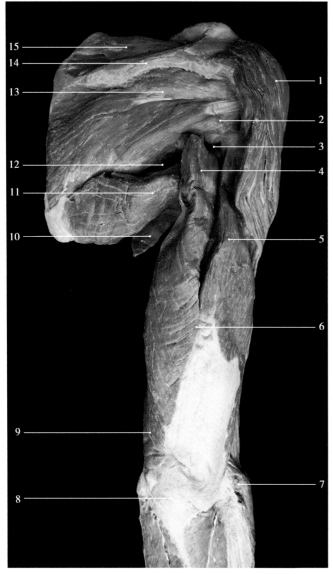

◀ 图 186

肩、臂部肌（后面观）

Muscles of shoulder and upper arm. Posterior aspect

1. 三角肌 deltoid
2. 小圆肌 teres minor
3. 四边孔 quadrilateral foramen
4. 肱三头肌长头 long head of triceps brachii
5. 肱三头肌外侧头 lateral head of biceps brachii
6. 肱三头肌 triceps brachii
7. 肱桡肌 brachioradialis
8. 鹰嘴 olecranon
9. 肱三头肌内侧头 medial head of biceps brachii
10. 背阔肌 latissimus dorsi
11. 大圆肌 teres major
12. 三边孔 trilateral foramen
13. 冈下肌 infraspinatus
14. 肩胛冈 spine of scapula
15. 冈上肌 supraspinatus

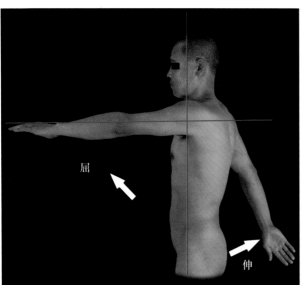

▲ 图 187 肩的屈和伸
Flexion and extension of shoulder

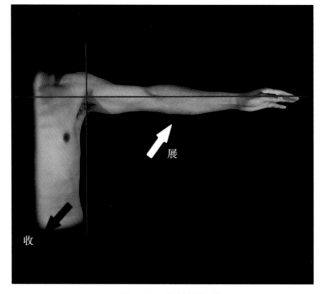

▲ 图 188 肩的展和收
Abduction and adduction of shoulder

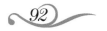

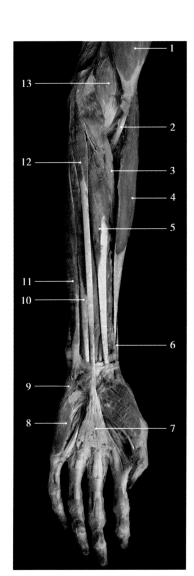

▲ 图 189　前臂肌（前面观 1）
Muscles of forearm. Anterior aspect（1）
1. 肱二头肌 biceps brachii
2. 肱二头肌腱 tendon of biceps brachii
3. 旋前圆肌 pronator teres
4. 肱桡肌 brachioradialis
5. 桡侧腕屈肌 flexor carpi radialis
6. 拇长展肌 abductor pollicis longus
7. 掌腱膜 palmar aponeurosis
8. 小指短屈肌 flexor digiti minimi brevis
9. 小指展肌 abductor digiti minimi
10. 指浅屈肌 flexor digitorum superiicialis
11. 尺侧腕屈肌 flexor carpi ulnaris
12. 掌长肌 palmaris longus
13. 肱肌 brachialis

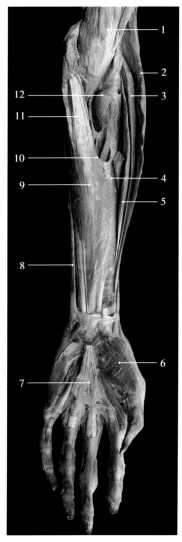

▲ 图 190　前臂肌（前面观 2）
Muscles of forearm. Anterior aspect（2）
1. 肱肌 brachialis
2. 肱桡肌 brachioradialis
3. 桡侧腕长伸肌 extensor carpi radialis longus
4. 指浅屈肌桡骨头 radial head of flexor digitorum superiicialis
5. 桡侧腕短伸肌 extensor carpi radialis brevis
6. 鱼际 thenar
7. 掌腱膜 palmar aponeurosis
8. 尺侧腕屈肌 flexor carpi ulnaris
9. 指浅屈肌 flexor digitorum superiicialis
10. 腱弓 arcus tendineus
11. 指浅屈肌肱尺骨头 humeroulnar head of flexor digitorum superiicialis
12. 肱二头肌腱 tendon of biceps brachii

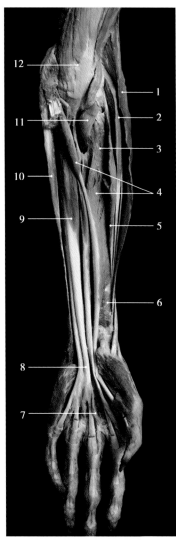

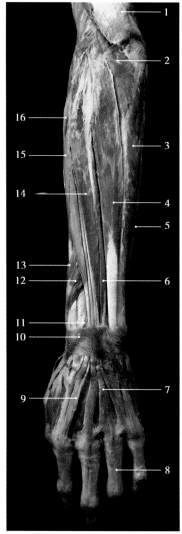

▲ 图191 前臂肌（前面观3）
Muscles of forearm. Anterior aspect（3）

1. 肱桡肌 brachioradialis
2. 桡侧腕长伸肌 extensor carpi radialis longus
3. 旋后肌 supinator
4. 拇长屈肌 flexor pollicis longus
5. 桡侧腕短伸肌 extensor carpi radialis brevis
6. 旋前方肌 pronator quadratus
7. 蚓状肌 lumbricales
8. 指深屈肌腱 tendon of flexor digitorum profundus
9. 指深屈肌 flexor digitorum profundus
10. 尺侧腕屈肌 flexor carpi ulnaris
11. 肱二头肌腱 tendon of biceps brachii
12. 肱肌 brachialis

▲ 图192 前臂肌（后面观1）
Muscles of forearm. Posterior aspect （1）

1. 肱三头肌 triceps brachii
2. 肘肌 anconeus
3. 指深屈肌 flexor digitorum profundus
4. 尺侧腕伸肌 extensor carpi ulnaris
5. 尺侧腕屈肌 flexor carpi ulnaris
6. 小指伸肌 extensor digiti minimi
7. 指伸肌腱 tendon of extensor digitorum
8. 指背腱膜 digital dorsal aponeurosis
9. 示指伸肌腱 tendon of extensor indicis
10. 伸肌支持带 extensor retinaculum
11. 拇长伸肌腱 tendon of extensor pollicis longus
12. 拇短伸肌 extensor pollicis brevis
13. 拇长展肌 abductor pollicis longus
14. 指伸肌 extensor digitorum
15. 桡侧腕短伸肌 extensor carpi radialis brevis
16. 桡侧腕长伸肌 extensor carpi radialis longus

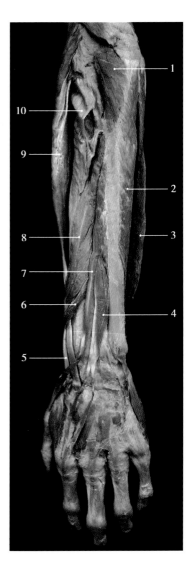

◀ 图 193

前臂肌（后面观 2）
Muscles of forearm. Posterior aspect（2）
1. 肘肌 anconeus
2. 指深屈肌 flexor digitorum profundus
3. 尺侧腕屈肌 flexor carpi ulnaris
4. 示指伸肌 extensor indicis
5. 桡侧腕长伸肌腱 tendon of extensor carpi radialis longus
6. 拇短伸肌 extensor pollicis brevis
7. 拇长伸肌 extensor pollicis longus
8. 拇长展肌 abductor pollicis longus
9. 桡侧腕短伸肌 extensor carpi radialis brevis
10. 旋后肌 supinator

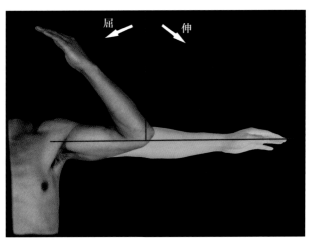

▲ 图 194 肘的屈和伸
Flexion and extension of elbow

95

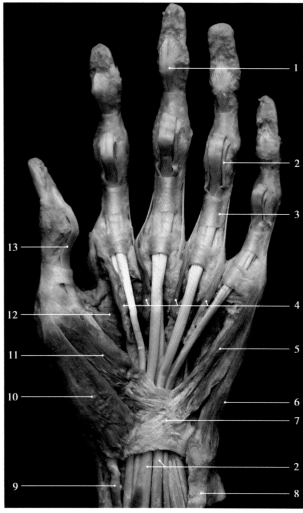 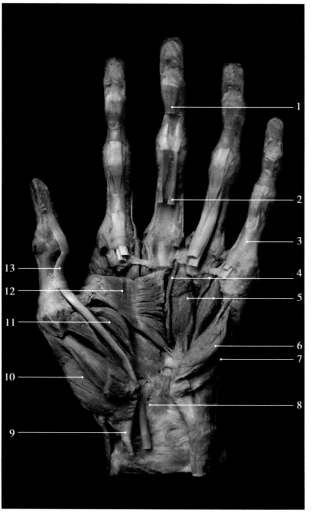

▲ 图 195　手肌（前面观 1）
Muscles of hand. Anterior aspect（1）
1. 指深屈肌腱 tendon of flexor digitorum profundus
2. 指浅屈肌腱 tendon of flexor digitorum superficialis
3. 指纤维鞘 fibrous sheaths of fingers
4. 蚓状肌 lumbricales
5. 小指短屈肌 flexor digiti minimi brevis
6. 小指展肌 abductor digiti minimi
7. 屈肌支持带 flexor retinaculum
8. 尺侧腕屈肌腱 tendon of flexor carpi ulnaris
9. 桡侧腕屈肌腱 tendon of flexor carpi radialis
10. 拇短展肌 abductor pollicis brevis
11. 拇短屈肌 flexor pollicis brevis
12. 拇收肌 adductor pollicis
13. 拇长屈肌腱 tendon of flexor pollicis longus

▲ 图 196　手肌（前面观 2）
Muscles of hand. Anterior aspect（2）
1. 指深屈肌腱 tendon of flexor digitorum profundus
2. 指浅屈肌腱 tendon of flexor digitorum superficialis
3. 指纤维鞘 fibrous sheaths of fingers
4. 骨间背侧肌 dorsal interossei
5. 骨间掌侧肌 palmar interossei
6. 小指短屈肌 flexor digiti minimi brevis
7. 小指对掌肌 opponens digiti minimi
8. 腕辐状韧带 radiate carpal lig.
9. 桡侧腕屈肌腱 tendon of flexor carpi radialis
10. 拇对掌肌 opponens pollicis
11. 拇收肌斜头 oblique head of adductor pollicis
12. 拇收肌横头 transverse head of adductor pollicis
13. 拇长屈肌腱 tendon of flexor pollicis longus

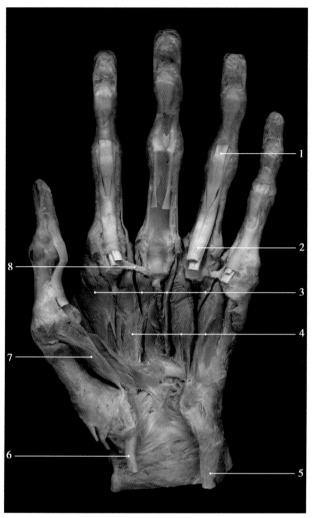

▲ 图197 手肌（前面观3）
Muscles of hand. Anterior aspect（3）
1. 指深屈肌腱 tendon of flexor digitorum profundus
2. 指浅屈肌腱 tendon of flexor digitorum superficialis
3. 骨间背侧肌 dorsal interossei
4. 骨间掌侧肌 palmar interossei
5. 尺侧腕屈肌腱 tendon of flexor carpi ulnaris
6. 桡侧腕屈肌腱 tendon of flexor carpi radialis
7. 拇收肌斜头 oblique head of adductor pollicis
8. 掌骨深横韧带 deep transverse metacarpal lig.

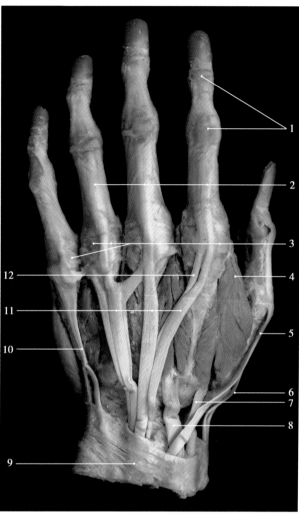

▲ 图198 手肌（后面观1）
Muscles of hand. Posterior aspect（1）
1. 指骨间关节 interphalangeal joints of hand
2. 指背腱膜 dorsal aponeurosis of fingers
3. 掌指关节 metacarpophalangeal joints
4. 第1骨间背侧肌 1st dorsal interossei
5. 拇长伸肌腱 tendon of extensor pollicis longus
6. 拇短伸肌腱 tendon of extensor pollicis brevis
7. 桡侧腕长伸肌腱 tendon of extensor carpi radialis longus
8. 桡侧腕短伸肌腱 tendon of extensor carpi radialis brevis
9. 伸肌支持带 extensor retinaculum
10. 小指伸肌腱 tendon of extensor digiti minimi
11. 指伸肌腱 tendon of extensor digitorum
12. 示指伸肌腱 tendon of extensor indicis

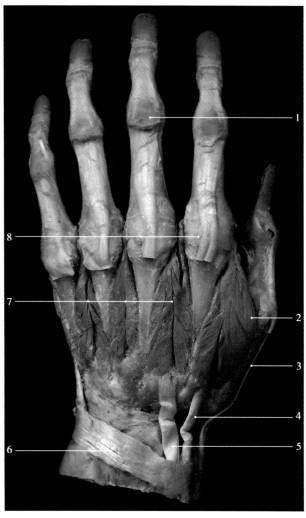

▲ 图 199　手肌（后面观 2）
Muscles of hand. Posterior aspect（2）

1. 指骨间关节 interphalangeal joints of hand
2. 第 1 骨间背侧肌 1st dorsal interossei
3. 拇短伸肌腱 tendon of extensor pollicis brevis
4. 桡侧腕长伸肌腱 tendon of extensor carpi radialis longus
5. 桡侧腕短伸肌腱 tendon of extensor carpi radialis brevis
6. 伸肌支持带 extensor retinaculum
7. 骨间背侧肌 dorsal interossei
8. 掌指关节 metacarpophalangeal joint

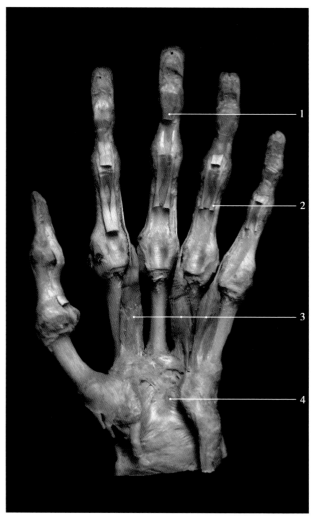

▲ 图 200　骨间掌侧肌（前面观）
Palmar interossei. Anterior aspect

1. 指深屈肌腱 tendon of flexor digitorum profundus
2. 指浅屈肌腱 tendon of flexor digitorum superficialis
3. 骨间掌侧肌 palmar interossei
4. 腕辐状韧带 radiate carpal lig.

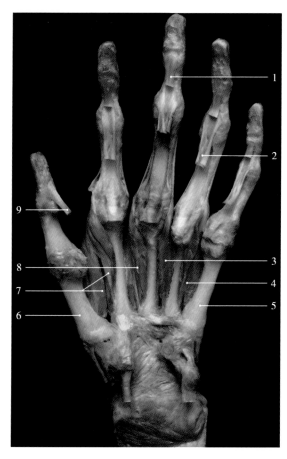

◀ 图 201

骨间背侧肌(前面观)

Dorsal interossei. Anterior aspect

1. 指深屈肌腱 tendon of flexor digitorum profundus
2. 指浅屈肌腱 tendon of flexor digitorum superficialis
3. 第 3 骨间背侧肌 3rd dorsal interossei
4. 第 4 骨间背侧肌 4th dorsal interossei
5. 第 5 掌骨 5th metacarpal bone
6. 第 1 掌骨 1st metacarpal bone
7. 第 1 骨间背侧肌 1st dorsal interossei
8. 第 2 骨间背侧肌 2nd dorsal interossei
9. 拇长屈肌腱 tendon of flexor pollicis longus

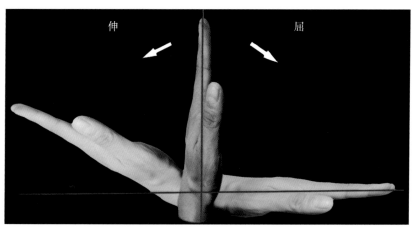

◀ 图 202

腕的屈和伸

Flexion and extension of wrist

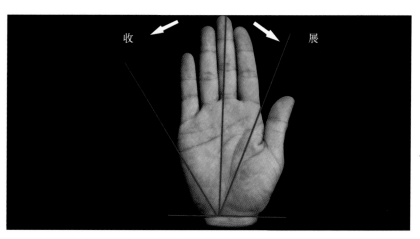

◀ 图 203

腕的收和展

Adduction and abduction of wrist

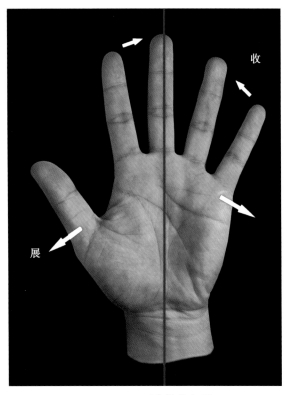

▲ 图204 手指的收和展
Adduction and abduction of fingers

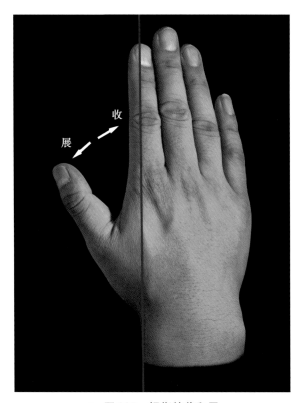

▲ 图205 拇指的收和展
Adduction and abduction of thumb

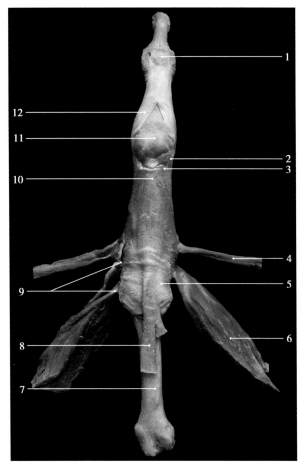

◀ 图206

指伸肌腱
Tendon of extensor digitorum

1. 终腱 terminal extensor tendon
2. 外侧束 lateral band
3. 内侧束 medial band
4. 蚓状肌 lumbricales
5. 腱帽 tendon hood
6. 骨间肌 interosseus
7. 掌骨 metacarpus
8. 指伸肌腱 tendon of extensor digitorum
9. 骨间肌止点 insertion of interosseous
10. 中间束 intermediate extensor band
11. 中间腱 intermediate extensor tendon
12. 外侧腱 lateral extensor tendon

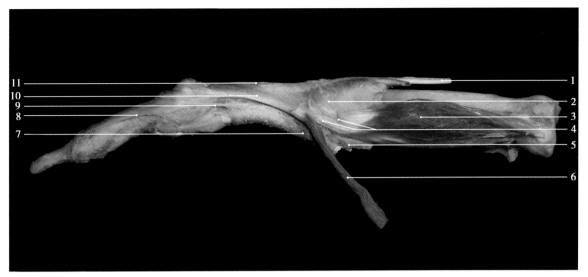

▲ 图 207　骨间肌和蚓状肌的止点
Insertion of interosseus and lumbrical

1. 指伸肌腱 tendon of extensor digitorum
2. 腱帽 tendon hood
3. 骨间肌 interosseous
4. 骨间肌腱 tendon of interosseus
5. 掌深横韧带 deep transverse metacarpal lig.
6. 蚓状肌 lumbricales

7. 指纤维鞘 fibrous sheaths of fingers
8. 外侧腱 lateral extensor tendon
9. 支持带(斜束)retinaculum (diagonal beam)
10. 外侧束 lateral extensor band
11. 中间束 intermediate extensor band

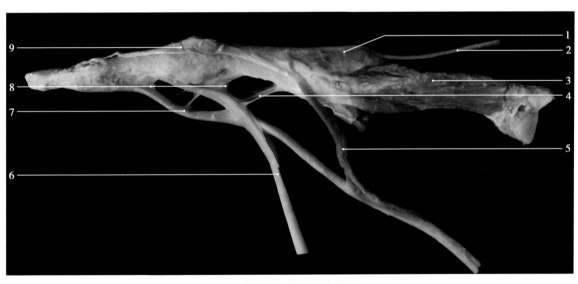

▲ 图 208　屈肌腱和腱纽
Flexor tendons and vincula tendinum

1. 腱帽 tendon hood
2. 指伸肌腱 tendon of extensor digitorum
3. 骨间肌 interosseus
4. 长纽 vinculum longum
5. 蚓状肌 lumbricales

6. 指浅屈肌腱 tendon of flexor digitorum superficialis
7. 指深屈肌腱 tendon of flexor digitorum profundus
8. 短纽 vinculum breve
9. 指背腱膜 dorsal aponeurosis of fingers

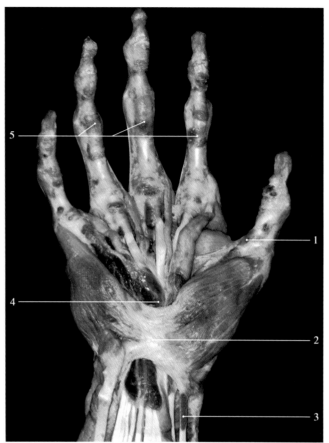

◀ 图 209

手腱鞘（前面观）
Tendinous sheaths of hand. Anterior aspect

1. 拇长屈肌腱鞘 tendinous sheath of flexor pollicis longus
2. 屈肌支持带 flexor retinaculum
3. 桡侧腕屈肌腱鞘 tendinous sheath of flexor carpi radialis
4. 屈肌总腱鞘 common flexor sheath
5. 指腱鞘 tendinous sheaths of fingers

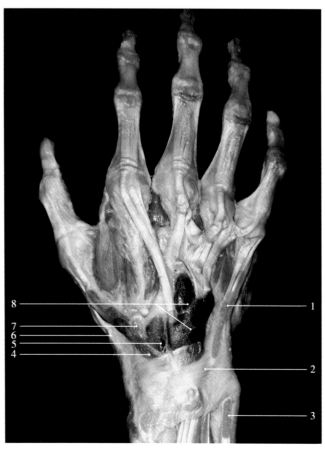

◀ 图 210

手腱鞘（后面观）
Tendinous sheaths of hand. Posterior aspect

1. 小指伸肌腱鞘 tendinous sheath of extensor digiti minimi
2. 伸肌支持带 extensor retinaculum
3. 尺侧腕伸肌腱鞘 tendinous sheath of extensor carpi ulnaris
4. 拇长伸肌腱鞘 tendinous sheath of extensor pollicis longus
5. 桡侧腕短伸肌腱鞘 tendinous sheath of extensor carpi radialis brevis
6. 拇长展肌和拇短伸肌腱鞘 tendinous sheath of abductor pollicis longus and extensor pollicis brevis
7. 桡侧腕长伸肌腱鞘 tendinous sheath of extensor carpi radialis longus
8. 指伸肌和示指伸肌腱鞘 tendinous sheath of extensor digitorum and extensor indicis

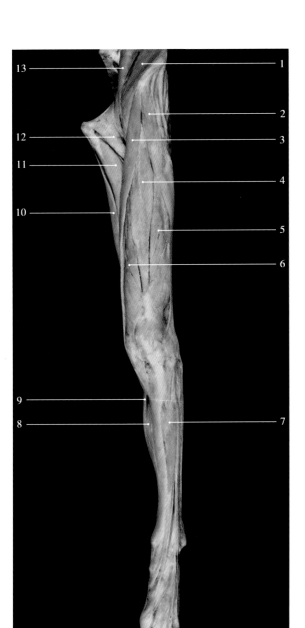

13 — 1
12 — 2
11 — 3
10 — 4
— 5
— 6
9 —
8 — 7

▲ 图 211　下肢肌（前面观）
Muscles of lower limb. Anterior aspect
1. 髂肌 iliacus
2. 阔筋膜张肌 tensor fasciae latae
3. 缝匠肌 sartorius
4. 股直肌 rectus femoris
5. 股外侧肌 vastus lateralis
6. 股内侧肌 vastus medialis
7. 胫骨前肌 tibialis anterior
8. 比目鱼肌 soleus
9. 腓肠肌 gastrocnemius
10. 股薄肌 gracilis
11. 长收肌 adductor longus
12. 耻骨肌 pectineus
13. 腰大肌 psoas major

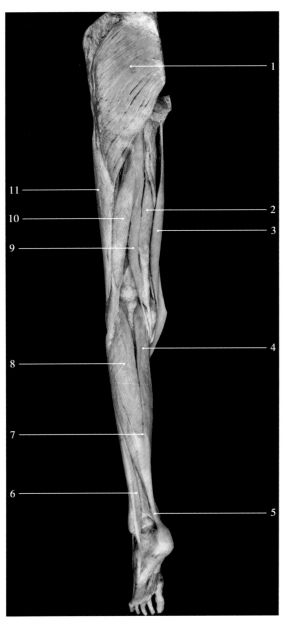

— 1
11 —
10 — 2
9 — 3
— 4
8 —
7 —
6 — 5

▲ 图 212　下肢肌（后面观）
Muscles of lower limb. Posterior aspect
1. 臀大肌 gluteus maximus
2. 半膜肌 semimembranosus
3. 股薄肌 gracilis
4. 腓肠肌内侧头 medial head of gastrocnemius
5. 跟腱 tendo calcaneus
6. 腓骨短肌 peroneus brevis
7. 腓肠肌 gastrocnemius
8. 腓肠肌外侧头 lateral head of gastrocnemius
9. 半腱肌 semitendinosus
10. 股二头肌长头 long head of biceps femoris
11. 髂胫束 iliotibial tract

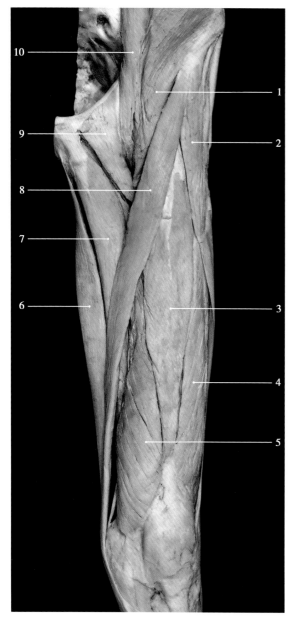

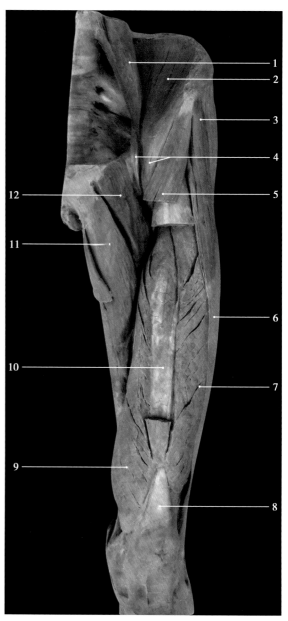

▲ 图 213　股部肌（前面观 1）
Muscles of thigh. Anterior aspect（1）
1. 髂肌 iliacus
2. 阔筋膜张肌 tensor fasciae latae
3. 股直肌 rectus femoris
4. 股外侧肌 vastus lateralis
5. 股内侧肌 vastus medialis
6. 股薄肌 gracilis
7. 长收肌 adductor longus
8. 缝匠肌 sartorius
9. 耻骨肌 pectineus
10. 腰大肌 psoas major

▲ 图 214　股部肌（前面观 2）
Muscles of thigh. Anterior aspect（2）
1. 腰大肌 psoas major
2. 髂肌 iliacus
3. 阔筋膜张肌 tensor fasciae latae
4. 髂腰肌 iliopsoas
5. 缝匠肌 sartorius
6. 髂胫束 iliotibial tract
7. 股外侧肌 vastus lateralis
8. 股四头肌腱 tendon of quadriceps
9. 股内侧肌 vastus medialis
10. 股中间肌 vastus intermedius
11. 长收肌 adductor longus
12. 耻骨肌 pectineus

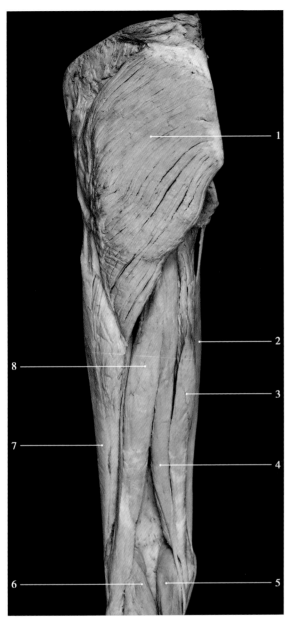

▲ 图 215　股部肌（后面观 1）
Muscles of thigh. Posterior aspect（1）
1. 臀大肌 gluteus maximus
2. 股薄肌 gracilis
3. 半膜肌 semimembranosus
4. 半腱肌 semitendinosus
5. 腓肠肌内侧头 medial head of gastrocnemius
6. 腓肠肌外侧头 lateral head of gastrocnemius
7. 髂胫束 iliotibial tract
8. 股二头肌长头 long head of biceps femoris

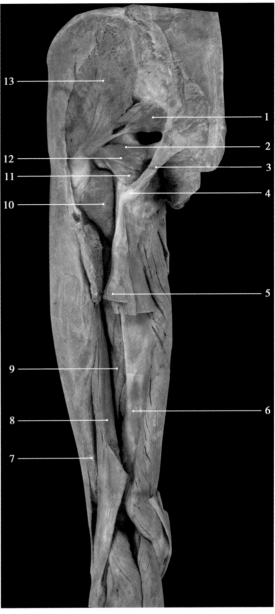

▲ 图 216　股部肌（后面观 2）
Muscles of thigh. Posterior aspect（2）
1. 梨状肌 piriformis
2. 上孖肌 gemellus superior
3. 骶结节韧带 sacrotuberous lig.
4. 坐骨结节 ischial tuberosity
5. 股二头肌长头 long head of biceps femoris
6. 半膜肌 semimembranosus
7. 股外侧肌 vastus lateralis
8. 股二头肌短头 short head of biceps femoris
9. 大收肌 adductor magnus
10. 股方肌 quadratus femoris
11. 下孖肌 gemellus inferior
12. 闭孔内肌 obturator internus
13. 臀中肌 gluteus medius

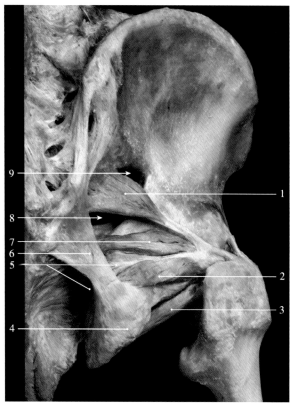

◀ 图 217

臀肌深层
Deep layer of glutcus

1. 梨状肌 piriformis
2. 下孖肌 gemellus inferior
3. 闭孔外肌 obturator externus
4. 坐骨结节 ischial tuberosity
5. 闭孔内肌 obturator internus
6. 骶结节韧带 sacrotuberous lig.
7. 上孖肌 gemellus superior
8. 梨状肌下孔 infrapiriformis foramen
9. 梨状肌上孔 suprapiriformis foramen

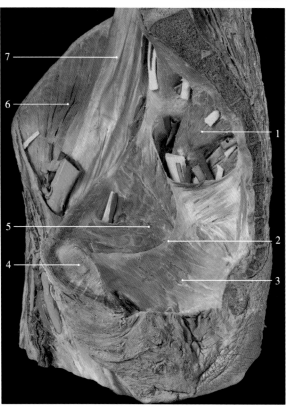

▲ 图 218　盆壁肌（1）
Muscles of pelvic wall（1）

1. 梨状肌 piriformis
2. 肛提肌腱弓 tendinous arch of levator ani
3. 肛提肌 levator ani
4. 耻骨联合面 symphysial surface
5. 闭孔内肌 obturator internus
6. 髂肌 iliacus
7. 腰大肌 psoas major

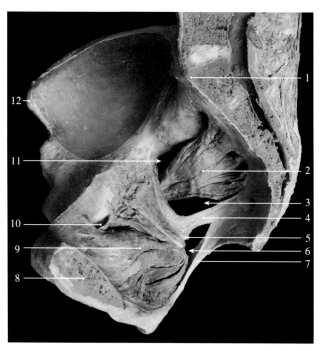

▲ 图 219　盆壁肌（2）
Muscles of pelvic wall（2）

1. 岬 promontory
2. 梨状肌 piriformis
3. 梨状肌下孔 infrapiriformis foramen
4. 骶棘韧带 sacrospinous lig.
5. 坐骨棘 ischial spine
6. 坐骨小孔 lesser sciatic foramen
7. 骶结节韧带 sacrotuberous lig.
8. 耻骨联合面 symphysial surface
9. 闭孔内肌 obturator internus
10. 闭膜管 obturator canal
11. 梨状肌上孔 suprapiriformis foramen
12. 髂前上棘 anterior superior iliac spine

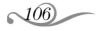

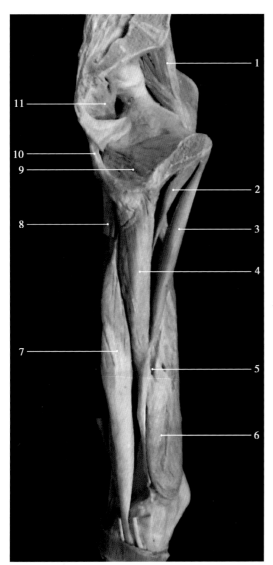

◀ 图 220

股部肌（内侧面观）
Muscles of thigh. Medial aspect
1. 腰大肌 psoas major
2. 短收肌 adductor brevis
3. 长收肌 adductor longus
4. 大收肌 adductor magnus
5. 收肌管 adductor canal
6. 股内侧肌 vastus medialis
7. 半膜肌 semimembranosus
8. 半腱肌 semitendinosus
9. 闭孔内肌 obturator internus
10. 骶结节韧带 sacrotuberous lig.
11. 梨状肌 piriformis

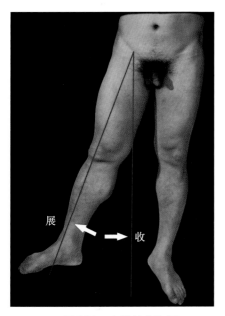

▲ 图 221　大腿的收和展
Adduction and abduction of thigh

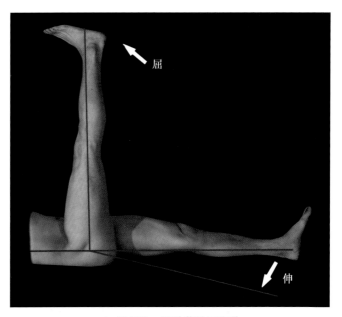

▲ 图 222　髋关节的屈和伸
Flexion and extension of hip joint

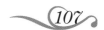

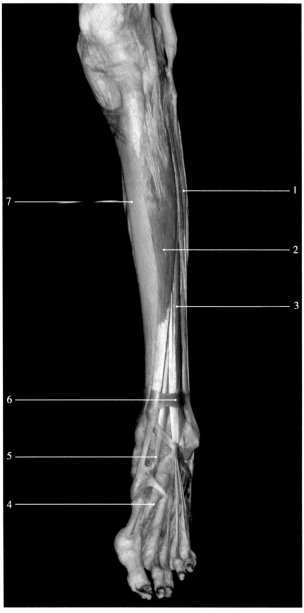

▲ 图 223　小腿肌 (前面观)
Muscles of leg. Anterior aspect

1. 腓骨长肌 peroneus longus
2. 胫骨前肌 tibialis anterior
3. 趾长伸肌 extensor digitorum longus
4. 跨短伸肌腱 tendon of extensor hallucis brevis
5. 跨长伸肌腱 tendon of extensor hallucis longus
6. 伸肌上支持带 superior extensor retinaculum
7. 胫骨 tibia

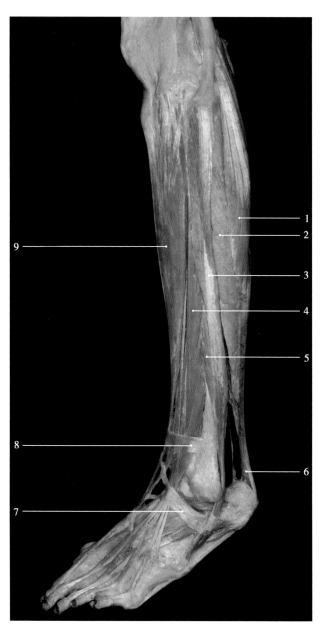

▲ 图 224　小腿肌 (外侧面观)
Muscle of leg. Lateral aspect

1. 腓肠肌外侧头 lateral head of gastrocnemius
2. 比目鱼肌 soleus
3. 腓骨长肌 peroneus longus
4. 趾长伸肌 extensor digitorum longus
5. 腓骨短肌 peroneus brevis
6. 跟腱 tendo calcaneus
7. 伸肌下支持带 inferior extensor retinaculum
8. 伸肌上支持带 superior extensor retinaculum
9. 胫骨前肌 tibialis anterior

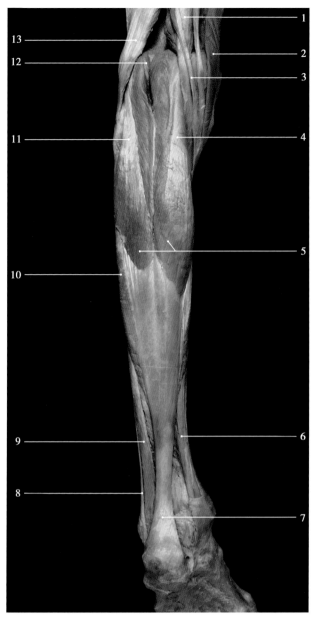

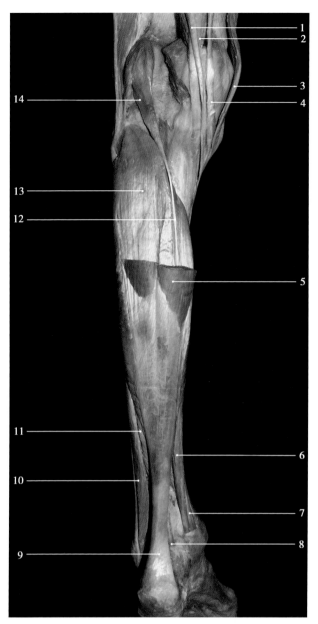

▲ 图 225　小腿肌（后面观 1）
Muscles of leg. Posterior aspect（1）

1. 半膜肌 semimembranosus
2. 缝匠肌 sartorius
3. 半腱肌腱 tendon of semitendinosus
4. 腓肠肌内侧头 medial head of gastrocnemius
5. 腓肠肌 gastrocnemius
6. 趾长屈肌 flexor digitorum longus
7. 跟腱 tendo calcaneus
8. 腓骨长肌腱 tendon of peroneus longus
9. 腓骨短肌 peroneus brevis
10. 比目鱼肌 soleus
11. 腓肠肌外侧头 lateral head of gastrocnemius
12. 跖肌 plantaris
13. 股二头肌 biceps femoris

▲ 图 226　小腿肌（后面观 2）
Muscles of leg. Posterior aspect（2）

1. 半腱肌 semitendinosus
2. 半膜肌 semimembranosus
3. 缝匠肌 sartorius
4. 股薄肌腱 tendon of gracilis
5. 腓肠肌 gastrocnemius
6. 趾长屈肌 flexor digitorum longus
7. 胫骨后肌腱 tendon of tibialis posterior
8. 踇长屈肌腱 tendon of flexor hallucis longus
9. 跟腱 tendo calcaneus
10. 腓骨短肌 peroneus brevis
11. 踇长屈肌 flexor hallucis longus
12. 跖肌腱 tendon of plantaris
13. 比目鱼肌 soleus
14. 跖肌 plantaris

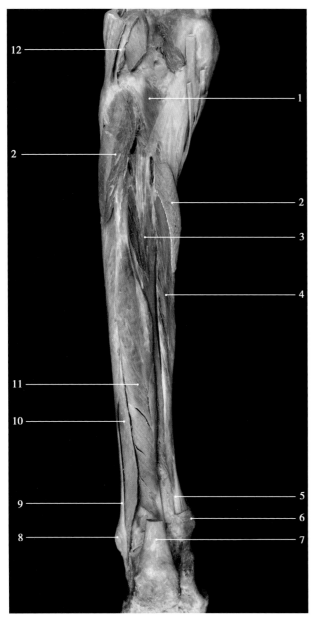

▲ 图 227　小腿肌（后面观 3）
Muscles of leg. Posterior aspect（3）

1. 腘肌 popliteus
2. 比目鱼肌 soleus
3. 胫骨后肌 tibialis posterior
4. 趾长屈肌 flexor digitorum longus
5. 趾长屈肌腱 tendon of flexor digitorum longus
6. 内踝 medial malleolus
7. 跟腱 tendo calcaneus
8. 外踝 lateral malleolus
9. 腓骨长肌腱 tendon of peroneus longus
10. 腓骨短肌 peroneus brevis
11. 踇长屈肌 flexor hallucis longus
12. 腓肠肌外侧头 lateral head of gastrocnemius

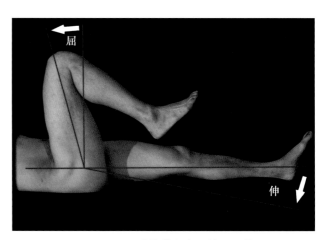

▲ 图 228　膝关节和大腿的屈和伸
Flexion and extension of knee and thigh

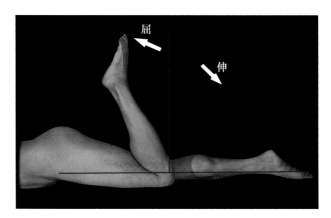

▲ 图 229　膝的屈和伸
Flexion and extension of knee

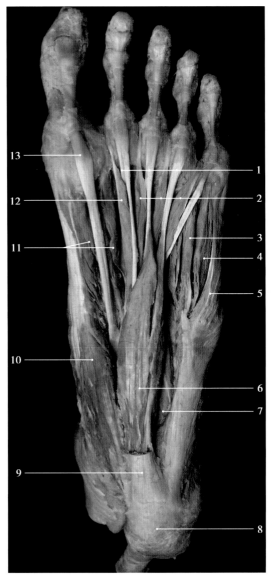

▲ 图230　足底肌（1）
Plantar muscles（1）
1. 趾长屈肌腱 tendon of flexor digitorum longus
2. 蚓状肌 lumbricales
3. 骨间足底肌 plantar interossei
4. 小趾短屈肌 flexor digiti minimi brevis
5. 小趾展肌 abductor digiti minimi
6. 趾短屈肌 flexor digitorum brevis
7. 足底方肌 quadratus plantae
8. 跟骨 calcaneus
9. 足底腱膜 plantar aponeurosis
10. 踇展肌 abductor hallucis
11. 踇短屈肌 flexor hallucis brevis
12. 第1蚓状肌 1st lumbricales
13. 踇长屈肌腱 tendon of flexor hallucis longus

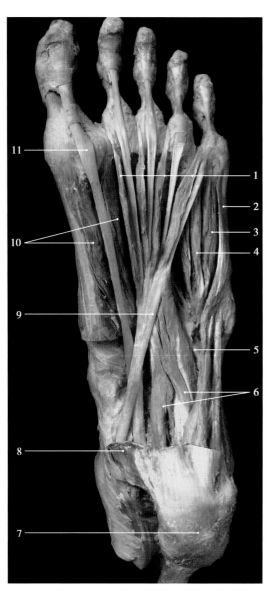

▲ 图231　足底肌（2）
Plantar muscles（2）
1. 蚓状肌 lumbricales
2. 小趾展肌 abductor digiti minimi
3. 小趾短屈肌 flexor digiti minimi brevis
4. 骨间足底肌 plantar interossei
5. 腓骨长肌腱 tendon of peroneus longus
6. 足底方肌 quadratus plantae
7. 跟骨 calcaneus
8. 踇展肌 abductor hallucis
9. 趾长屈肌腱 tendon of flexor digitorum longus
10. 踇短屈肌 flexor hallucis brevis
11. 踇长屈肌腱 tendon of flexor hallucis longus

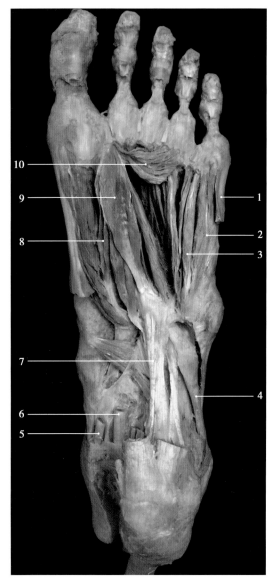

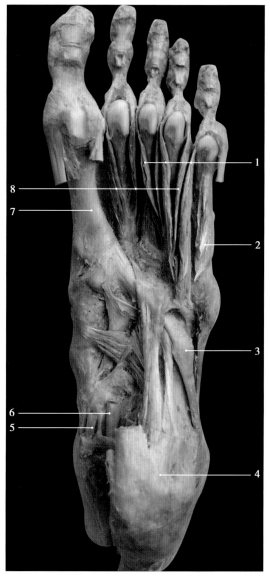

▲ 图 232　足底肌（3）
Plantar muscles（3）

1. 小趾展肌 abductor digiti minimi
2. 小趾短屈肌 flexor digiti minimi brevis
3. 骨间足底肌 plantar interossei
4. 腓骨长肌腱 tendon of peroneus longus
5. 趾长屈肌腱 tendon of flexor digitorum longus
6. 蹈长屈肌腱 tendon of flexor hallucis longus
7. 足底长韧带 long plantar lig.
8. 蹈短屈肌 flexor hallucis brevis
9. 蹈收肌斜头 oblique head of adductor hallucis
10. 蹈收肌横头 transverse head of adductor hallucis

▲ 图 233　足底肌（4）
Plantar muscles（4）

1. 骨间足底肌 plantar interossei
2. 小趾短屈肌 flexor digiti minimi brevis
3. 腓骨长肌腱 tendon of peroneus longus
4. 跟骨 calcaneus
5. 趾长屈肌腱 tendon of flexor digitorum longus
6. 蹈长屈肌腱 tendon of flexor hallucis longus
7. 第 1 跖骨 1st metatarsal bone
8. 骨间背侧肌 dorsal interossei

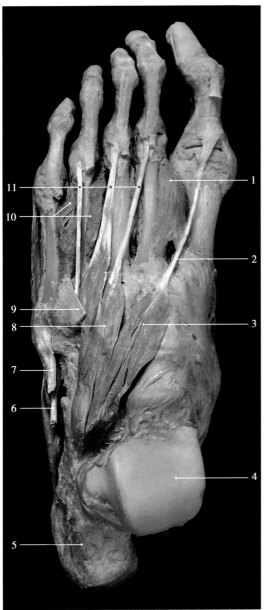

◀ 图 234

足背肌
Muscles of dorsum of foot
1. 第 1 骨间背侧肌 1st dorsal interossei
2. 踇短伸肌腱 tendon of extensor hallucis brevis
3. 踇短伸肌 extensor hallucis brevis
4. 距骨 talus
5. 跟骨 calcaneus
6. 腓骨长肌腱 tendon of peroneus longus
7. 腓骨短肌腱 tendon of peroneus brevis
8. 趾短伸肌 extensor digitorum brevis
9. 第 3 腓骨肌腱 tendon of peroneus tertius
10. 骨间背侧肌 dorsal interossei
11. 趾短伸肌腱 tendon of extensor digitorum brevis

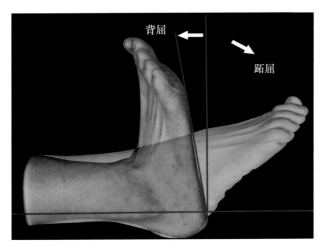

▲ 图 235 足的背屈和跖屈
Dorsiflexion and plantar flexion of foot

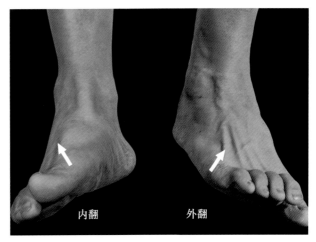

▲ 图 236 足的内翻和外翻
Inversion and eversion of foot

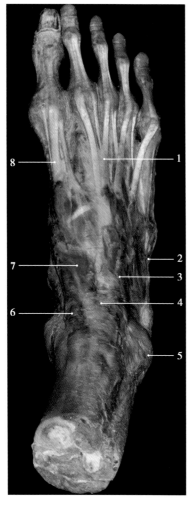

◄ 图 237

足腱鞘（前面观）
Tendinous sheaths of foot. Anterior aspect
1. 趾长伸肌腱 tendon of extensor digitorum longus
2. 腓骨短肌腱鞘 tendinous sheaths of peroneus brevis
3. 趾长伸肌腱鞘 tendinous sheath of extensor digitorum longus
4. 伸肌支持带 extensor retinaculum
5. 外踝 lateral malleolus
6. 胫骨前肌腱鞘 tendinous sheath of tibialis anterior
7. 踇长伸肌腱鞘 tendinous sheath of extensor hallucis longus
8. 踇长伸肌腱 tendon of extensor hallucis longus

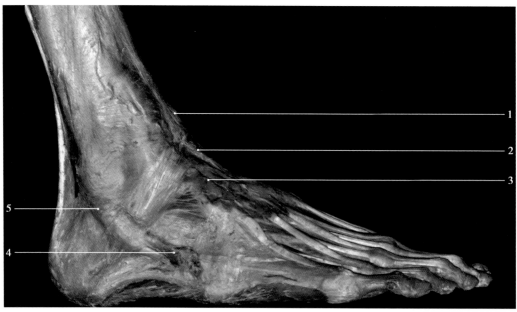

▲ 图 238　足腱鞘（外侧面观）
Tendinous sheaths of foot. Lateral aspect

1. 胫骨前肌腱鞘 tendinous sheath of tibialis anterior
2. 踇长伸肌腱鞘 tendinous sheath of extensor hallucis longus
3. 趾长伸肌腱鞘 tendinous sheath of extensor digitorum longus
4. 腓骨短肌腱鞘 tendinous sheath of peroneus brevis
5. 腓骨肌总腱鞘 common sheath of peronei

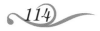

第五章 消化系统
Alimentary System

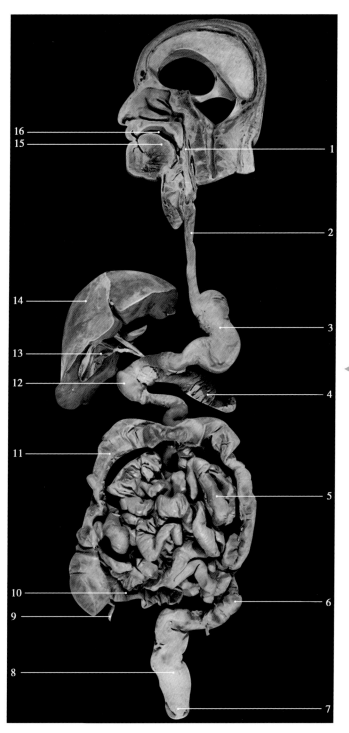

◀ 图 239

消化系统全貌
General arrangement of the
alimentary system

1. 口咽 oropharynx
2. 食管 esophagus
3. 胃 stomach
4. 胰 pancreas
5. 空肠 jejunum
6. 乙状结肠 sigmoid colon
7. 肛管 anal canal
8. 直肠 rectum
9. 阑尾 vermiform appendix
10. 回肠 ileum
11. 结肠 colon
12. 十二指肠 duodenum
13. 胆囊 gallbladder
14. 肝 liver
15. 舌 tongue
16. 口腔 oral cavity

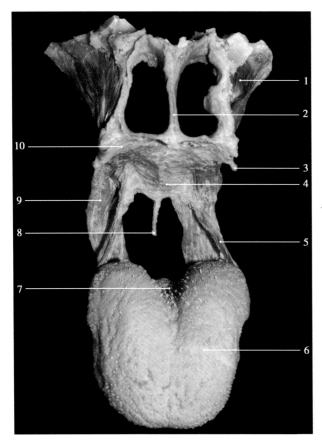

◀ 图 240　腭肌 (前面观)
Palatine muscles. Anterior aspect
1. 腭帆张肌 tensor veli palatini
2. 鼻中隔 nasal septum
3. 翼钩 pterygoid hamulus
4. 软腭 soft palate
5. 腭舌肌 palatoglossus
6. 舌 tongue
7. 舌根 lingual root
8. 腭垂肌 musculus uvulae
9. 腭咽肌 palatopharyngeus
10. 腭腱膜 palatine aponeurosis

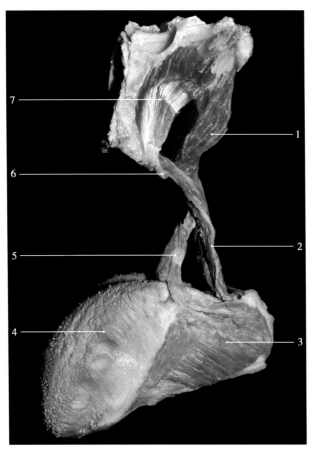

◀ 图 241
腭肌 (侧面观)
Palatine muscles. Lateral aspect
1. 腭帆提肌 levator veli palatini
2. 腭咽肌 palatopharyngeus
3. 舌骨舌肌 hyoglossus
4. 舌 tongue
5. 腭舌肌 palatoglossus
6. 翼钩 pterygoid hamulus
7. 腭帆张肌 tensor veli palatini

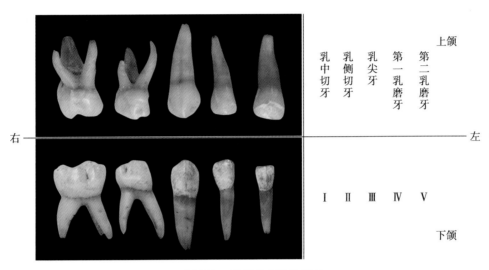

上颌

乳中切牙　乳侧切牙　乳尖牙　第一乳磨牙　第二乳磨牙

右 ——————————————— 左

Ⅰ　Ⅱ　Ⅲ　Ⅳ　Ⅴ

下颌

▲ 图242　乳牙的名称和符号
Name and notation of deciduous teeth

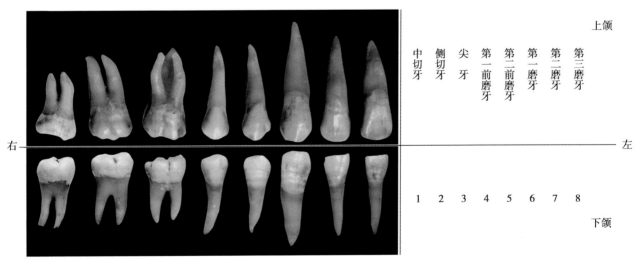

上颌

中切牙　侧切牙　尖牙　第一前磨牙　第二前磨牙　第一磨牙　第二磨牙　第三磨牙

右 ——————————————— 左

1　2　3　4　5　6　7　8

下颌

▲ 图243　恒牙的名称和符号
Name and notation of permanent teeth

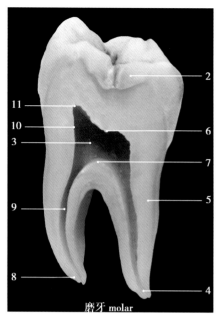

切牙 incisor

磨牙 molar

▲ 图244　牙的切面
Section of teeth

1. 切缘 incisal margin
2. 釉质 enamel
3. 牙腔 dental cavity
4. 牙根尖孔 apical foramen

5. 牙质 dentinum
6. 髓室顶 roof of pulp chamber
7. 髓室底 floor of pulp chamber
8. 牙根尖 root of tooth

9. 牙根管 root canal
10. 髓室壁 wall of pulp chamber
11. 髓角 pulp horn

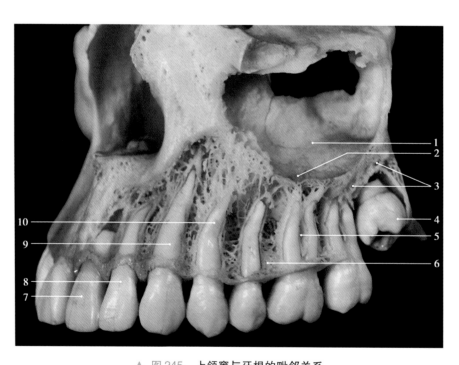

▲ 图245　上颌窦与牙根的毗邻关系
Relations between the maxillary sinus and root of teeth

1. 上颌窦 maxillary sinus
2. 上颌窦底 floor of maxillary sinus
3. 上牙槽后管 posterio superior alveolar canals
4. 第3磨牙 3rd molar
5. 牙根间隔 interradicular septa

6. 牙槽间隔 interalveolar septa
7. 中切牙 central incisor
8. 侧切牙 lateral incisor
9. 尖牙根 root of canine tooth
10. 第1前磨牙根 root of the 1st premolar

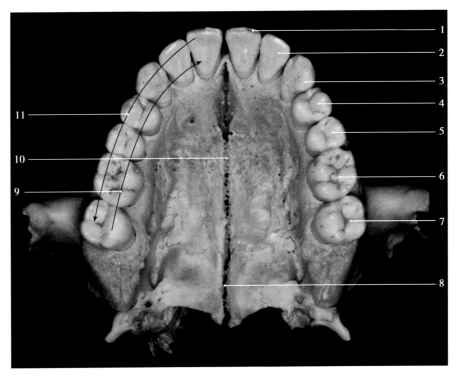

▲ 图 246　**上颌恒牙**
Maxillary permanent teeth

1. 中切牙 central incisor
2. 侧切牙 lateral incisor
3. 尖牙 canine tooth
4. 第 1 前磨牙 1st premolar
5. 第 2 前磨牙 2nd premolar
6. 第 1 磨牙 1st molar
7. 第 2 磨牙 2nd molar
8. 腭正中缝 median palatine suture
9. 近中方向 medial direction
10. 上颌间缝 intermaxillary suture
11. 远中方向 diasal direction

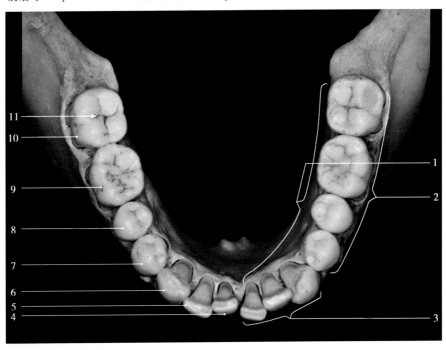

▲ 图 247　**下颌恒牙**
Mandibular permanent teeth

1. 舌面 lingual surface
2. 颊面 buccal surface
3. 唇面 labial surface
4. 中切牙 central incisor
5. 侧切牙 lateral incisor
6. 尖牙 canine tooth
7. 第 1 前磨牙 1st premolar
8. 第 2 前磨牙 2nd premolar
9. 第 1 磨牙 1st molar
10. 第 2 磨牙 2nd molar
11. 𬌗面 occlusal surface

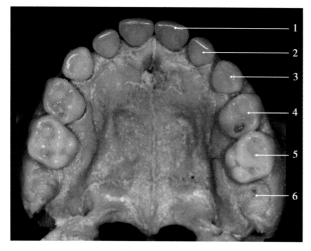

▲ 图 248　上颌乳牙
Maxillary deciduous teeth
1. 乳中切牙 central deciduous incisor
2. 乳侧切牙 lateral deciduous incisor
3. 乳尖牙 canine deciduous tooth
4. 第 1 乳磨牙 1st deciduous molar
5. 第 2 乳磨牙 2nd deciduous molar
6. 第 1 磨牙胚 dental germ of the 1st molar

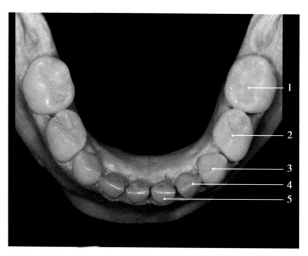

▲ 图 249　下颌乳牙
Mandibular deciduous teeth
1. 第 2 乳磨牙 2nd deciduous molar
2. 第 1 乳磨牙 1st deciduous molar
3. 乳尖牙 canine deciduous tooth
4. 乳侧切牙 lateral deciduous incisor
5. 乳中切牙 medial deciduous incisor

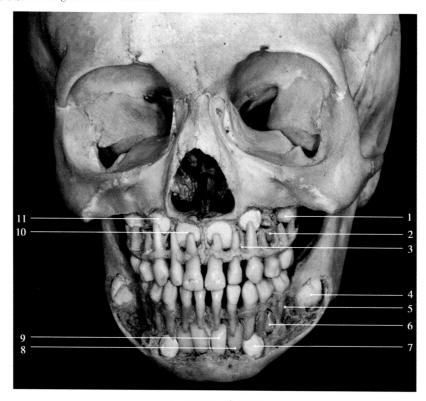

▲ 图 250　恒牙胚
Bud of permanent teeth

1. 上颌第 1 磨牙胚（9 岁）dental germ of the 1st molar of maxilla（9th year）
2. 上颌第 2 前磨牙胚（10 岁）dental germ of the 2nd premolar of maxilla（10th year）
3. 上颌侧切牙胚（8 岁）dental germ of lateral incisor of maxilla（8th year）
4. 第 1 磨牙胚（6 岁）dental germ of the 1st molar（6th year）
5. 第 2 前磨牙胚（10 岁）dental germ of the 2nd premolar（10th year）
6. 第 1 前磨牙胚（9 岁）dental germ of the 1st premolar（9th year）
7. 尖牙胚（11～12 岁）dental germ of canine tooth（11～12th year）
8. 侧切牙胚（8 岁）dental germ of lateral incisor（8th year）
9. 中切牙胚（7 岁）dental germ of central incisor（7th year）
10. 上颌中切牙胚（7 岁）dental germ of central incisor of maxilla（7th year）
11. 上颌尖牙胚（11～12 岁）dental germ of canine tooth of maxilla（11～12th year）

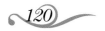

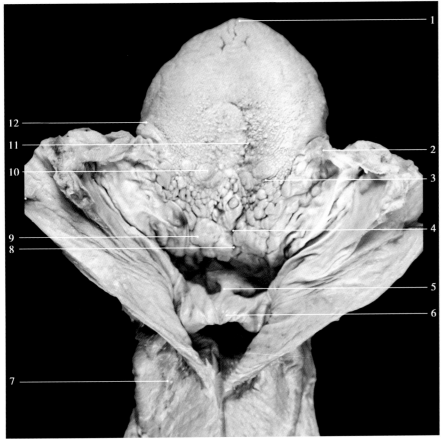

◀ 图 251

舌（背面观）

Tongue. Dorsal aspect

1. 舌尖 apex of tongue
2. 腭舌弓 palatoglossus arch
3. 界沟 terminal sulcus
4. 舌盲孔 foramen cecum of tongue
5. 舌会厌正中襞 median glossoepiglottic fold
6. 会厌 epiglottis
7. 咽缩肌 constrictor of pharynx
8. 舌根 lingual root
9. 舌扁桃体 lingual tonsil
10. 轮廓乳头 vallate papillae
11. 舌正中沟 median sulcus of tongue
12. 叶状乳头 foliate papillae

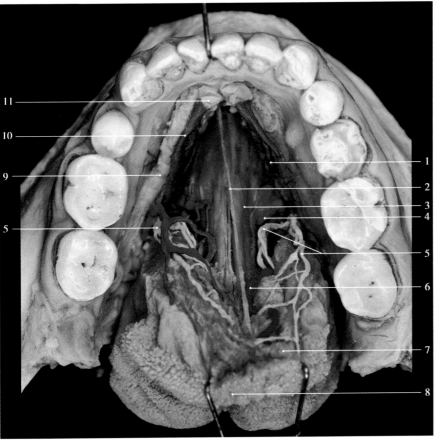

◀ 图 252

舌下面

Inferior surface of tongue

1. 舌下腺大管 major sublingual duct
2. 舌系带 frenulum of tongue
3. 颏舌肌 genioglossus
4. 舌深静脉 deep lingual v.
5. 舌神经 lingual n.
6. 舌深动脉 deep lingual a.
7. 舌前腺 anterior lingual gland
8. 舌尖 apex of tongue
9. 舌下腺 sublingual gland
10. 下颌下腺管 submandibular duct
11. 舌下阜 sublingual caruncle

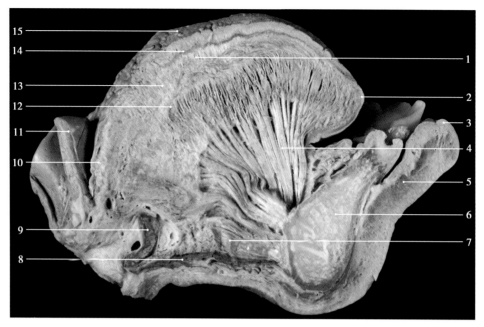

▲ 图 253　舌肌（纵切面）
Muscles of tongue. Longitudinal section

1. 舌垂直肌 vertical muscle of tongue
2. 舌尖 apex of tongue
3. 下唇 lower lip
4. 颏舌肌 genioglossus
5. 口轮匝肌 orbicularis oris

6. 下颌骨 mandible
7. 颏舌骨肌 geniohyoid
8. 下颌舌骨肌 mylohyoid
9. 舌骨 hyoid bone
10. 舌扁桃体 lingual tonsil

11. 会厌 epiglottis
12. 下纵肌 inferior longitudinal m.
13. 舌横肌 transverse muscle of tongue
14. 上纵肌 superior longitudinal m.
15. 舌粘膜 lingual mucous membrane

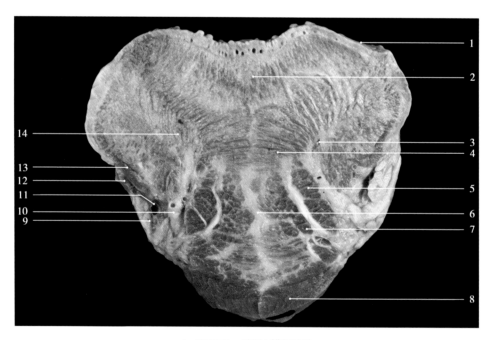

▲ 图 254　舌肌（横切面）
Muscles of tongue. Transverse section

1. 舌粘膜 lingual mucous membrane
2. 上纵肌 superior longitudinal m.
3. 舌深动脉 deep lingual a.
4. 舌横肌 transverse muscle of tongue
5. 下纵肌 inferior longitudinal m.

6. 舌中隔 septum of tongue
7. 颏舌肌 genioglossus
8. 颏舌骨肌 geniohyoid
9. 舌下腺 sublingual gland
10. 舌动脉 lingual a.

11. 舌静脉 lingual v.
12. 茎突舌肌 styloglossus
13. 舌骨舌肌 hyoglossus
14. 舌垂直肌 vertical muscle of tongue

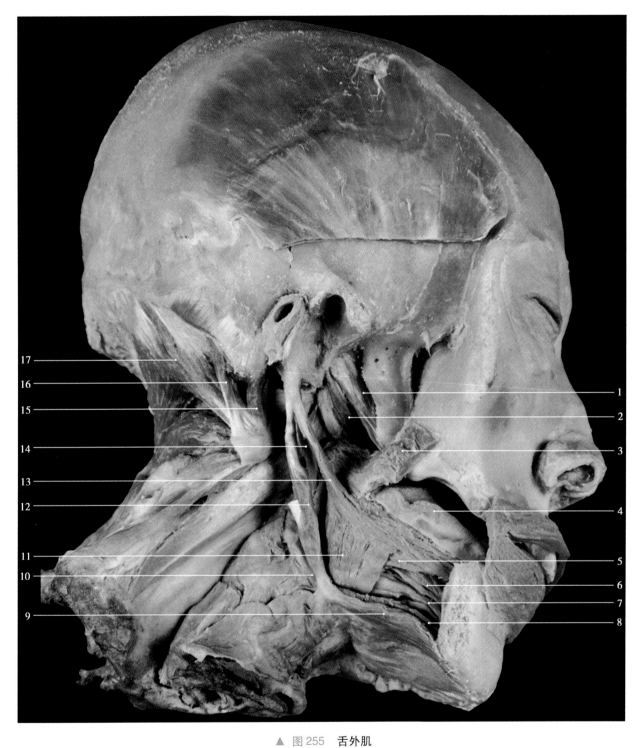

▲ 图 255　舌外肌
Extrinsic muscles of tongue

1. 腭帆张肌 tensor veli palatini
2. 腭帆提肌 levator veli palatini
3. 颊肌 buccinator
4. 舌 tongue
5. 下纵肌 inferior longitudinal m.
6. 颏舌肌 genioglossus
7. 颏舌骨肌 geniohyoid
8. 下颌舌骨肌 mylohyoid
9. 二腹肌（前腹）digastric（anterior belly）
10. 舌骨大角 greater horn of hyoid bon
11. 舌骨舌肌 hyoglossus
12. 茎突舌骨肌 stylohyoid
13. 茎突舌肌 styloglossus
14. 茎突咽肌 stylopharyngeus
15. 头前直肌 rectus capitis anterior
16. 头外侧直肌 rectus capitis lateralis
17. 头上斜肌 obliquus capitis superior

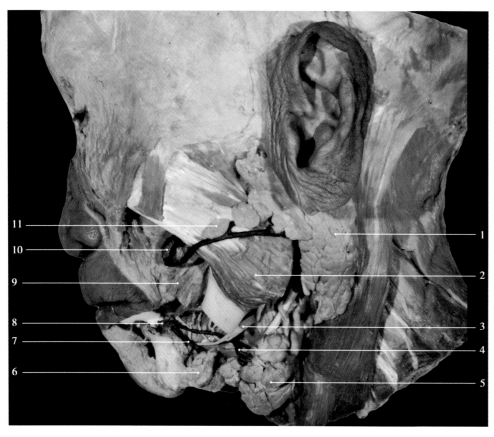

◀ 图 256

口腔腺（外侧面观）
Glands of oral cavity.
Lateral aspect

1. 腮腺 parotid gland
2. 咬肌 masseter
3. 舌下神经 hypoglossal n.
4. 下颌下腺管 submandibular duct
5. 下颌下腺 submandibular gland
6. 舌下腺 sublingual gland
7. 舌下腺管 sublingual duct
8. 舌下阜 sublingual caruncle
9. 颊肌 buccinator
10. 腮腺管 parotid duct
11. 副腮腺 accessory parotid gland

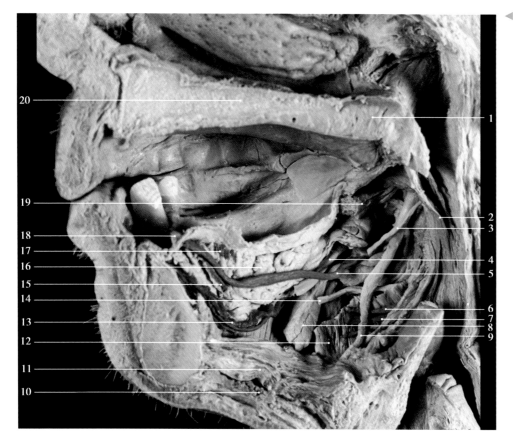

◀ 图 257

口腔腺（内侧面观）
Gland of oral cavity.
Medial aspect

1. 软腭 soft palate
2. 腭咽肌 palatopharyngeus
3. 舌咽神经 glossopharyngeal n.
4. 舌神经 lingual n.
5. 下颌下腺管 submandibular duct
6. 舌静脉 lingual v.
7. 舌动脉 lingual a
8. 下颌下腺 submandibular gland
9. 茎突舌骨韧带 stylohyoid lig.
10. 下颌舌骨肌 mylohyoid
11. 颏舌骨肌 geniohyoid
12. 舌骨舌肌 hyoglossus
13. 舌下动脉 sublingual a.
14. 舌下神经 hypoglossal n.
15. 舌下腺大管 major sublingual duct
16. 舌下腺 sublingual gland
17. 舌下腺小管 minor sublingual ducts
18. 舌下阜 sublingual caruncle
19. 腭舌肌 palatoglossus
20. 硬腭 hard palate

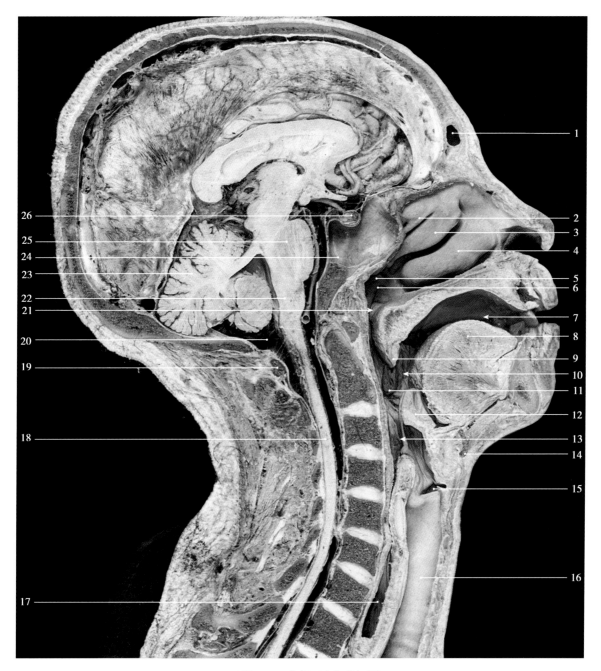

▲ 图 258 头部正中矢状切面
Median sagittal section of head

1. 额窦 frontal sinus
2. 上鼻甲 superior nasal concha
3. 中鼻甲 middle nasal concha
4. 下鼻甲 inferior nasal concha
5. 咽鼓管圆枕 tubal torus
6. 咽鼓管咽口 pharyngeal opening of auditory tube
7. 口腔 oral cavity
8. 舌 tongue

9. 腭垂 uvula
10. 口咽 oropharynx
11. 腭扁桃体 palatine tonsil
12. 会厌 epiglottis
13. 喉咽 laryngopharynx
14. 舌骨 hyoid bone
15. 喉室 ventricle of larynx
16. 气管 trachea
17. 食管 esophagus

18. 脊髓 spinal cord
19. 寰椎后弓 posterior arch of atlas
20. 小脑延髓池 cerebellomedullary cistern
21. 鼻咽 nasopharynx
22. 延髓 medulla oblongata
23. 小脑 cerebellum
24. 蝶窦 sphenoidal sinus
25. 脑桥 pons
26. 垂体 hypophysis

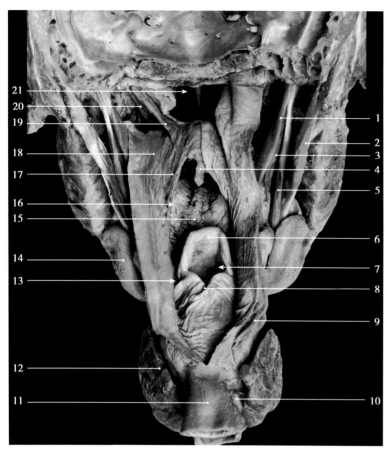

◀ 图 259

咽腔（后面观）
Pharyngeal cavity. Posterior aspect
1. 茎突咽肌 stylopharyngeus
2. 二腹肌（后腹）digastric（posterior belly）
3. 茎突舌肌 styloglossus
4. 腭垂肌 musculus uvulae
5. 茎突舌骨肌 stylohyoid
6. 会厌 epiglottis
7. 喉口 aperture of larynx
8. 杓间切迹 interarytenoid notch
9. 咽下缩肌 inferior constrictor of pharynx
10. 气管 trachea
11. 食管 esophagus
12. 甲状腺 thyroid gland
13. 喉咽 laryngopharynx
14. 下颌下腺 submandibular gland
15. 舌 tongue
16. 口咽 oropharynx
17. 腭咽肌 palatopharyngeus
18. 咽缩肌 constrictor of pharynx
19. 腭帆提肌 levator veli palatini
20. 腭帆张肌 tensor veli palatini
21. 鼻咽 nasopharynx

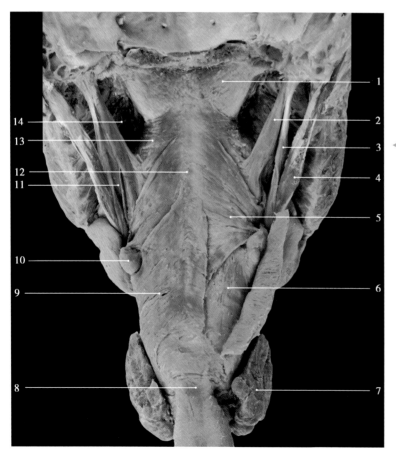

◀ 图 260

咽肌（后面观）
Pharyngeal muscles. Posterior aspect
1. 咽颅底筋膜 pharyngobasilar fascia
2. 茎突咽肌 stylopharyngeus
3. 茎突舌骨肌 stylohyoid
4. 二腹肌（后腹）digastric（posterior belly）
5. 咽中缩肌 middle constrictor of pharynx
6. 咽纵肌 longitudinal pharyngeal m.
7. 甲状腺 thyroid gland
8. 食管第 1 狭窄 1st narrow of esophagus
9. 咽下缩肌 inferior constrictor of pharyn
10. 舌骨大角 greater horn of hyoid bone
11. 茎突舌肌 styloglossus
12. 咽缝 raphe pharynx
13. 咽上缩肌 superior constrictor of pharynx
14. 翼内肌 medial pterygoid

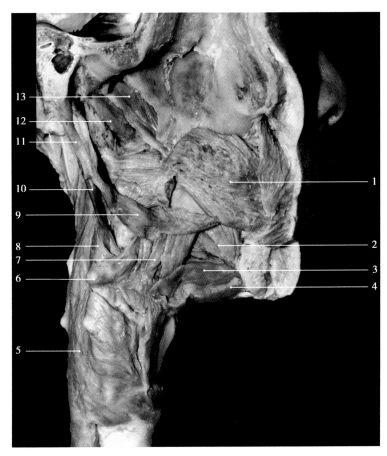

◀ 图 261

咽肌(外侧面观)
Pharyngeal muscles. Lateral aspect

1. 颊肌 buccinator
2. 颏舌肌 genioglossus
3. 颏舌骨肌 geniohyoid
4. 下颌舌骨肌 mylohyoid
5. 咽下缩肌 inferior constrictor of pharynx
6. 舌骨大角 greater horn of hyoid bone
7. 舌骨舌肌 hyoglossus
8. 咽中缩肌 middle constrictor of pharynx
9. 茎突舌肌 styloglossus
10. 茎突咽肌 stylopharyngeus
11. 茎突 styloid process
12. 腭帆提肌 levator veli palatini
13. 腭帆张肌 tensor veli palatini

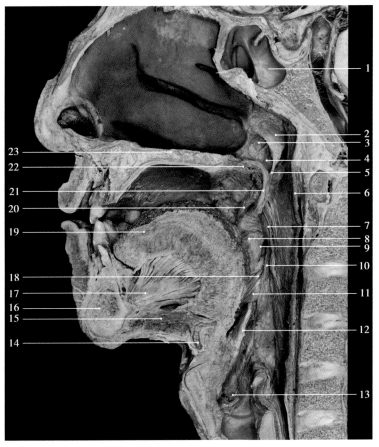

◀ 图 262

咽肌(内侧面观)
Pharyngeal muscles. Medial aspect

1. 蝶窦 sphenoidal sinus
2. 咽鼓管软骨 cartilage of auditory tube
3. 腭帆张肌 tensor veli palatini
4. 腭帆提肌 levator veli palatini
5. 咽鼓管咽肌 salpingopharyngeus
6. 咽后壁 posterior wall of pharynx
7. 腭咽肌 palatopharyngeus
8. 茎突舌肌 styloglossus
9. 咽上缩肌 superior constrictor of pharynx
10. 茎突咽肌 stylopharyngeus
11. 咽中缩肌 middle constrictor of pharynx
12. 会厌 epiglottis
13. 喉腔 laryngeal cavity
14. 舌骨体 body of hyoid bone
15. 颏舌骨肌 geniohyoid
16. 下颌骨 mandible
17. 颏舌肌 genioglossus
18. 舌咽神经 glossopharyngeal n.
19. 舌 tongue
20. 腭舌肌 palatoglossus
21. 腭垂肌 musculus uvulae
22. 软腭 soft palate
23. 硬腭 hard palate

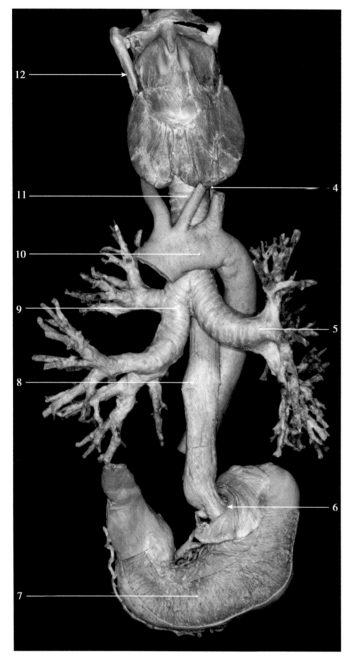
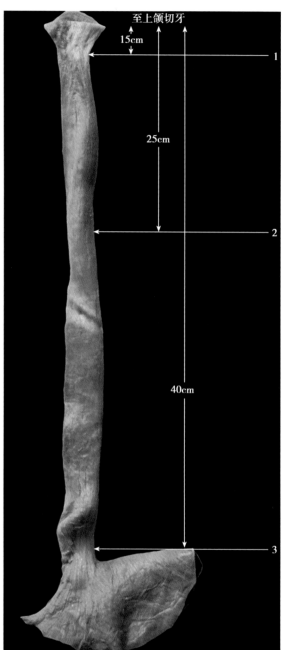

▲ 图 263　食管的狭窄
Esophageal narrow

1. 第一狭窄 the 1st narrow
2. 第二狭窄 the 2nd narrow
3. 第三狭窄 the 3rd narrow
4. 食管颈部 cervical part of esophagus
5. 左主支气管 left principal bronchus
6. 膈食管裂孔 esophageal hiatus of diaphragm

7. 胃 stomach
8. 食管胸部 thoracic part of esophagus
9. 右主支气管 right principal bronchus
10. 主动脉弓 aortic arch
11. 气管 trachea
12. 喉 larynx

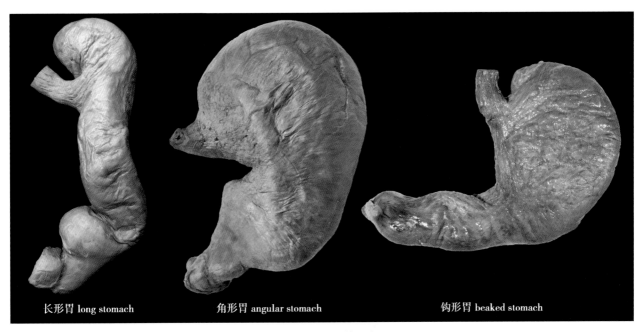

长形胃 long stomach　　　角形胃 angular stomach　　　钩形胃 beaked stomach

▲ 图 264　胃的形态
Shape of stomach

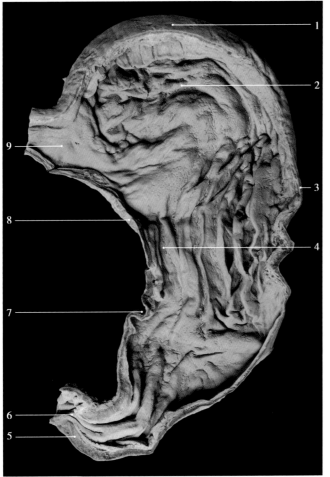

◀ 图 265

胃的黏膜
Mucous membrane of stomach
1. 胃底 fundus of stomach
2. 黏膜皱襞 mucous folds
3. 胃大弯 greater curvature of stomach
4. 胃道 ventricular canal
5. 幽门括约肌 pyloric sphincter
6. 幽门 pylorus
7. 角切迹 angular incisure
8. 胃小弯 lesser curvature of stomach
9. 贲门 cardia

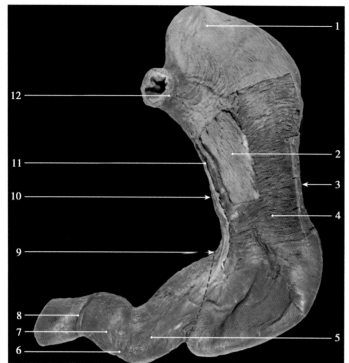

◀ 图 266

胃的肌层
Muscular layer of stomach
1. 胃底 fundus of stomach
2. 斜纤维 oblique fibers
3. 胃大弯 greater curvature of stomach
4. 环层 circular layer
5. 幽门窦 pyloric antrum
6. 中间沟 intermediate groove
7. 幽门管 pyloric canal
8. 幽门 pylorus
9. 角切迹 angular incisure
10. 胃小弯 lesser curvature of stomach
11. 纵层 longitudinal layer
12. 贲门 cardia

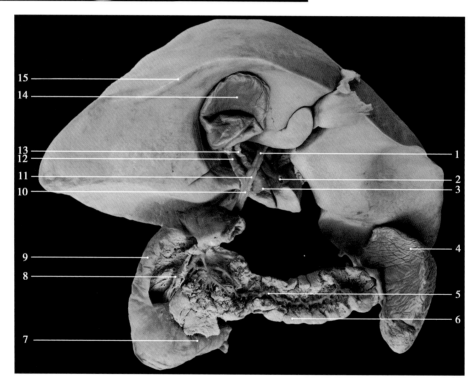

▲ 图 267 胆道、十二指肠和胰
Biliary tract, duodenum and pancreas

1. 肝左管 left hepatic duct
2. 肝固有动脉 proper hepatic a.
3. 肝门静脉 hepatic portal v.
4. 脾 spleen
5. 胰管 pancreatic duct
6. 胰体 body of pancreas
7. 十二指肠水平部 horizontal part of duodenum
8. 十二指肠大乳头 major duodenal papilla
9. 十二指肠降部 descending part of duodenum
10. 胆总管 common bile duct
11. 肝总管 common hepatic duct
12. 胆囊管 cystic duct
13. 肝右管 right hepatic duct
14. 胆囊 gallbladder
15. 肝 live

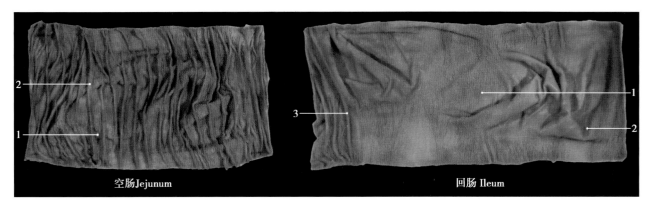

空肠 Jejunum   回肠 Ileum

▲ 图 268　**空肠与回肠**
Jejunum and ileum

1. 孤立淋巴滤泡 solitary lymphatic follicles　　1. 集合淋巴滤泡 aggregated lymphatic follicles
2. 环皱襞 circular fold　　　　　　　　　　　2. 孤立淋巴滤泡 solitary lymphatic follicles
　　　　　　　　　　　　　　　　　　　　　3. 环皱襞 circular fold

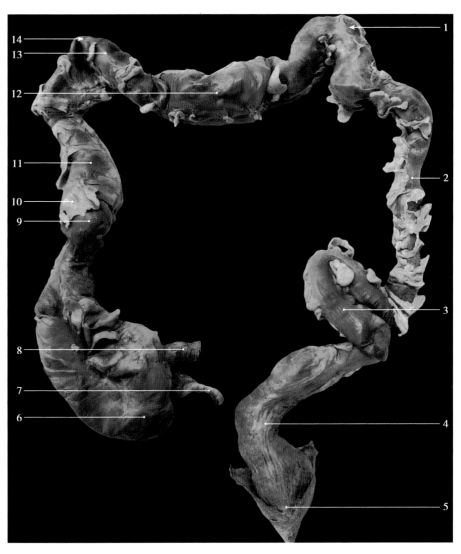

◀ 图 269

结肠
Colon
1. 结肠左曲 left colic flexure
2. 降结肠 descending colon
3. 乙状结肠 sigmoid colon
4. 直肠 rectum
5. 肛管 anal canal
6. 盲肠 cecum
7. 阑尾 vermiform appendix
8. 回肠 ileum
9. 结肠袋 haustra of colon
10. 肠脂垂 epiploic appendices
11. 升结肠 ascending colon
12. 横结肠 transverse colon
13. 结肠带 colic bands
14. 结肠右曲 right colic flexure

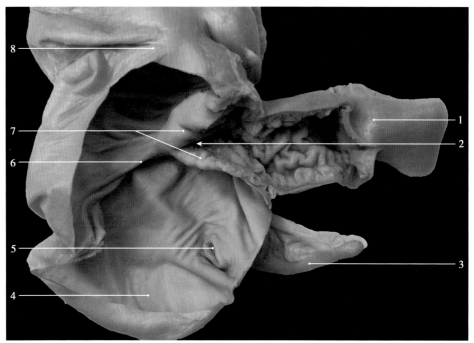

◀ 图 270

盲肠及阑尾

Cecum and vermiform appendix

1. 回肠 ileum
2. 回盲口 ileocecal orifice
3. 阑尾 vermiform appendix
4. 盲肠 cecum
5. 阑尾口 orifice of vermiform appendix
6. 回盲瓣系带 frenulum of ileocecal valve
7. 回盲瓣 ileocecal valve
8. 升结肠 ascending colon

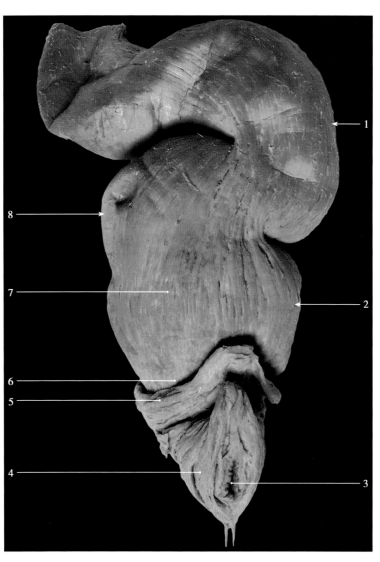

◀ 图 271

直肠及肛管

Rectum and anal canal

1. 直肠上方侧曲 flexura superior lateralis recti
2. 直肠下方侧曲 flexura inferior lateralis recti
3. 肛门 anus
4. 肛门外括约肌 sphincter ani externus
5. 肛提肌 levator ani
6. 肛管 anal canal
7. 直肠壶腹 ampulla of rectum
8. 直肠中间侧曲 flexura intermedia lateralis recti

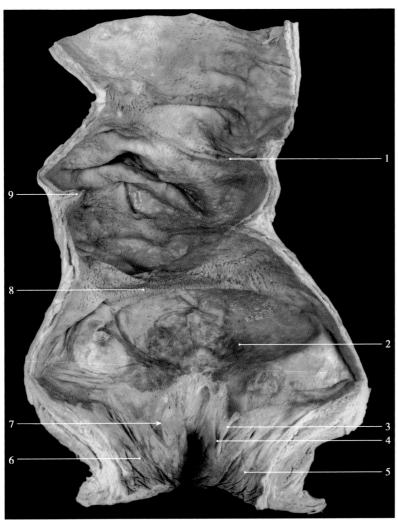

◀ 图 272

直肠及肛管（冠状切面）
Rectum and anal canal. Coronal section

1. 上直肠横襞 superior transverse folds of rectum
2. 直肠壶腹 ampulla of rectum
3. 肛柱 anal columns
4. 肛窦 anal sinuses
5. 白线 white line
6. 肛瓣 anal valves
7. 肛管 anal canal
8. 下直肠横襞 inferior transverse folds of rectum
9. 中直肠横襞 median transverse folds of rectum

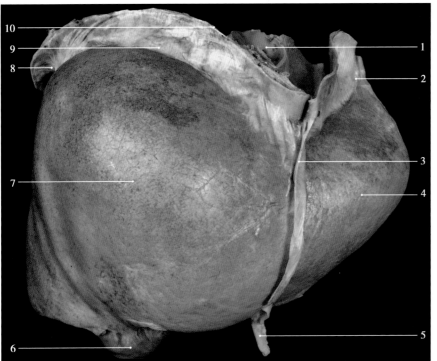

◀ 图 273

肝的前面
Anterior surface of liver

1. 下腔静脉 inferior vena cava
2. 左三角韧带 left triangular lig.
3. 肝镰状韧带 falciform ligament of liver
4. 肝左叶 left lobe of liver
5. 肝圆韧带 ligamentum teres hepatis
6. 胆囊 gallbladder
7. 肝右叶 right lobe of liver
8. 右三角韧带 right triangular lig.
9. 冠状韧带 coronary lig.
10. 膈 diaphragm

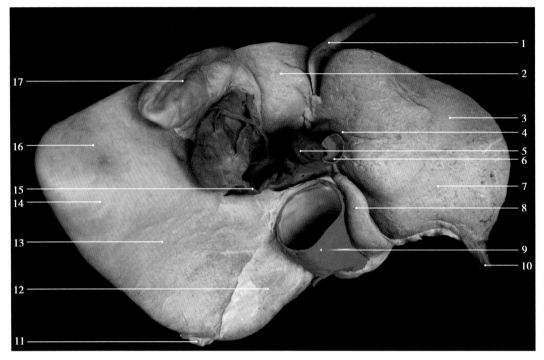

▲ 图 274　肝的脏面
Visceral surface of liver

1. 肝圆韧带 ligamentum teres hepatis
2. 方叶 quadrate lobe
3. 胃压迹 gastric impression
4. 肝固有动脉 proper hepatic a.
5. 胆总管 common bile duct
6. 肝门静脉 hepatic portal v.
7. 肝左叶 left lobe of liver
8. 尾状叶 caudate lobe
9. 下腔静脉 inferior vena cava
10. 肝纤维附件 fibrous appendix of liver
11. 右三角韧带 right triangular lig.
12. 肝裸区 bare area of liver
13. 肾压迹 renal impression
14. 肝右叶 right lobe of liver
15. 胆囊管 cystic duct
16. 结肠压迹 colic impression
17. 胆囊 gallbladder

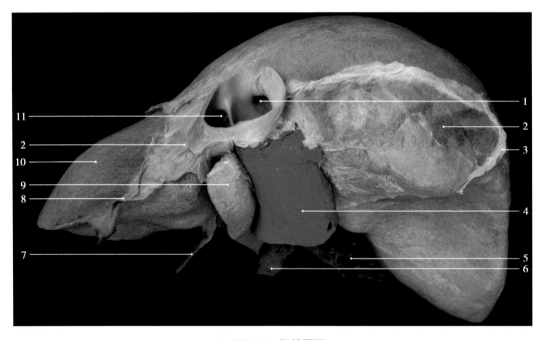

▲ 图 275　肝的膈面
Diaphragmatic surface of liver

1. 肝右静脉 right hepatic v.
2. 肝裸区 bare area of liver
3. 右三角韧带 right triangular lig.
4. 下腔静脉 inferior vena cava
5. 胆囊 gallbladder
6. 胆总管 common bile duct
7. 肝圆韧带 ligamentum teres hepatis
8. 左三角韧带 left triangular lig.
9. 尾状叶 caudate lobe
10. 肝左叶 left lobe of liver
11. 肝左静脉 left hepatic v.

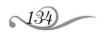

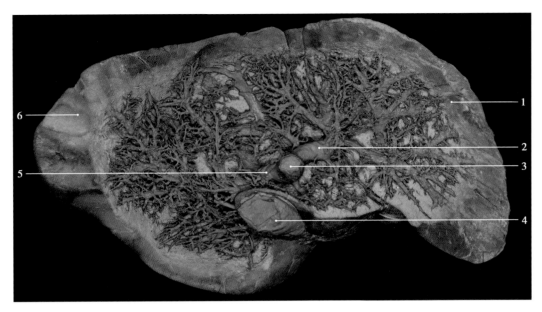

▲ 图 276 肝门静脉
Hepatic portal vein

1. 肝左叶 left lobe of liver
2. 肝门静脉左支 left branch of hepatic portal v.
3. 肝门静脉 hepatic portal v.
4. 下腔静脉 inferior vena cava
5. 肝门静脉右支 right branch of hepatic portal v.
6. 肝右叶 right lobe of liver

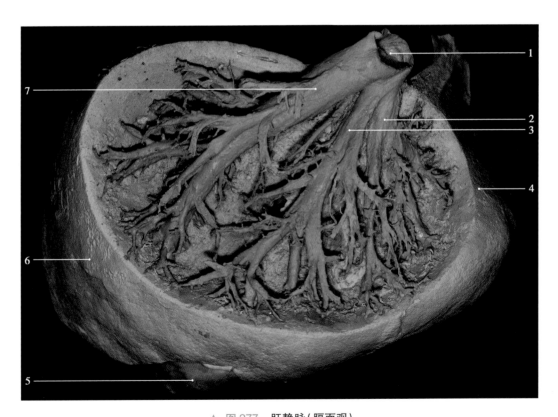

▲ 图 277 肝静脉 (膈面观)
Hepatic vein. Diaphragmatic aspect

1. 下腔静脉 inferior vena cava
2. 肝左静脉 left hepatic v.
3. 肝中间静脉 intermediate hepatic v.
4. 肝左叶 left lobe of liver
5. 胆囊 gallbladder
6. 肝右叶 right lobe of liver
7. 肝右静脉 right hepatic v.

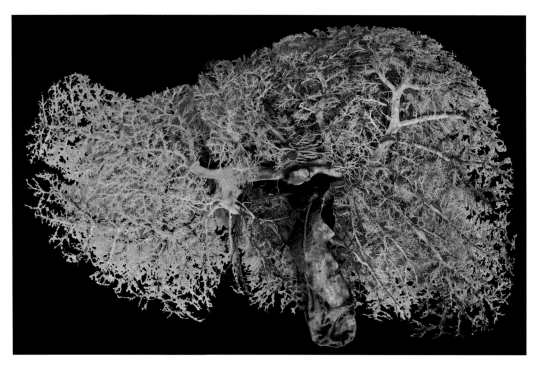

▲ 图 278　肝脏管道铸型（脏面观）
Cast of hepatic duct. Visceral aspect

黄色：肝门静脉 hepatic portal v.
红色：肝动脉 hepatic a.
绿色：胆囊和肝内胆管 gall bladder and intrahepatic bile duct

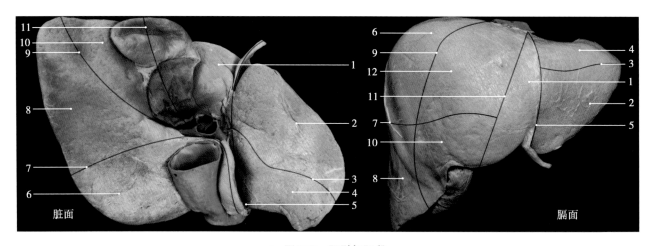

▲ 图 279　肝裂与肝段
Hepatic fissure and hepatic segments

1. 左内叶 left internal lobe
2. 左外叶下段 inferior segment of left external lobe
3. 左段间裂 left intersegmental fissure
4. 左外叶上段 superior segment of left external lobe
5. 左叶间裂 left interlobar fissure
6. 右后叶上段 superior segment of right posterior lobe
7. 右段间裂 right intersegmental fissure
8. 右后叶下段 inferior segment of right posterior lobe
9. 右叶间裂 right interlobar fissure
10. 右前叶下段 inferior segment of right anterior lobe
11. 正中裂 median fissure
12. 右前叶上段 superior segment of right anterior lobe

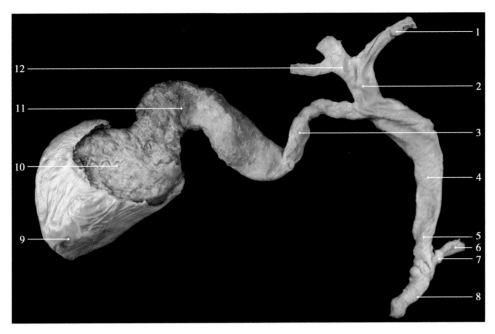

▲ 图 280　胆囊与输胆管道（1）
Gallbladder and biliary pore（1）

1. 肝左管 left hepatic duct
2. 肝总管 common hepatic duct
3. 胆囊管 cystic duct
4. 胆总管 common bile duct
5. 胆总管括约肌 sphincter of common bile duct
6. 胰管 pancreatic duct
7. 胰管括约肌 sphincter of pancreatic duct
8. 肝胰壶腹括约肌 sphincter of hepatopancreatic ampulla
9. 胆囊底 fundus of gallbladder
10. 胆囊体 body of gallbladder
11. 胆囊颈 neck of gallbladder
12. 肝右管 right hepatic duct

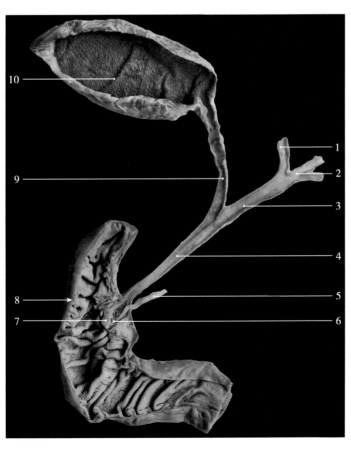

◀ 图 281
胆囊与输胆管道（2）
Gallbladder and biliary pore（2）

1. 肝右管 right hepatic duct
2. 肝左管 left hepatic duct
3. 肝总管 common hepatic duct
4. 胆总管 common bile duct
5. 胰管 pancreatic duct
6. 肝胰壶腹 hepatopancreatic ampulla
7. 十二指肠大乳头 major duodenal papilla
8. 十二指肠降部 descending part of duodenum
9. 胆囊管 cystic duct
10. 胆囊 gallbladder

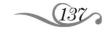

第六章 呼吸系统
Respiratory System

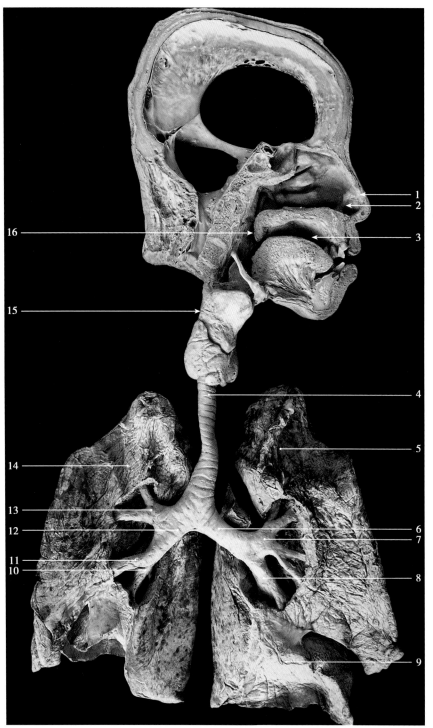

◀ 图 282

呼吸系统全貌
General arrangement of respiratory system

1. 鼻 nose
2. 鼻腔 nasal cavity
3. 口腔 oral cavity
4. 气管 trachea
5. 左肺上叶 superior lobe of left lung
6. 左主支气管 left principal bronchus
7. 左肺上叶支气管 left superior lobar bronchus
8. 左肺下叶支气管 left inferior lobar bronchus
9. 左肺下叶 inferior lobe of left lung
10. 右肺下叶支气管 right inferior lobar bronchus
11. 右肺中叶支气管 right middle lobar bronchus
12. 右主支气管 right principal bronchus
13. 右肺上叶支气管 right superior lobar bronchus
14. 右肺上叶 superior lobe of right lung
15. 喉 larynx
16. 咽 pharynx

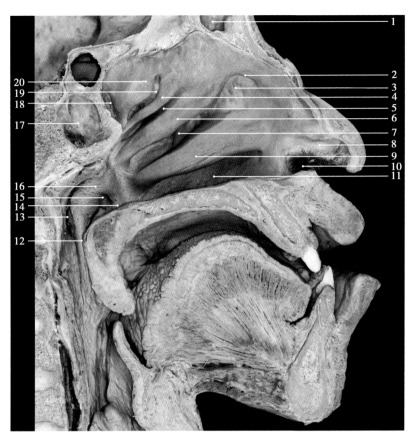

◀ 图283

鼻腔外侧壁（1）
Lateral wall of nasal cavity（1）
1. 额窦 frontal sinus
2. 鼻堤 agger nasi
3. 中鼻道前房 atrium of middle meatus
4. 上鼻甲 superior nasal concha
5. 上鼻道 superior nasal meatus
6. 中鼻甲 middle nasal concha
7. 中鼻道 middle nasal meatus
8. 鼻阈 limen nasi
9. 下鼻甲 inferior nasal concha
10. 鼻前庭 nasal vestibule
11. 下鼻道 inferior nasal meatus
12. 咽鼓管咽襞 salpingopharyngeal fold
13. 咽隐窝 pharyngeal recess
14. 咽鼓管腭襞 salpingopalatine fold
15. 咽鼓管咽口 pharyngeal opening of auditory tube
16. 咽鼓管圆枕 tubal torus
17. 蝶窦 sphenoidal sinus
18. 蝶筛隐窝 sphenoethmoidal recess
19. 最上鼻道 supreme nasal meatus
20. 最上鼻甲 supreme nasal concha

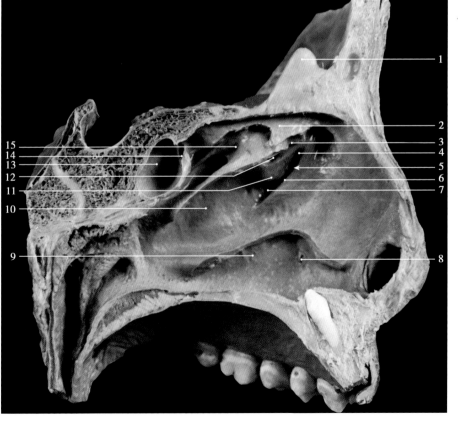

◀ 图284

鼻腔外侧壁（2）
Lateral wall of nasal cavity（2）
1. 鸡冠 crista galli
2. 上鼻甲 superior nasal concha
3. 前筛窦口 aperture of anterior ethmoidal sinuses
4. 额窦口 aperture of frontal sinus
5. 半月裂孔 hiatus semilunaris
6. 筛骨钩突 uncinate process of ethmoid bone
7. 上颌窦口 opening of maxillary sinus
8. 鼻泪管口 orifice of nasolacrimal duct
9. 下鼻道 inferior nasal meatus
10. 中鼻道 middle nasal meatus
11. 筛泡 ethmoidal bulla
12. 中筛窦口 aperture of middle ethmoidal sinuses
13. 蝶窦 sphenoidal sinus
14. 蝶窦口 aperture of sphenoidal sinus
15. 后筛窦口 aperture of posterior ethmoidal sinuses

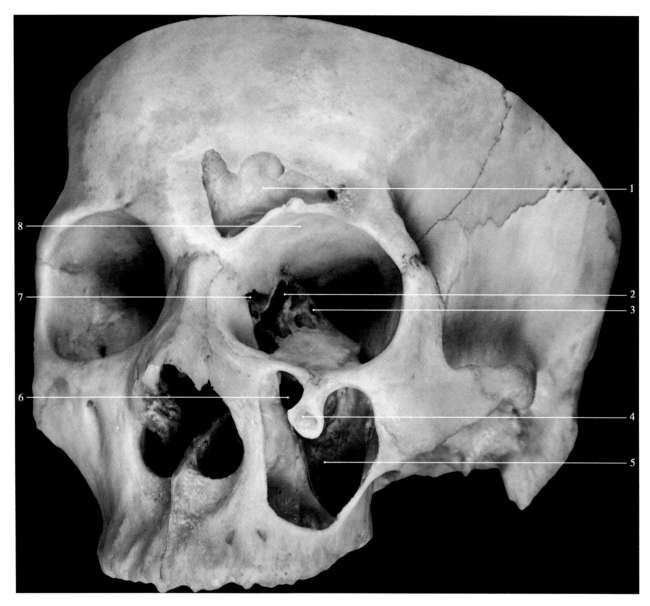

▲ 图 285 鼻旁窦
Paranasal sinuses

1. 额窦 frontal sinus
2. 中筛窦 middle ethmoidal sinuses
3. 后筛窦 posterior ethmoidal sinuses
4. 眶下孔 infraorbital foramen
5. 上颌窦 maxillary sinus
6. 上颌窦口 opening of maxillary sinus
7. 前筛窦 anterior ethmoidal sinuses
8. 额骨眶面 orbital surface of frontal bone

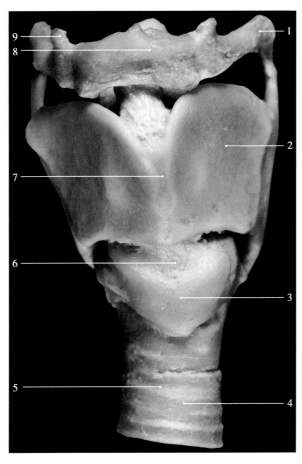

◀ 图 286

喉软骨（前面观）
Laryngeal cartilages. Anterior aspect

1. 舌骨大角 greater horn of hyoid bone
2. 甲状软骨 thyroid cartilage
3. 环状软骨 cricoid cartilage
4. 气管软骨 tracheal cartilages
5. 环韧带 annular lig.
6. 环甲正中韧带 median cricothyroid lig.
7. 喉结 laryngeal prominence
8. 舌骨体 body of hyoid bone
9. 舌骨小角 lesser horn of hyoid bone

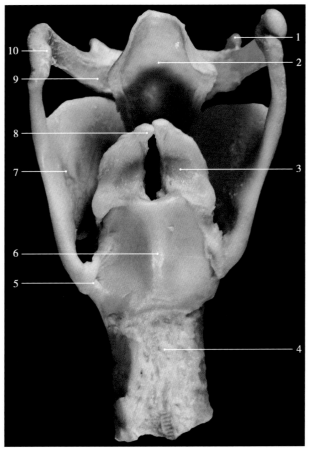

◀ 图 287

喉软骨（后面观）
Laryngeal cartilages. Posterior aspect

1. 舌骨小角 lesser horn of hyoid bone
2. 会厌软骨 epiglottic cartilage
3. 杓状软骨 arytenoid cartilage
4. 气管膜壁 membranous wall of trachea
5. 环甲关节 cricothyroid joint
6. 环状软骨 cricoid cartilage
7. 甲状软骨 thyroid cartilage
8. 小角软骨 corniculate cartilage
9. 舌骨 hyoid bone
10. 麦粒软骨 triticeal cartilage

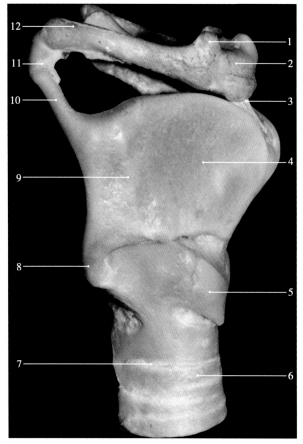

◀ 图 288

喉软骨（侧面观）
Larygeal cartilages. Lateral aspect
1. 舌骨小角 lesser horn of hyoid bone
2. 舌骨体 body of hyoid bone
3. 甲状舌骨正中韧带 median thyrohyoid lig.
4. 右板 right lamina
5. 环状软骨 cricoid cartilage
6. 气管软骨 tracheal cartilage
7. 环韧带 annular lig.
8. 下角 inferior cornu
9. 斜线 oblique line
10. 上角 superior cornu
11. 甲状舌骨外侧韧带 lateral thyrohyoid lig.
12. 舌骨大角 greater horn of hyoid bone

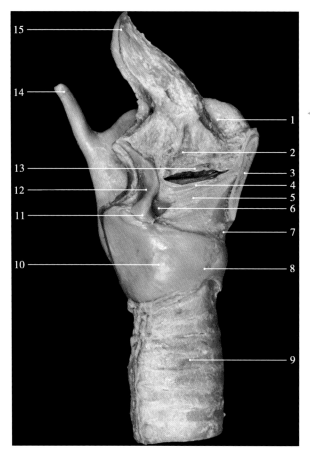

◀ 图 289

弹性圆锥和方形膜（侧面观）
Elastic cone and quadrangular membrane.
Lateral aspect
1. 会厌软骨前脂体 preepiglottic adipose body
2. 方形膜 quadrangular membrane
3. 甲状软骨 thyroid cartilage
4. 声韧带 vocal lig.
5. 弹性圆锥 conus elasticus
6. 声带突 vocal process
7. 环甲正中韧带 median cricothyroid lig.
8. 环状软骨 cricoid cartilage
9. 气管 trachea
10. 甲关节面 thyroid articular surface
11. 肌突 muscular process
12. 杓状软骨 arytenoid cartilage
13. 前庭韧带 vestibular lig.
14. 上角 superior cornu
15. 会厌软骨 epiglottic cartilage

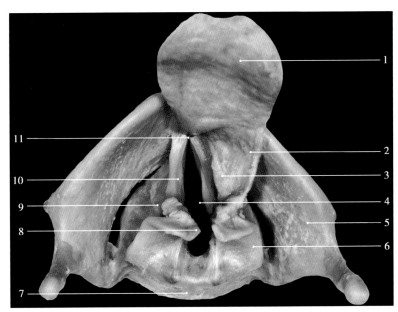

◀ 图290

弹性圆锥和方形膜（上面观）
Elastic cone and quadrangular membrane.
Superior aspect

1. 会厌软骨 epiglottic cartilage
2. 方形膜 quadrangular membrane
3. 前庭韧带 vestibular lig.
4. 声门裂 fissure of glottis
5. 甲状软骨 thyroid cartilage
6. 杓状软骨 arytenoid cartilage
7. 环状软骨 cricoid cartilage
8. 小角软骨 corniculate cartilage
9. 弹性圆锥 elastic cone
10. 声韧带 vocal lig.
11. 甲状会厌韧带 thyroepiglottic lig.

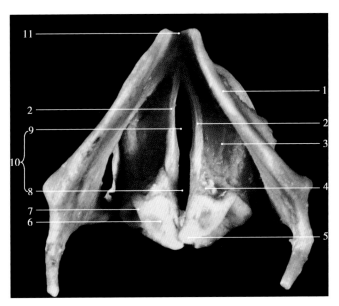

▲ 图291 **弹性圆锥（上面观）**
Elastic cone. Superior aspect

1. 甲状软骨 thyroid cartilage
2. 声韧带 vocal lig.
3. 弹性圆锥 elastic cone
4. 杓状软骨声带突 vocal process of arytenoid cartilage
5. 小角软骨 corniculate cartilage
6. 杓状软骨 arytenoid cartilage
7. 杓状软骨肌突 muscular process of arytenoid cartilage
8. 声门裂软骨间部 intercartilaginous part of fissure of glottis
9. 声门裂膜间部 intermembranous part of fissure of glottis
10. 声门裂 fissure of glottis
11. 甲状软骨上切迹 superior thyroid notch

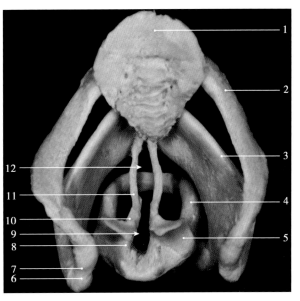

▲ 图292 **喉软骨及声韧带（上面观）**
Laryngeal cartilage and vocal ligament. Superior aspect

1. 会厌软骨 epiglottic cartilage
2. 舌骨 hyoid bone
3. 甲状软骨 thyroid cartilage
4. 环状软骨 cricoid cartilage
5. 杓状软骨肌突 muscular process of arytenoid cartilage
6. 甲状舌骨外侧韧带 lateral thyrohyoid lig.
7. 麦粒软骨 triticeal cartilage
8. 杓状软骨 arytenoid cartilage
9. 声门裂软骨间部 intercartilaginous part of fissure of glottis
10. 杓状软骨声带突 vocal process of arytenoid cartilage
11. 声韧带 vocal lig.
12. 声门裂膜间部 intermembranous part of fissure of glottis

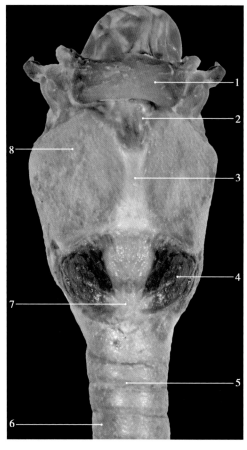

◀ 图 293

喉肌（前面观）

Muscles of larynx. Anterior aspect

1. 舌骨 hyoid bone
2. 甲状舌骨膜 hyrothyroid membrane
3. 喉结 laryngeal prominence
4. 环甲肌 cricothyroid
5. 环韧带 annular lig.
6. 气管软骨 tracheal cartilage
7. 环状软骨 cricoid cartilage
8. 甲状软骨板 lamina of thyroid cartilage

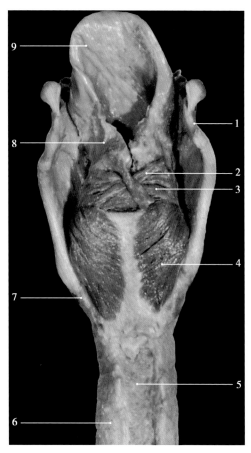

◀ 图 294

喉肌（后面观）

Muscles of larynx. Posterior aspect

1. 麦粒软骨 triticeal cartilage
2. 杓斜肌 oblique arytenoid
3. 杓横肌 transverse arytenoid
4. 环杓后肌 posterior cricoarytenoid
5. 气管膜壁 membranous wall of trachea
6. 气管软骨 tracheal cartilages
7. 环甲关节 cricothyroid joint
8. 杓会厌肌 aryepiglottic m.
9. 会厌 epiglottis

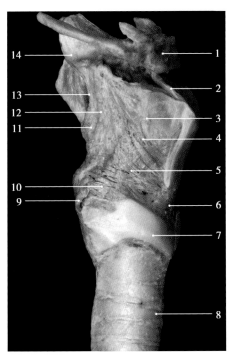

◀ 图 295

喉肌（侧面观）
Muscles of larynx. Lateral aspect
1. 舌骨 hyoid bone
2. 甲状舌骨正中韧带 median thyrohyoid lig.
3. 方形膜 quadrangular membrane
4. 甲状会厌肌 thyroepiglottideus
5. 甲杓肌 thyroarytenoid
6. 环甲正中韧带 median cricothyroid lig.
7. 环状软骨 cricoid cartilage
8. 气管软骨 tracheal cartilages
9. 环杓后肌 posterior cricoarytenoid
10. 环杓侧肌 lateral cricoarytenoid
11. 楔结节软骨 cuneiform cartilage
12. 杓会厌肌 aryepiglottic m.
13. 杓状会厌襞 aryepiglottic fold
14. 会厌 epiglottis

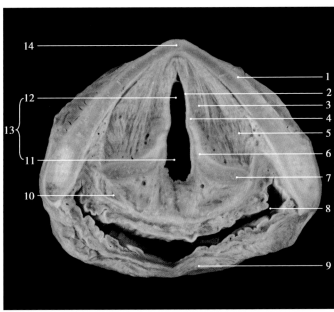

▲ 图 296　**喉的横切面（通过声门裂）**
Transverse section of larynx. Through the level
of fissure of glottis

1. 甲状软骨 thyroid cartilage
2. 声襞 vocal fold
3. 声带肌 vocalis
4. 声韧带 vocal lig.
5. 甲杓肌 thyroarytenoid
6. 声带突 vocal process
7. 肌突 muscular process
8. 喉咽 laryngopharynx
9. 咽后壁 posterior wall of pharynx
10. 杓横肌 transverse arytenoid
11. 声门裂软骨间部 intercartilaginous part of fissure of glottis
12. 声门裂膜间部 intermembranous part of fissure of glottis
13. 声门裂 fissure of glottis
14. 喉结 laryngeal prominence

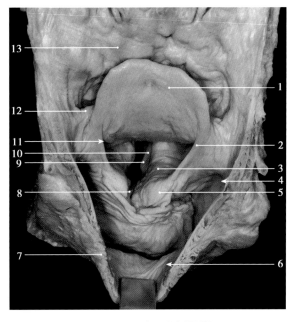

▲ 图 297　**喉口（上面观）**
Aperture of larynx. Superior aspect

1. 会厌 epiglottis
2. 杓状会厌襞 aryepiglottic fold
3. 前庭襞 vestibular fold
4. 梨状隐窝 piriform recess
5. 小角结节 corniculate tubercle
6. 喉咽 laryngopharynx
7. 咽后壁 posterior wall of pharynx
8. 杓间切迹 interarytenoid notch
9. 声襞 vocal fold
10. 喉室 ventricle of larynx
11. 喉口 aperture of larynx
12. 舌会厌外侧襞 lateral glossoepiglottic fold
13. 舌根 root of tongue

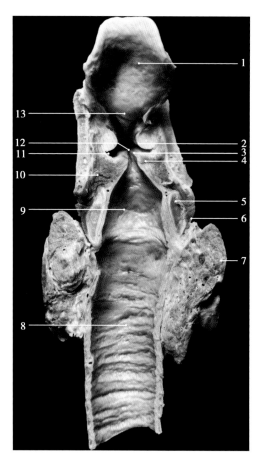

◀ 图 298

喉冠状切（后面观）
Coronal section of larynx. Posterior aspect
1. 会厌 epiglottis
2. 前庭襞 vestibular fold
3. 声襞 vocal fold
4. 声带肌 vocalis
5. 环状软骨 cricoid cartilage
6. 环甲肌 cricothyroid
7. 甲状腺 thyroid gland
8. 气管 trachea
9. 声门下腔 infraglottic cavity
10. 甲杓肌 thyroarytehoid
11. 喉室 ventricle of larynx
12. 喉中间腔 intermedial cavity of larynx
13. 会厌结节 tubercle of epiglottis

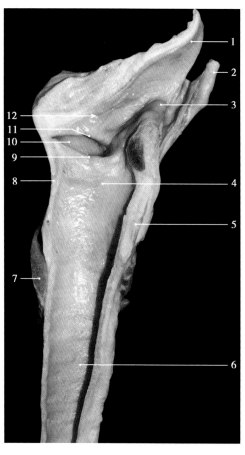

◀ 图 299

喉（矢状切面）
Larynx. Sagittal section
1. 会厌 epiglottis
2. 甲状软骨上角 superior cornu of thyroid cartilage
3. 杓会厌襞 aryepiglottic fold
4. 声门下腔 infraglottic cavity
5. 环状软骨板 lamina of cricoid cartilage
6. 气管 trachea
7. 甲状腺 thyroid gland
8. 甲状软骨 thyroid cartilage
9. 声襞 vocal fold
10. 喉室 ventricle of larynx
11. 前庭襞 vestibular fold
12. 喉前庭 laryngeal vestibule

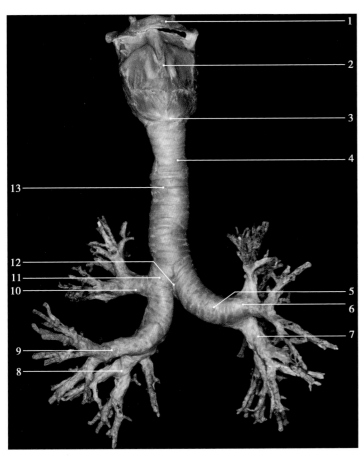

 图 300

气管与支气管（前面观）
Trachea and bronchi. Anterior aspect

1. 舌骨 hyoid bone
2. 甲状软骨 thyroid cartilage
3. 环状软骨 cricoid cartilage
4. 气管软骨 tracheal cartilage
5. 左主支气管 left principal bronchus
6. 左肺上叶支气管 left superior lobar bronchus
7. 左肺下叶支气管 left inferior lobar bronchus
8. 右肺下叶支气管 right inferior lobar bronchus
9. 右肺中叶支气管 right middle lobar bronchus
10. 右肺上叶支气管 right superior lobar bronchus
11. 右主支气管 right principal bronchus
12. 气管杈 bifurcation of trachea
13. 环韧带 annular lig.

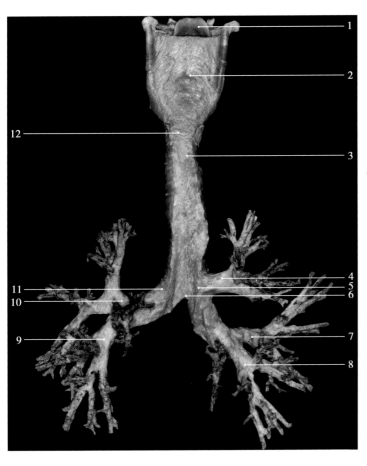

 图 301

气管与支气管（后面观）
Trachea and bronchi. Posterior aspect

1. 会厌 epiglottis
2. 咽后壁 posterior wall of pharynx
3. 气管膜壁 membranous wall of trachea
4. 右肺上叶支气管 right superior lobar bronchus
5. 右主支气管 right principal bronchus
6. 气管杈 bifurcation of trachea
7. 右肺中叶支气管 right middle lobar bronchus
8. 右肺下叶支气管 right inferior lobar bronchus
9. 左肺下叶支气管 left inferior lobar bronchus
10. 左肺上叶支气管 left superior lobar bronchus
11. 左主支气管 left principal bronchus
12. 食管 esophagus

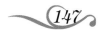

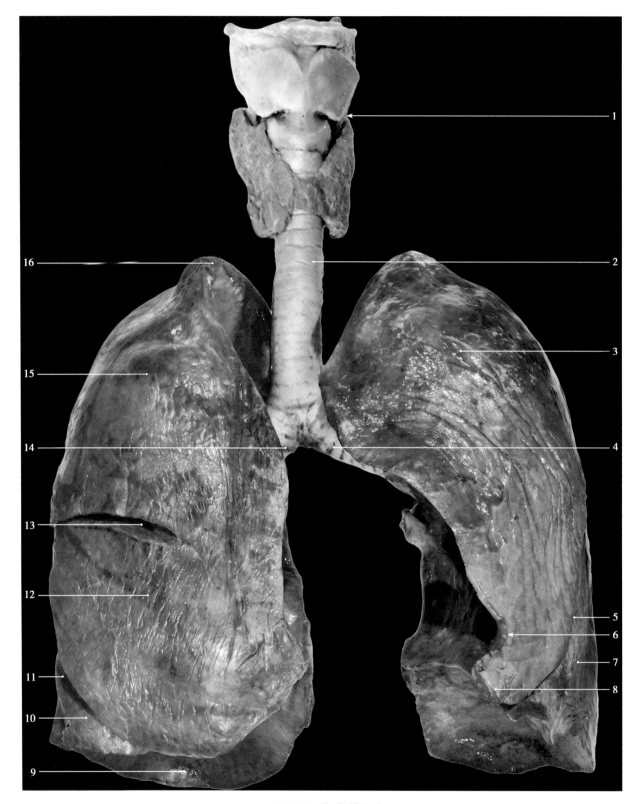

▲ 图 302　喉、气管和肺
Larynx, trachea and lungs

1. 喉 larynx
2. 气管 trachea
3. 左肺上叶 superior lobe of left lung
4. 左主支气管 left principal bronchus
5. 斜裂 oblique fissure
6. 心压迹 cardiac impression
7. 左肺下叶 inferior lobe of left lung
8. 左肺小舌 lingula of left lung
9. 右肺底 base of right lung
10. 右肺下叶 inferior lobe of right lung
11. 斜裂 oblique fissure
12. 右肺中叶 middle lobe of right lung
13. 右肺水平裂 horizontal fissure of right lung
14. 右主支气管 right principal bronchus
15. 右肺上叶 superior lobe of right lung
16. 右肺尖 apex of right lung

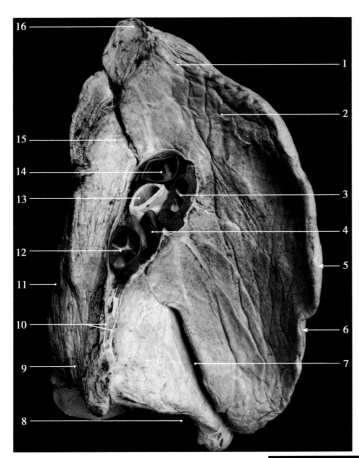

左肺门
1. 锁骨下动脉沟 sulcus for subclavian a.
2. 左肺上叶 superior lobe of left lung
3. 左上肺静脉 left superior pulmonary v.
4. 左支气管肺门淋巴结 left bronchopulmonary hilar lymph nodes
5. 左肺前缘 anterior border of left lung
6. 心压迹 cardiac impression
7. 斜裂 oblique fissure
8. 肺底 base of lung
9. 左肺下叶 inferior lobe of left lung
10. 肺韧带 pulmonary lig.
11. 左肺后缘 posterior border of left lung
12. 左下肺静脉 left inferior pulmonary v.
13. 左主支气管 left principal bronchus
14. 左肺动脉 left pulmonary a.
15. 主动脉沟 sulcus for aorta
16. 肺尖 apex of lung

右肺门
1. 肺尖 apex of lung
2. 右肺上叶 superior lobe of right lung
3. 右主支气管 right principal bronchus
4. 右肺后缘 posterior border of right lung
5. 右支气管肺门淋巴结 right bronchopulmonary hilar lymph node
6. 右上肺静脉 right superior pulmonary v.
7. 右下肺静脉 left inferior pulmonary v.
8. 肺韧带 pulmonary lig.
9. 右肺下叶 inferior lobe of right lung
10. 肺底 base of lung
11. 斜裂 oblique fissure
12. 右肺中叶 middle lobe of right lung
13. 右肺水平裂 horizontal fissure of right lung
14. 右肺前缘 anterior border of right lung
15. 右肺动脉 right pulmonary a.
16. 锁骨下动脉沟 sulcus for subclavian a.

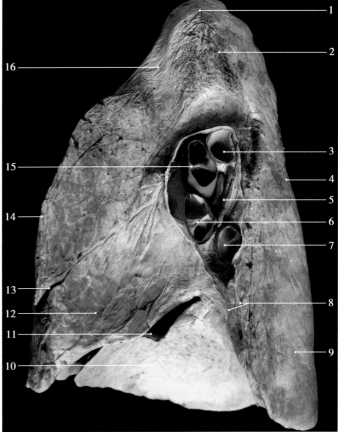

▲ 图 303 肺门
Hilum of lung

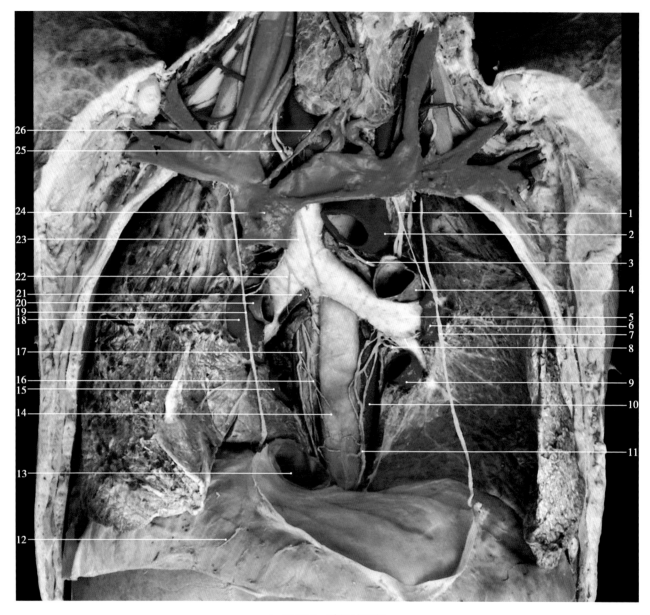

▲ 图304　肺根的结构
Structures of pedicle of lung

1. 左迷走神经 left vagus n.
2. 主动脉弓 aortic arch
3. 左喉返神经 left recurrent laryngeal n.
4. 左肺动脉 left pulmonary a.
5. 左主支气管 left principal bronchus
6. 左上肺静脉 left superior pulmonary v.
7. 左膈神经 left phrenic n.
8. 迷走神经肺支 pulmonary branches of vagus n.
9. 左下肺静脉 left inferior pulmonary v.
10. 胸主动脉 thoracic aorta
11. 迷走神经前干 anterior vagal trunk
12. 膈 diaphragm
13. 下腔静脉 inferior vena cava

14. 食管 esophagus
15. 右下肺静脉 right inferior pulmonary v.
16. 迷走神经食管支 esophageal branches of vagus n.
17. 奇静脉 azygos v.
18. 右上肺静脉 right superior pulmonary v.
19. 右膈神经 right phrenic n.
20. 右肺动脉 right pulmonary a.
21. 气管支气管下淋巴结 inferior tracheobronchial lymph nodes
22. 右主支气管 right principal bronchus
23. 气管 trachea
24. 上腔静脉 superior vena cava
25. 右迷走神经 right vagus n.
26. 头臂干 brachiocephalic trunk

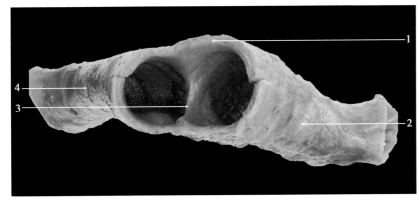

◀ 图 305

气管隆嵴
Carina of trachea
1. 气管 trachea
2. 右主支气管 right principal bronchus
3. 气管隆嵴 carina of trachea
4. 左主支气管 left principal bronchus

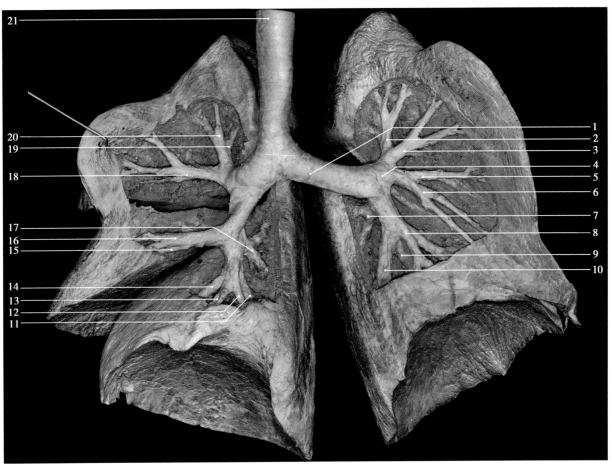

▲ 图 306 **肺段支气管**
Segmental bronchi

1. 左主支气管 left principal bronchus
2. 尖后段支气管 apicoposterior segmental bronchus
3. 前段支气管 anterior segmenta bronchus
4. 左肺上叶支气管 left superior lobar bronchus
5. 上舌段支气管 superior lingular bronchus
6. 下舌段支气管 inferior lingular bronchus
7. 上段支气管 superior segmental bronchus
8. 内前底段支气管 medioanterior basal segmental bronchus
9. 外侧底段支气管 lateral basal segmental bronchus
10. 后底段支气管 posterior basal segmental bronchus
11. 右肺后底段支气管 posterior basal segmental bronchus of right lung

12. 右肺内侧底段支气管 medial basal segmental bronchus of right lung
13. 右肺前底段支气管 anterior basal segmental bronchus of right lung
14. 右肺外侧底段支气管 lateral basal segmental bronchus of right lung
15. 外侧段支气管 lateral segmental bronchus
16. 内侧段支气管 medial segmental bronchus
17. 上段支气管（右肺）superior segmental bronchus
18. 前段支气管（右肺）anterior segmental bronchus
19. 后段支气管 posterior segmental bronchus
20. 尖段支气管 apical segmental bronchus
21. 气管 trachea

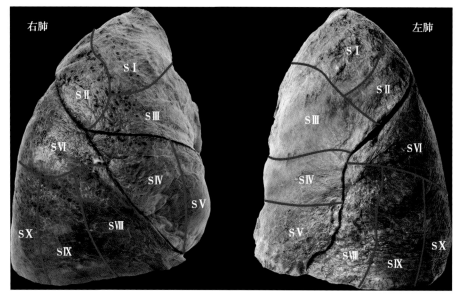

右肺　　　　　　　　　　　　　　左肺

▲ 图307　支气管肺段（外侧面观）
Bronchopulmonary segments. Lateral aspect

尖段 apical segment（S I ）　　　　　　　尖段 apical segment（S I ）
后段 posterior segment（S II ）　　　　　　后段 posterior segment（S II ）
前段 anterior segment（S III ）　　　　　　前段 anterior segment（S III ）
外侧段 lateral segment（S IV ）　　　　　　上舌段 superior lingular segment（S IV ）
内侧段 medial segment（S V ）　　　　　　下舌段 inferior lingular segment（S V ）
上段 superior segment（S VI ）　　　　　　上段 superior segment（S VI ）
前底段 anterior basal segment（S VIII ）　　　前底段 anterior basal segment（S VIII ）
外侧底段 lateral basal segment（S IX ）　　　外侧底段 lateral basal segment（S IX ）
后底段 posterior basal segment（S X ）　　　后底段 posterior basal segment（S X ）

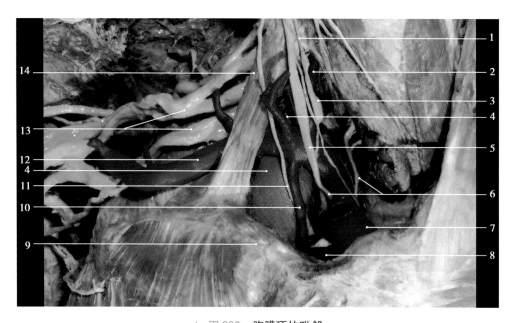

▲ 图308　胸膜顶的毗邻
Adjacent structures of cupula of pleura

1. 交感干 sympathetic trunk
2. 椎动脉 vertebral a.
3. 颈胸神经节 cervicothoracic ganglion
4. 胸膜顶 cupula of pleura
5. 右迷走神经 right vagus n.
6. 喉返神经 recurrent laryngeal n.
7. 头臂干 brachiocephalic trunk
8. 右头臂静脉 right brachiocephalic v.
9. 第 1 肋 1st rib
10. 胸廓内动脉 internal thoracic a.
11. 右膈神经 right phrenic n.
12. 锁骨下动脉 subclavian a.
13. 臂丛 brachial plexus
14. 前斜角肌 scalenus anterior

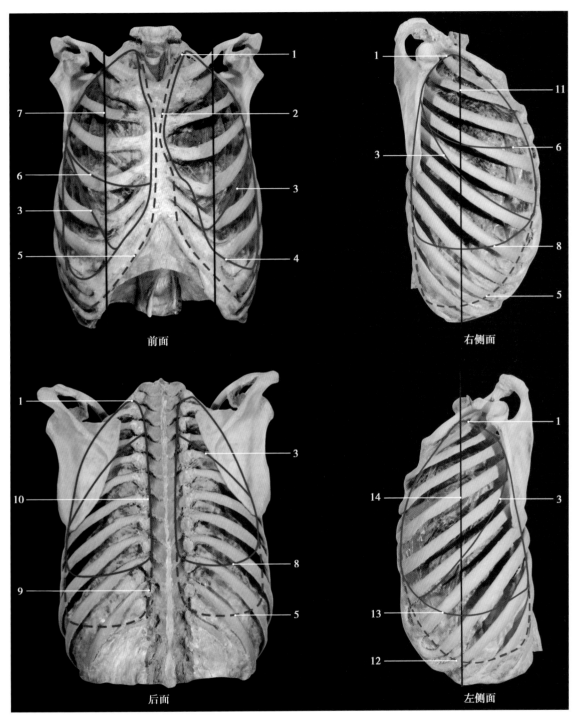

前面

右侧面

后面

左侧面

▲ 图 309 胸膜与肺的体表投影
Body surface projection of pleura and lung

1. 胸膜顶 cupula of pleura
2. 胸膜前界 anterior border of pleura
3. 斜裂 oblique fissure
4. 左肺下缘 inferior border of left lung
5. 右胸膜下界 inferior border of right pleura
6. 水平裂 horizontal fissure
7. 锁骨中线 medioclavicular line

8. 右肺下缘 inferior border of right lung
9. 胸膜后界 posterior border of pleura
10. 左肺后缘 posterior border of left lung
11. 右腋中线 right midaxillary line
12. 左胸膜下界 inferior border of left pleura
13. 左肺下缘 inferior border of left lung
14. 左腋中线 left midaxillary line

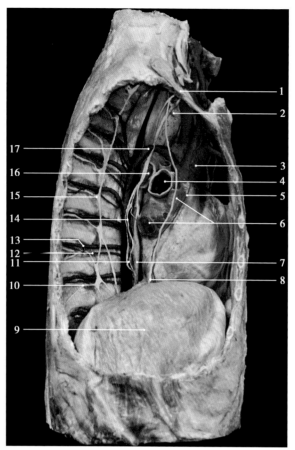

◀ 图 310

纵隔 (右侧面观)
Mediastinum. Right aspect

1. 第 1 肋 the 1st rib
2. 气管 trachea
3. 上腔静脉 superior vena cava
4. 右肺动脉 right pulmonary a.
5. 心包膈动脉 pericardiacophrenic a.
6. 右肺静脉 right pulmonary v.
7. 食管 esophagus
8. 膈神经 phrenic n.
9. 膈 diaphragm
10. 肋间神经 intercostal n.
11. 胸导管 thoracic duct
12. 肋间后动脉 posterior intercostal a.
13. 肋间后静脉 posterior intercostal v.
14. 迷走神经 vagus n.
15. 交感干 sympathetic trunk
16. 右主支气管 right principal bronchus
17. 奇静脉 azygos v.

图 311 ▶

纵隔 (左侧面观)
Mediastinum. Left aspect

1. 胸导管 thoracic duct
2. 左肺动脉 left pulmonary a.
3. 交感干 sympathetic trunk
4. 左主支气管 left principal bronchus
5. 膈神经 phrenic n.
6. 肋间神经 intercostal n.
7. 胸主动脉 thoracic aorta
8. 肋间后动脉 posterior intercostal a.
9. 肋间后静脉 posterior intercostal v.
10. 膈 diaphragm
11. 心包 pericardium
12. 左肺静脉 left pulmonary v.
13. 心包膈动脉 pericardiacophrenic a.
14. 主动脉弓 aortic arch
15. 迷走神经 vagus n.
16. 左锁骨下动脉 left subclavian a.

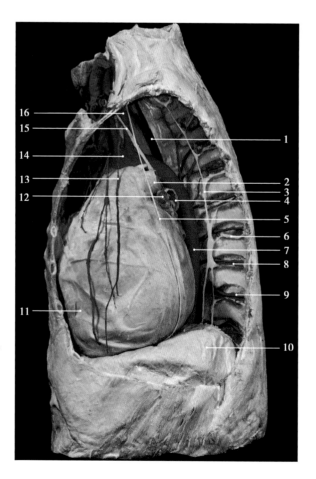

第七章　泌尿生殖系统
Urogenital System

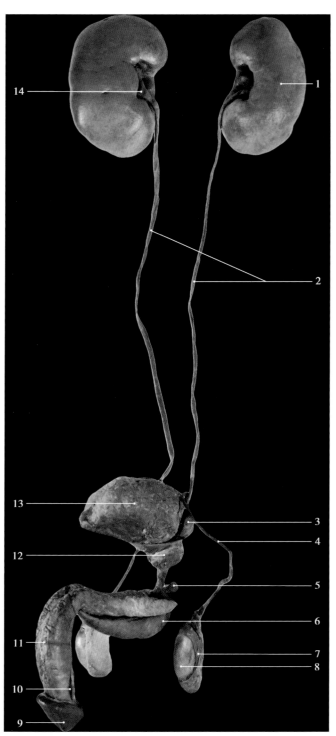

◀ 图312

男性泌尿生殖系统全貌
General arrangement of the male urogenital
system

1. 肾 kidney
2. 输尿管 ureter
3. 精囊 seminal vesicle
4. 输精管 ductus deferens
5. 尿道球腺 bulbourethral gland
6. 尿道球 bulb of urethra
7. 附睾体 body of epididymis
8. 睾丸 testis
9. 阴茎头 glans penis
10. 尿道海绵体 cavernous body of urethra
11. 阴茎海绵体 cavernous body of penis
12. 前列腺 prostate
13. 膀胱 urinary bladder
14. 肾盂 renal pelvis

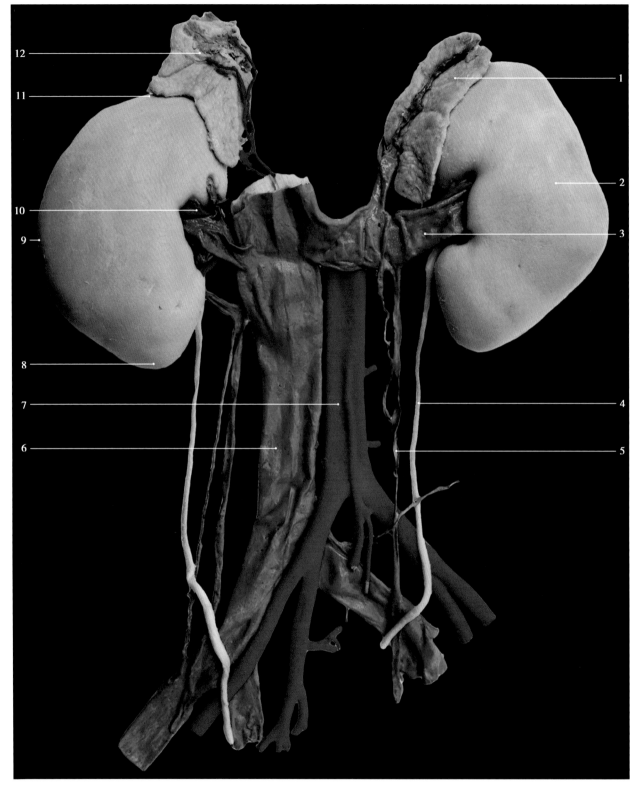

▲ 图313　肾与输尿管
Kidney and ureter

1. 左肾上腺 left suprarenal gland　　7. 腹主动脉 abdominal aorta
2. 左肾 left kidney　　8. 右肾下端 inferior extremity of right kidney
3. 左肾静脉 left renal v.　　9. 右肾外侧缘 lateral border of right kidney
4. 输尿管 ureter　　10. 肾动脉 renal a.
5. 睾丸静脉 testicular v.　　11. 右肾上端 superior extremity of right kidney
6. 下腔静脉 inferior vena cava　　12. 右肾上腺 right suprarenal gland

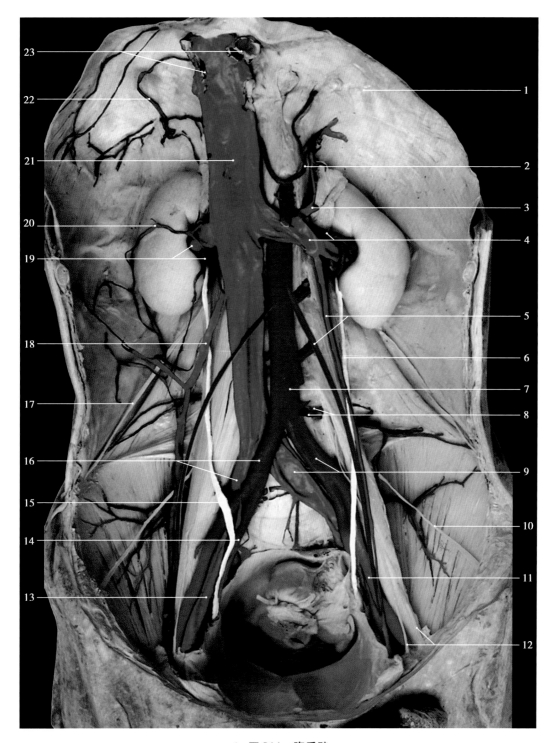

▲ 图314　腹后壁
Posterior abdominal wall

1. 膈 diaphragm
2. 膈下动脉 inferior phrenic a.
3. 左肾上腺静脉 left suprarenal v.
4. 左肾动、静脉 left renal a. and v.
5. 左睾丸动、静脉 left testicular a. and v.
6. 左输尿管 left ureter
7. 腹主动脉 abdominal aorta
8. 左腰动、静脉 left lumbar a. and v.

9. 左髂总动、静脉 left common iliac a. and v.
10. 股外侧皮神经 lateral femoral cutaneous n.
11. 左髂外动脉 left external iliac a.
12. 生殖股神经 genitofemoral n.
13. 右髂外静脉 right external iliac v.
14. 右髂内动脉 right internal iliac a.
15. 右输尿管 right ureter

16. 右髂总动、静脉 right common iliac a. and v.
17. 髂腹下神经 iliohypogastric n.
18. 右睾丸静脉 right testicular v.
19. 右肾动、静脉 right renal a. and v.
20. 肾囊静脉 capsular v.
21. 下腔静脉 inferior vena cava
22. 膈下静脉 inferior phrenic v.
23. 肝静脉 hepatic v.

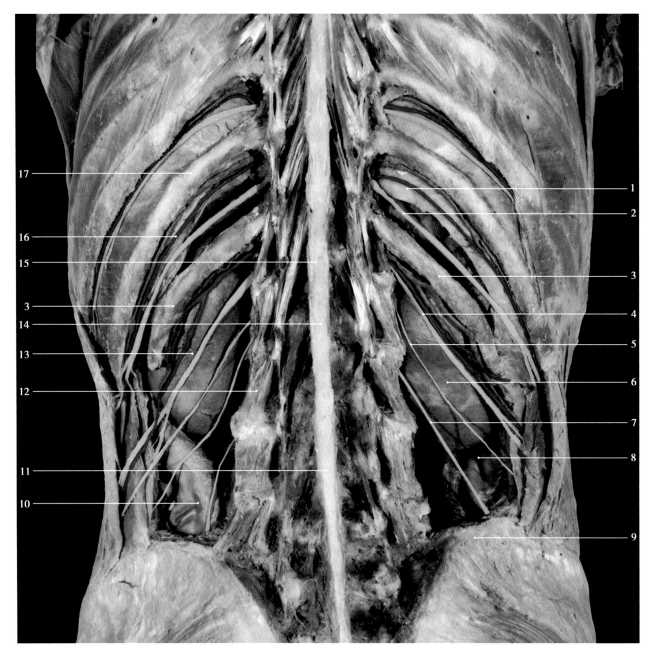

▲ 图 315　肾的体表投影（后面观）
Body surface projection of kidney. Posterior aspect

1. 壁胸膜 parietal pleura
2. 第 11 肋间神经 the 11th intercostal n.
3. 第 12 肋 the 12th rib
4. 肋下神经 subcostal n.
5. 髂腹下神经 iliohypogastric n.
6. 右肾 right kidney
7. 髂腹股沟神经 ilioinguinal n.
8. 结肠右曲 right colic flexure
9. 髂嵴 iliac crest

10. 降结肠 descending colon
11. 第 3 腰椎棘突 spinous process of the 3rd lumbar vertebra
12. 横突间肌 intertransversarii
13. 左肾 left kidney
14. 第 1 腰椎棘突 spinous process of the 1st lumbar vertebra
15. 第 12 胸椎棘突 spinous process of the 12th thoracic vertebra
16. 肋间后动脉 posterior intercostal a.
17. 第 11 肋 the 11th rib

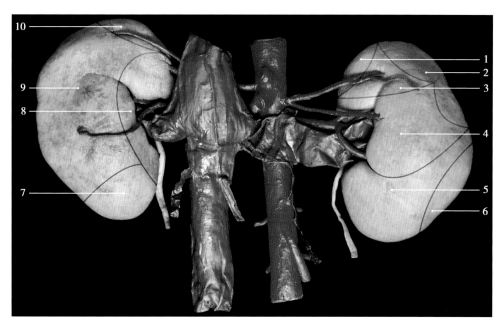

▲ 图316　肾周围的关系（前面观）
Relation of kidney with peripheral organs. Anterior aspect

1. 左肾上腺 left suprarenal gland
2. 脾 spleen
3. 胃 stomach
4. 胰 pancreas
5. 空肠 jejunum
6. 降结肠 descending colon
7. 结肠右曲 right colic flexure
8. 十二指肠 duodenum
9. 肝 liver
10. 右肾上腺 right suprarenal gland

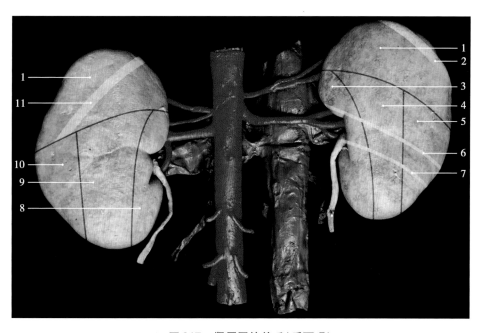

▲ 图317　肾周围的关系（后面观）
Relation of kidney with peripheral organs. Posterior aspect

1. 膈 diaphragm
2. 右侧第12肋 right the 12th rib
3. 右侧腰大肌 right psoas major
4. 右侧腰方肌 right quadratus lumborum
5. 右侧腹横肌 right transverses abdominis
6. 髂腹下神经 iliohypogastric n.
7. 髂腹股沟神经 ilioinguinal n.
8. 左侧腰大肌 left psoas major
9. 左侧腰方肌 left quadratus lumborum
10. 左侧腹横肌 left transverses abdominis
11. 左侧第12肋 left the 12th rib

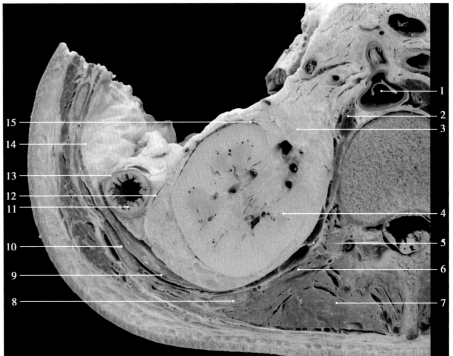

◀ 图 318

肾的被膜 (横切面)
Coverings of kidney. Transverse section

1. 腹主动脉 abdominal aorta
2. 左脚 left crus
3. 脂肪囊 fatty renal capsule
4. 肾 kidney
5. 肾后筋膜 retrorenal fascia
6. 腰方肌 quadratus lumborum
7. 竖脊肌 erector spinae
8. 第 12 肋 12th rib
9. 膈 diaphragm
10. 第 11 肋 11th rib
11. 降结肠 descending colon
12. 肾前筋膜 prerenal fascia
13. 脏腹膜 visceral peritoneum
14. 壁腹膜 parietal peritoneum
15. 纤维囊 fibrous capsule

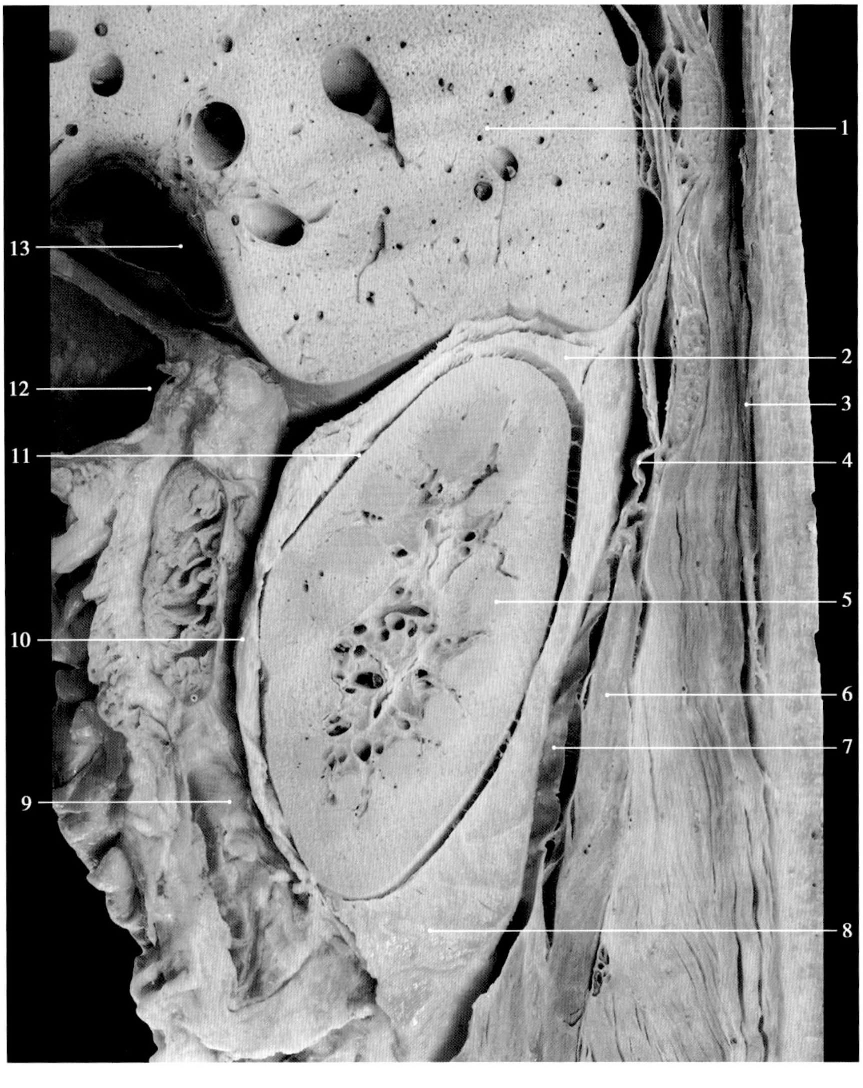

◀ 图 319

肾的被膜 (矢状切面)
Coverings of kidney. Sagittal section

1. 肝 liver
2. 肾上腺 suprarenal gland
3. 背阔肌 latissimus dorsi
4. 膈 diaphragm
5. 肾 kidney
6. 腰方肌 quadratus lumborum
7. 肾后筋膜 retrorenal fascia
8. 脂肪囊 fatty renal capsule
9. 升结肠 ascending colon
10. 肾前筋膜 prerenal fascia
11. 纤维囊 fibrous capsule
12. 结肠右曲 right colic flexure
13. 胆囊 gallbladder

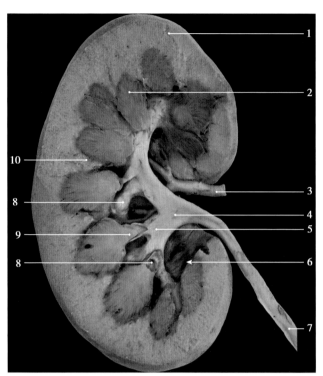

◀ 图 320

肾冠状切面
Coronal section of kidney
1. 肾皮质 renal cortex
2. 肾锥体 renal pyramid
3. 肾动脉 renal a.
4. 肾盂 renal pelvis
5. 肾大盏 major renal calices
6. 肾窦 renal sinus
7. 输尿管 ureter
8. 肾小盏 minor renal calices
9. 肾乳头 renal papillae
10. 肾柱 renal columns

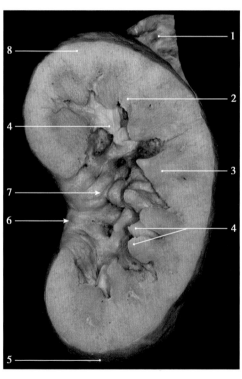

▲ 图 321 **肾窦**
Renal sinus
1. 纤维囊 fibrous capsule
2. 肾柱 renal columns
3. 肾锥体 renal pyramid
4. 肾乳头 renal papillae
5. 肾下端 inferior extremity of kidney
6. 肾门 renal hilus
7. 肾窦 renal sinus
8. 肾皮质 renal cortex

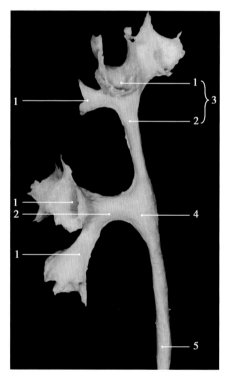

▲ 图 322 **肾盂和肾盏**
Renal pelvis and renal calices
1. 肾小盏 minor renal calices
2. 肾大盏 major renal calices
3. 肾盏 renal calices
4. 肾盂 renal pelvis
5. 输尿管 ureter

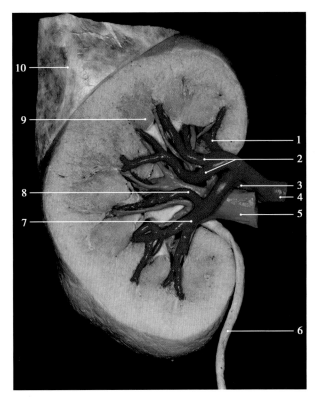

◀ 图 323

肾动脉
Renal artery
1. 上段动脉 superior segmental a.
2. 上前段动脉 superior anterior segmental a.
3. 后段动脉 posterior segmental a.
4. 肾动脉 renal a.
5. 肾静脉 renal v.
6. 输尿管 ureter
7. 下段动脉 inferior segmental a.
8. 下前段动脉 inferior anterior segmental a.
9. 肾乳头 renal papillae
10. 纤维囊 fibrous capsule

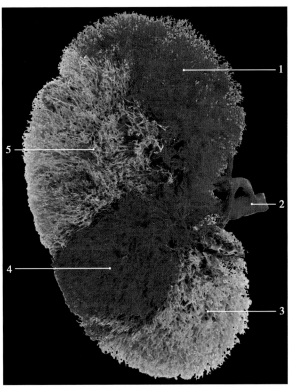

▲ 图 324　肾段铸型(前面观)
Cast of renal segments. Anterior aspect
1. 上段 superior segment
2. 肾动脉 renal a.
3. 下段 inferior segment
4. 下前段 inferior anterior segment
5. 上前段 superior anterior segment

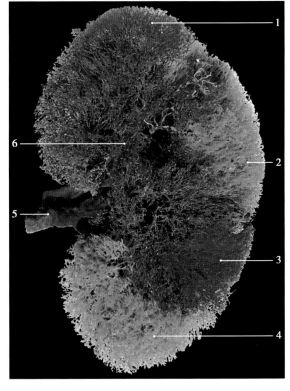

▲ 图 325　肾段铸型(后面观)
Cast of renal segments. Posterior aspect
1. 上段 superior segment
2. 上前段 superior anterior segment
3. 下前段 inferior anterior segment
4. 下段 inferior segment
5. 肾动脉 renal a.
6. 后段 posterior segment

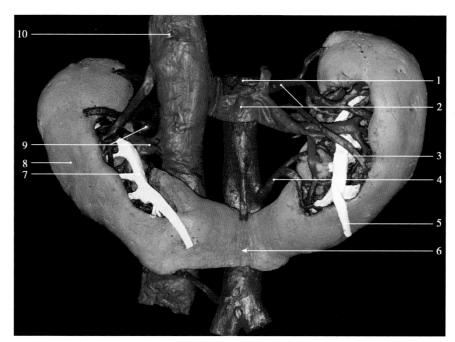

◀ 图 326　马蹄肾
Horseshoe kidney. Anterior aspect
1. 腹主动脉 abdominal aorta
2. 左肾动、静脉 left renal a. and v.
3. 左肾盂 left renal pelvis
4. 副肾动脉 accessory renal a.
5. 左输尿管 left ureter
6. 融合部 confluence part
7. 右肾盂 right renal pelvis
8. 右肾 right kidney
9. 右肾动、静脉 right renal a. and v.
10. 下腔静脉 inferior vena cava

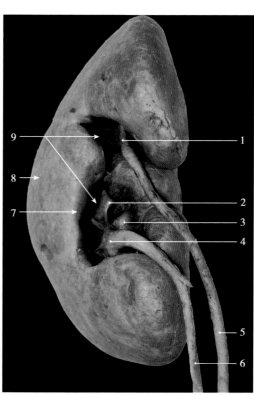

▲ 图 327　不完全性重复肾
Incomplete renal duplication
1. 上位肾盂 superior renal pelvis
2. 肾小盏 minor renal calices
3. 肾大盏 major renal calices
4. 下位肾盂 inferior renal pelvis
5. 上位输尿管 superior ureter
6. 下位输尿管 inferior ureter
7. 肾门 renal hilum
8. 肾前面 anterior surface of kidney
9. 肾窦 renal sinus

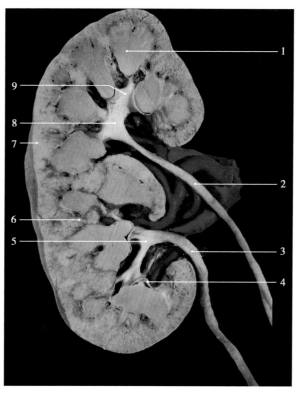

▲ 图 328　不完全性重复肾（冠状切面）
Incomplete renal duplication. Coronal section
1. 肾锥体 renal pyramid
2. 上位输尿管 superior ureter
3. 下位输尿管 inferior ureter
4. 肾小盏 minor renal calices
5. 下位肾盂 inferior renal pelvis
6. 肾柱 renal columns
7. 肾皮质 renal cortex
8. 上位肾盂 superior renal pelvis
9. 肾大盏 major renal calices

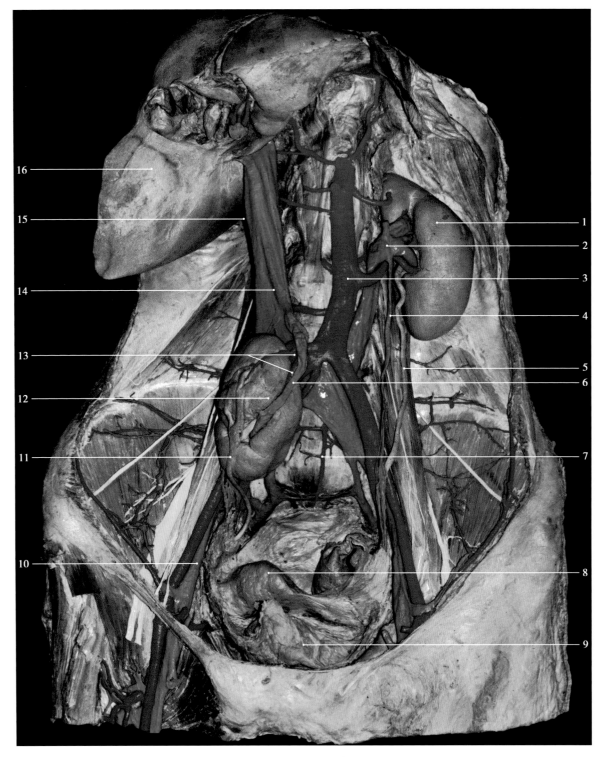

▲ 图 329　**移位肾**
Renal ectopia

1. 左肾 left kidney
2. 左肾静脉 left renal v.
3. 腹主动脉 abdominal aorta
4. 左卵巢静脉 left ovarian v.
5. 左输尿管 left ureter
6. 右肾静脉 right renal v.
7. 骶正中动脉 median sacral a.
8. 子宫 uterus
9. 膀胱 urinary bladder
10. 右髂外静脉 right external iliac v.
11. 右输尿管 right ureter
12. 右肾 right kidney
13. 右肾动脉 right renal a.
14. 下腔静脉 inferior vena cava
15. 右肾上腺 right suprarenal gland
16. 肝 liver

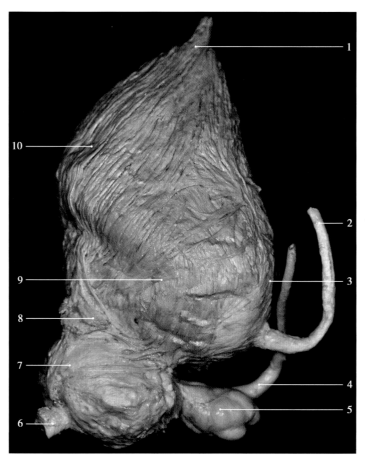

◀ 图 330

膀胱（侧面观）
Urinary bladder. Lateral aspect
1. 膀胱尖 apex of bladder
2. 输尿管 ureter
3. 后纵行肌 posterior longitudinal m.
4. 输精管 ductus deferens
5. 精囊 seminal vesicle
6. 尿道膜部 membranous part of urethra
7. 前列腺 prostate
8. 膀胱括约肌 vesical sphincter
9. 环行肌 circular m.
10. 前纵行肌 anterior longitudinal m.

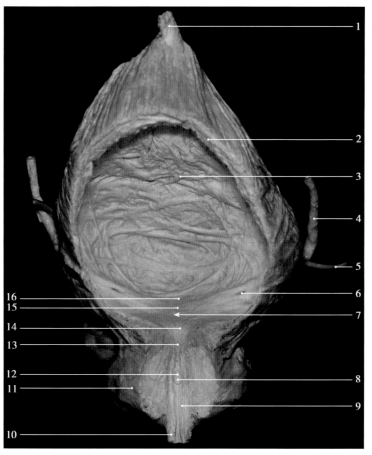

◀ 图 331

膀胱（前面观）
Urinary bladder. Anterior aspect
1. 膀胱尖 apex of bladder
2. 肌层 muscular layer
3. 黏膜襞 mucosal fold
4. 输尿管 ureter
5. 输精管 ductus deferens
6. 输尿管口 ureteric orifice
7. 膀胱三角 trigone of bladder
8. 前列腺小囊开口 orifice of prostatic utricle
9. 前列腺窦 prostatic sinus
10. 尿道膜部 membranous part of urethra
11. 前列腺 prostate
12. 精阜 seminal colliculus
13. 尿道内口 internal urethral orifice
14. 膀胱垂 vesical uvula
15. 输尿管间襞 interureteric fold
16. 输尿管后窝 posterior fovea of ureter

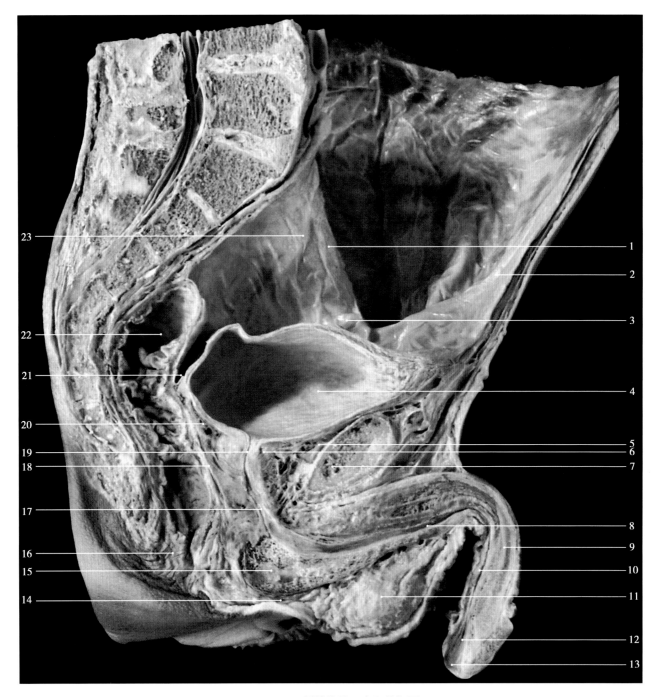

▲ 图 332　男性盆腔正中矢状切面
Median sagittal section of the male pelvic cavity

1. 髂外动脉 external iliac a.
2. 脐内侧襞 medial umbilical fold
3. 输精管 ductus deferens
4. 膀胱 urinary bladder
5. 耻骨后间隙 retropubic space
6. 前列腺 prostate
7. 耻骨 pubis
8. 尿道海绵体部 cavernous part of urethra
9. 阴茎海绵体 cavernous body of penis
10. 尿道海绵体 cavernous body of urethra
11. 阴囊中隔 septum of scrotum
12. 尿道舟状窝 navicular fossa of urethra
13. 尿道外口 external orifice of urethra
14. 球海绵体肌 bulbocavernosus
15. 尿道球 bulb of urethra
16. 肛门 anus
17. 尿道膜部 membranous part of urethra
18. 直肠膀胱隔 rectovesical septum
19. 尿道前列腺部 prostatic part of urethra
20. 精囊 seminal vesicle
21. 直肠膀胱陷凹 rectovesical pouch
22. 直肠 rectum
23. 输尿管 ureter

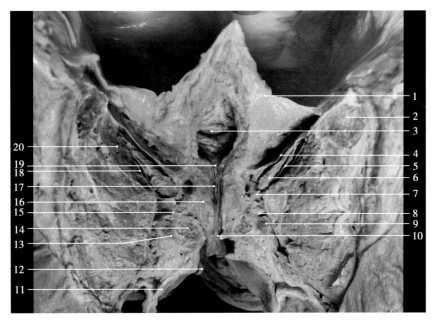

▲ 图333　**女性尿道**
Female urethra

1. 膀胱筋膜 urocystic fascia
2. 耻骨上支 superior ramus of pubis
3. 膀胱 urinary bladder
4. 盆膈上筋膜 superior fascia of pelvic diaphragm
5. 盆膈下筋膜 inferior fascia of pelvic diaphragm
6. 肛提肌 levator ani
7. 尿生殖膈上筋膜 superior fascia of urogenital diaphragm

8. 尿生殖膈下筋膜 inferior fascia of urogenital diaphragm
9. 阴蒂脚 crus of clitoris
10. 尿道外口 external orifice of urethra
11. 大阴唇 greater lip of pudendum
12. 小阴唇 lesser lip of pudendum
13. 会阴浅隙 superficial perineal space
14. 前庭球 bulb of vestibule

15. 会阴深隙 deep perineal space
16. 尿道肌层 muscular layer of urethra
17. 尿道嵴 urethral ridge
18. 闭孔筋膜 obturator fascia
19. 尿道内口 internal urethral orifice
20. 闭孔内肌 obturator internus

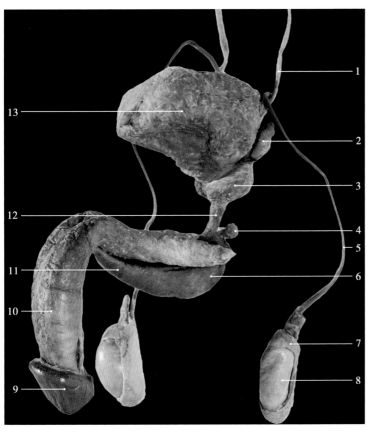

◀ 图334

男性生殖系统
Male genital system

1. 输尿管 ureter
2. 精囊 seminal vesicle
3. 前列腺 prostate
4. 尿道球腺 bulbourethral gland
5. 输精管 ductus deferens
6. 尿道球 bulb of urethra
7. 附睾 epididymis
8. 睾丸 testis
9. 阴茎头 glans penis
10. 阴茎海绵体 cavernous body of penis
11. 尿道海绵体 cavernous body of urethra
12. 尿道膜部 membranous part of urethra
13. 膀胱 urinary bladder

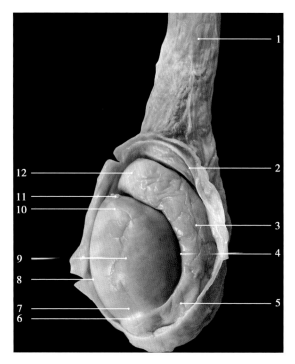

▲ 图 335　睾丸 (外侧面观)
Testis. Lateral aspect

1. 精索 spermatic cord
2. 睾丸鞘膜壁层 parietal layer of tunica vaginalis of testis
3. 附睾体 body of epididymis
4. 附睾窦 sinus of epididymis
5. 附睾尾 tail of epididymis
6. 附睾下韧带 inferior ligament of epididymis
7. 睾丸下端 inferior extremity of testis
8. 睾丸前缘 anterior border of testis
9. 睾丸外侧面 lateral surface of testis
10. 睾丸上端 superior extremity of testis
11. 睾丸附件 appendix of testis
12. 附睾头 head of epididymis

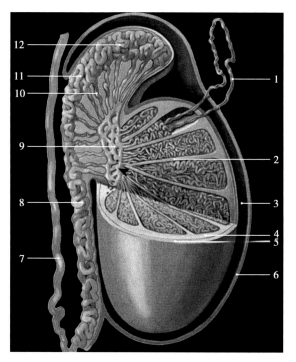

▲ 图 336　睾丸结构 (模式图)
Structures of testis. Diagram

1. 精曲小管 contorted seminiferous tubules
2. 睾丸小隔 septula testis
3. 鞘膜腔 vaginal cavity
4. 睾丸白膜 tunica albuginea of testis
5. 鞘膜脏层 visceral layer of tunica vaginalis
6. 鞘膜壁层 parietal layer of tunica vaginalis
7. 输精管 ductus deferens
8. 附睾体 body of epididymis
9. 睾丸网 rete testis
10. 睾丸输出小管 efferent ductules of testis
11. 附睾管 duct of epididymis
12. 附睾头 head of epididymis

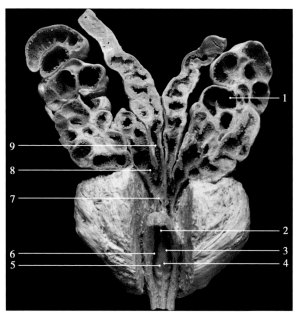

◀ 图 337

前列腺 (前面观)
Prostate. Anterior aspect

1. 精囊 seminal vesicle
2. 尿道嵴 urethral ridge
3. 精阜 seminal colliculus
4. 前列腺小囊开口 orifice of prostatic utricle
5. 射精管开口 orifice of ejaculatory duct
6. 前列腺窦 prostatic sinus
7. 射精管 ejaculatory duct
8. 精囊排泄管 excretory duct of seminal vesicle
9. 输精管 ductus deferens

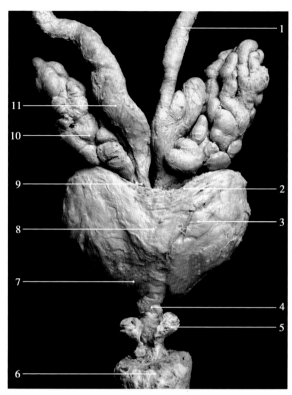

◄ 图 338

前列腺（后面观）
Prostate. Posterior aspect

1. 输精管 ductus deferens
2. 前列腺底 base of prostate
3. 前列腺后面 posterior surface of prostate
4. 尿道膜部 membranous part of urethra
5. 尿道球腺 bulbourethral gland
6. 尿道球 bulb of urethra
7. 前列腺尖 apex of prostate
8. 前列腺沟 prostatic groove
9. 射精管 ejaculatory duct
10. 精囊 seminal vesicle
11. 输精管壶腹 ampulla ductus deferentis

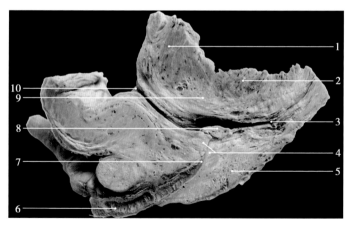

▲ 图 339 前列腺分区（矢状切面）
Zonation of prostate. Sagittal section

1. 膀胱环形肌 circular muscle of bladder
2. 纤维肌质区 fibro-muscular zone
3. 尿道 urethra
4. 中央区 central area
5. 外周区 peripheral area
6. 输精管壶腹 ampulla ductus deferentis
7. 射精管 ejaculatory duct
8. 精阜 seminal colliculus
9. 移行区 transitional area
10. 尿道内口 internal urethral orifice

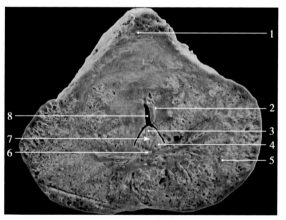

▲ 图 340 前列腺分区（横切面）
Zonation of prostate. Transverse section

1. 纤维肌质区 fibro-muscular zone
2. 移行区 transitional area
3. 前列腺小囊 prostatic utricle
4. 射精管 ejaculatory duct
5. 外周区 peripheral area
6. 中央区 central area
7. 精阜 seminal colliculus
8. 尿道 urethra

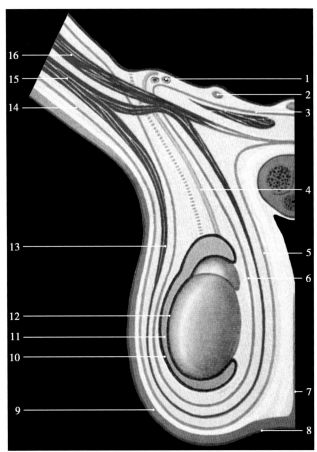

◀ 图 341

阴囊的结构（模式图）
Structure of scrotal. Diagram

1. 腹壁下动脉 inferior epigastric a.
2. 脐内侧韧带 medial umbilical lig.
3. 腹横筋膜 transverse fascia
4. 输精管 ductus deferens
5. 精索外筋膜 external spermatic fascia
6. 精索内筋膜 internal spermatic fascia
7. 阴囊中隔 septum of scrotum
8. 阴囊皮肤 skin of scrotum
9. 肉膜 dartos coat
10. 鞘膜壁层 parietal layer of tunica vaginalis
11. 鞘膜腔 vaginal cavity
12. 鞘膜脏层 visceral layer of tunica vaginalis
13. 提睾肌 cremaster
14. 腹外斜肌腱膜 aponeurosis of obliquus externus abdominis
15. 腹内斜肌 obliquus internus abdominis
16. 腹横肌 transversus abdominis

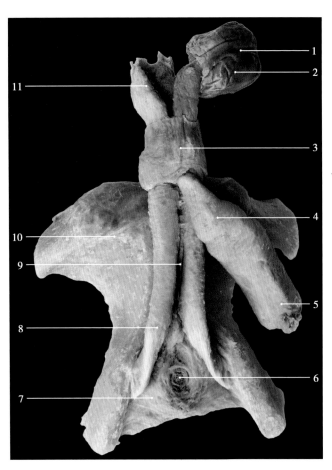

◀ 图 342

阴茎海绵体和尿道海绵体
Cavernous body of urethra and cavernous body of penis

1. 尿道外口 external orifice of urethra
2. 阴茎头 glans penis
3. 阴茎深筋膜 deep fascia of penis
4. 尿道海绵体 cavernous body of urethra
5. 尿道球 bulb of urethra
6. 尿道 urethra
7. 尿生殖膈下筋膜 inferior fascia of urogenital diaphragm
8. 阴茎脚 crus penis
9. 阴茎中隔 septum penis
10. 耻骨 pubis
11. 阴茎海绵体 cavernous body of penis

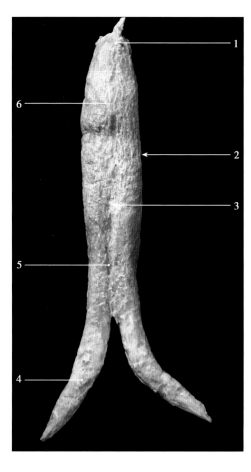

◀ 图 343

阴茎海绵体（背面观）
Cavernous body of penis. Dorsal aspect

1. 前端 anterior extremity
2. 阴茎海绵体 cavernous body of penis
3. 阴茎背侧沟 dorsal sulcus of penis
4. 阴茎脚 crus penis
5. 阴茎中隔 septum of penis
6. 阴茎海绵体背面 dorsum of cavernous body of penis

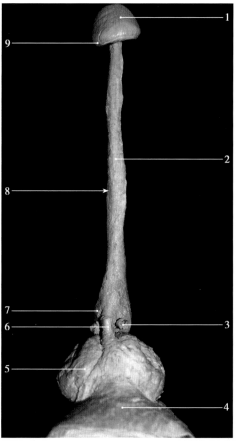

◀ 图 344

尿道海绵体（背面观）
Cavernous body of urethra. Dorsal aspect

1. 阴茎头 glans penis
2. 尿道海绵体白膜 albuginea of cavernous body of urethra
3. 尿道球腺 bulbourethral gland
4. 膀胱颈 neck of bladder
5. 前列腺 prostate
6. 尿道膜部 membranous part of urethra
7. 尿道球 bulb of urethra
8. 尿道海绵体 cavernous body of urethra
9. 阴茎头冠 corona glandis

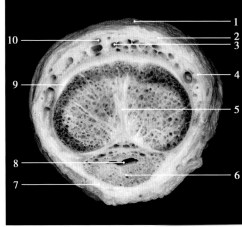

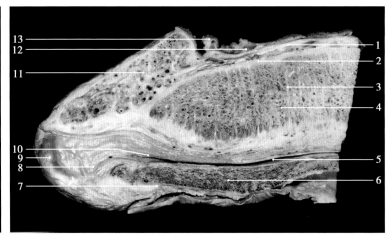

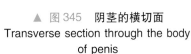

▲ 图345 阴茎的横切面
Transverse section through the body
of penis

1. 皮肤 skin
2. 阴茎浅筋膜 superficial fascia of penis
3. 阴茎背深静脉 deep dorsal vein of penis
4. 阴茎深筋膜 deep fascia of penis
5. 阴茎中隔 septum penis
6. 尿道海绵体 cavernous body of urethra
7. 尿道海绵体白膜 albuginea of cavernous body of urethra
8. 尿道 urethra
9. 阴茎海绵体白膜 albuginea of cavernous body of penis
10. 阴茎背浅静脉 superficial dorsal veins of penis

▲ 图346 阴茎正中矢状切面
Median sagittal section through penis

1. 阴茎深筋膜 deep fascia of penis
2. 阴茎海绵体白膜 albuginea of cavernous body of penis
3. 阴茎海绵体小梁 trabeculae of cavernous body of penis
4. 阴茎海绵体 cavernous body of penis
5. 尿道海绵体部 cavernous part of urethra
6. 尿道海绵体 cavernous body of urethra
7. 尿道海绵体白膜 albuginea of cavernous body of urethra
8. 尿道舟状窝 navicular fossa of urethra
9. 尿道外口 external orifice of urethra
10. 舟状窝瓣 valve of navicular fossa
11. 阴茎头 glans penis
12. 阴茎浅筋膜 superficial fascia of penis
13. 阴茎包皮 prepuce of penis

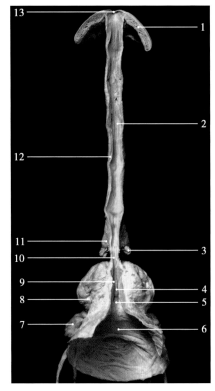

◀ 图347
男性尿道（背面观）
Male urethra. Dorsal aspect

1. 阴茎头 glans penis
2. 尿道海绵体部 cavernous part of urethra
3. 尿道球腺 bulbourethral gland
4. 精阜 seminal colliculus
5. 尿道内口 internal urethral orifice
6. 膀胱三角 trigone of bladder
7. 精囊 seminal vesicle
8. 前列腺 prostate
9. 尿道前列腺部 prostatic part of urethra
10. 尿道膜部 membranous part of urethra
11. 尿道球 bulb of urethra
12. 尿道海绵体 cavernous body of urethra
13. 尿道外口 external orifice of urethra

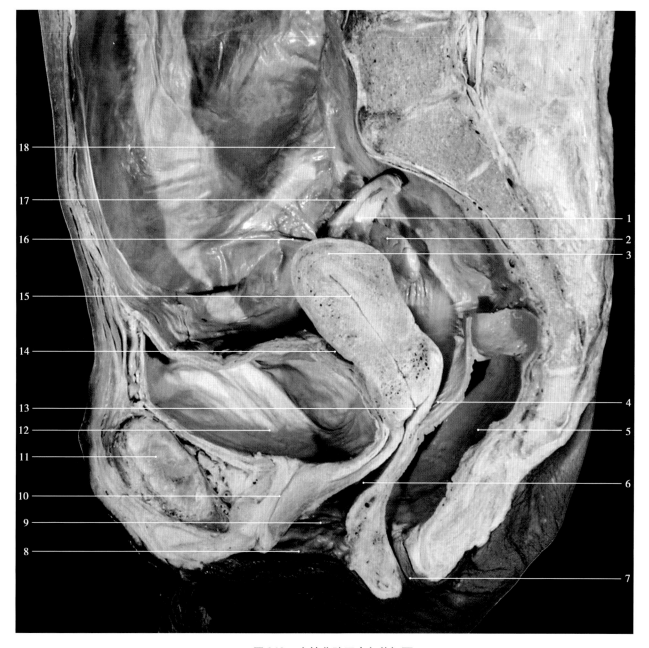

▲ 图 348　女性盆腔正中矢状切面
Median sagittal section of female pelvic cavity

1. 输卵管伞 fimbriae of uterine tube
2. 卵巢 ovary
3. 子宫底 fundus of uterus
4. 直肠子宫陷凹 rectouterine pouch
5. 直肠 rectum
6. 阴道 vagina
7. 肛门 anus
8. 小阴唇 lesser lip of pudendum
9. 阴道口 vaginal orifice
10. 尿道 urethra
11. 耻骨联合面 symphysial surface
12. 膀胱 urinary bladder
13. 子宫口 orifice of uterus
14. 膀胱子宫陷凹 vesicouterine pouch
15. 子宫腔 cavity of uterus
16. 子宫圆韧带 round ligament of uterus
17. 输卵管 uterine tube
18. 输尿管 ureter

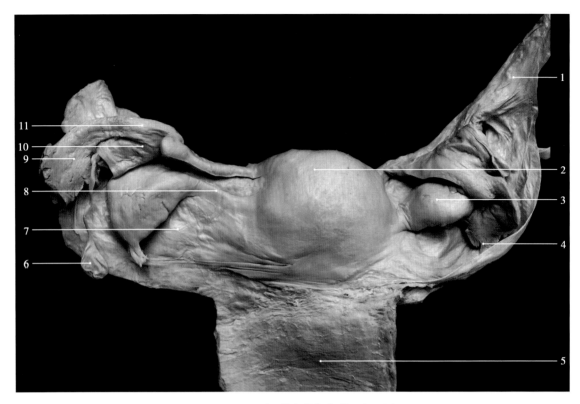

▲ 图 349　**子宫、输卵管与卵巢（后面观）**
Uterus, uterine tube and ovary. Posterior aspect

1. 卵巢悬韧带 suspensory ligament of ovary
2. 子宫 uterus
3. 卵巢 ovary
4. 输卵管伞 fimbriae of uterine tube
5. 阴道后壁 posterior wall of vagina
6. 囊状附件 vesicular appendage
7. 子宫阔韧带 broad ligament of uterus
8. 卵巢固有韧带 proper ligament of ovary
9. 输卵管漏斗 infundibulum of uterine tube
10. 输卵管系膜 mesosalpinx
11. 输卵管 uterine tube

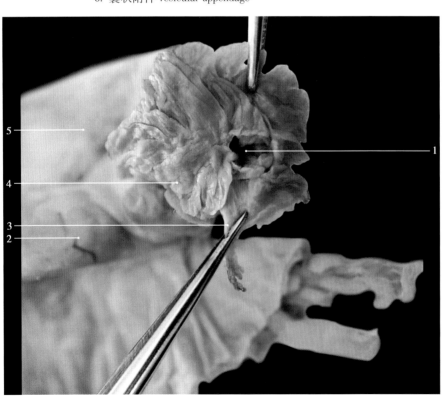

◀ 图 350

输卵管漏斗
Infundibulum of uterine tube

1. 输卵管腹腔口 abdominal orifice of uterine tube
2. 卵巢 ovary
3. 卵巢伞 ovarian fimbria
4. 输卵管伞 fimbriae of uterine tube
5. 输卵管 uterine duct

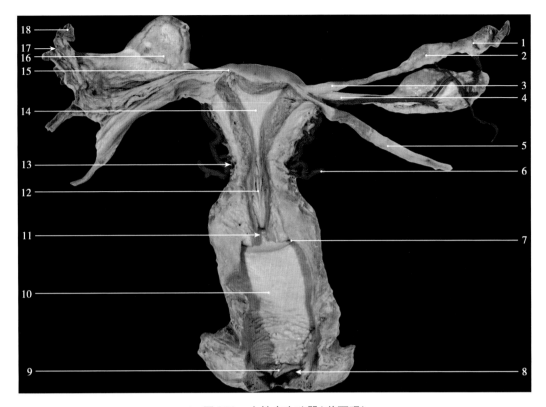

▲ 图 351　**女性内生殖器（前面观）**
Female internal genital organs. Anterior aspect

1. 输卵管漏斗 infundibulum of uterine tube
2. 输卵管壶腹 ampulla of uterine tube
3. 输卵管峡 isthmus of uterine tube
4. 卵巢固有韧带 proper ligament of ovary
5. 子宫圆韧带 round ligament of uterus
6. 子宫动脉 uterine a.
7. 阴道穹侧部 lateral part of fornix of vagina
8. 阴道口 vaginal orifice
9. 处女膜痕 carunculae hymenales

10. 阴道 vagina
11. 子宫口 orifice of uterus
12. 子宫颈管 canal of cervix of uterus
13. 子宫峡 isthmus of uterus
14. 子宫腔 cavity of uterus
15. 输卵管子宫部 uterine part of uterine tube
16. 卵巢 ovary
17. 输卵管腹腔口 abdominal orifice of uterine tube
18. 输卵管伞 fimbriae of uterine tube

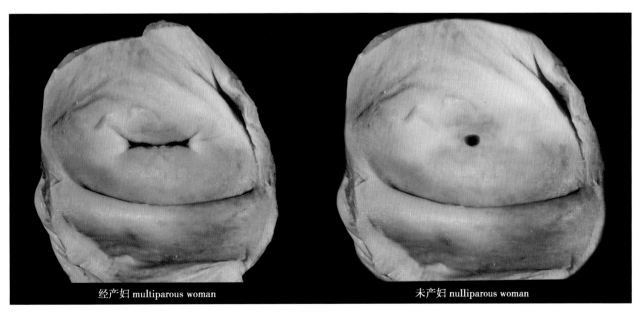

经产妇 multiparous woman　　　　　　　　未产妇 nulliparous woman

▲ 图 352　**子宫口的形态**
Shapes of orifice of uterus

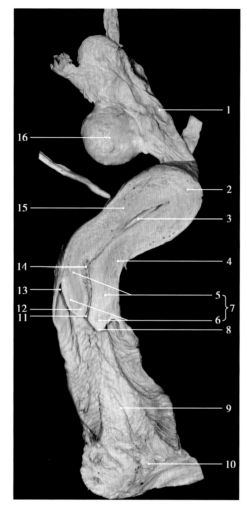

◀ 图 353

子宫的分部（矢状切面）
Distribution of uterus. Sagittal section

1. 输卵管 uterine tube
2. 子宫底 fundus of uterus
3. 子宫腔 cavity of uterus
4. 子宫峡 isthmus of uterus
5. 子宫颈阴道上部 supravaginal part of cervix
6. 子宫颈阴道部 vaginal part of cervix
7. 子宫颈 neck of uterus
8. 子宫口前唇 anterior lip of orifice of uterus
9. 阴道 vagina
10. 阴道口 vaginal orifice
11. 子宫口 orifice of uterus
12. 子宫口后唇 posterior lip of orifice of uterus
13. 阴道后穹 posterior fornix of vagina
14. 子宫颈管 canal of cervix of uterus
15. 子宫体 body of uterus
16. 卵巢 ovary

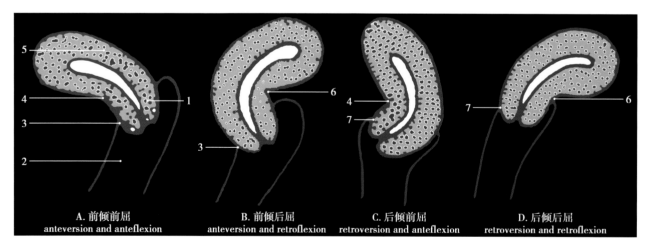

A. 前倾前屈
anteversion and anteflexion

B. 前倾后屈
anteversion and retroflexion

C. 后倾前屈
retroversion and anteflexion

D. 后倾后屈
retroversion and retroflexion

▲ 图 354　**子宫姿势的类型**
Types of uterine attitude

1. 子宫颈 neck of uterus
2. 阴道 vagina
3. 前倾 anteversion
4. 前屈 anteflexion
5. 子宫体 body of uterus
6. 后屈 retroflexion
7. 后倾 retroversion

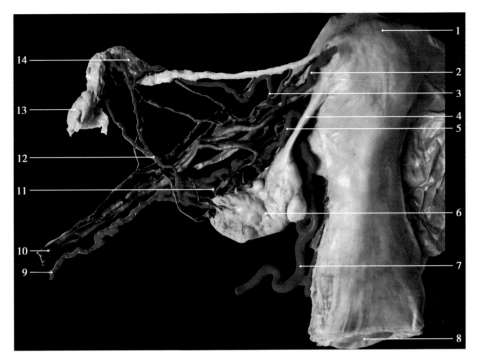

▲ 图 355　**子宫的血管**
Blood vessels of uterus

1. 子宫底 fundus of uterus
2. 宫底支 branch of fundus of uterus
3. 子宫动脉输卵管支 tubal branch of uterine a.
4. 卵巢固有韧带 proper ligament of ovary
5. 子宫动脉卵巢支 ovarian branch of uterine a.
6. 卵巢 ovary
7. 子宫动脉 uterine a.

8. 子宫口 orifice of uterus
9. 卵巢动脉 ovarian a.
10. 卵巢静脉 ovarian v.
11. 卵巢动脉卵巢支 ovarian branch of ovarian a.
12. 卵巢动脉输卵管支 tubal branch of ovarian a.
13. 输卵管伞 fimbriae of uterine tube
14. 输卵管壶腹 ampulla of uterine tube

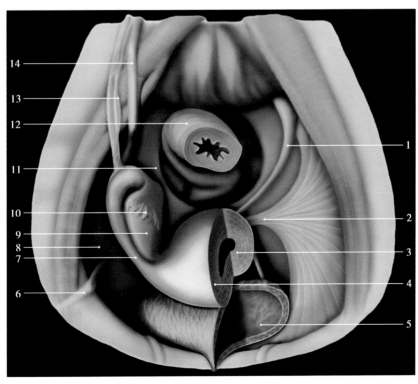

◄ 图 356

子宫的固定装置
Fixed structure of uterus
1. 子宫骶韧带 uterosacral lig.
2. 子宫主韧带 cardinal ligament of uterus
3. 子宫颈 neck of uterus
4. 子宫底 fundus of uterus
5. 膀胱 urinary bladder
6. 子宫圆韧带 round ligament of uterus
7. 输卵管 uterine tube
8. 子宫阔韧带 broad ligament of uterus
9. 卵巢 ovary
10. 输卵管伞 fimbriae of uterine tube
11. 直肠子宫襞 rectouterine fold
12. 直肠 rectum
13. 卵巢悬韧带 suspensory ligament of ovary
14. 输尿管 ureter

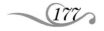

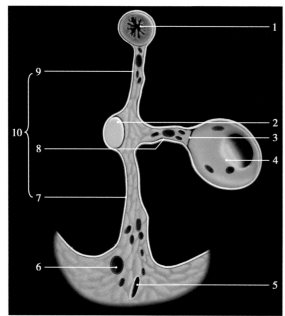

◀ 图 357
子宫阔韧带矢状切面（模式图）
Sagittal section of broad ligament of uterus.
Diagram
1. 输卵管 uterine tube
2. 子宫圆韧带 round ligament of uterus
3. 卵巢门 hilus of ovary
4. 卵巢 ovary
5. 输尿管 ureter
6. 子宫动脉 uterine a.
7. 子宫系膜 mesometrium
8. 卵巢系膜 mesovarium
9. 输卵管系膜 mesosalpinx
10. 子宫阔韧带 broad ligament of uterus

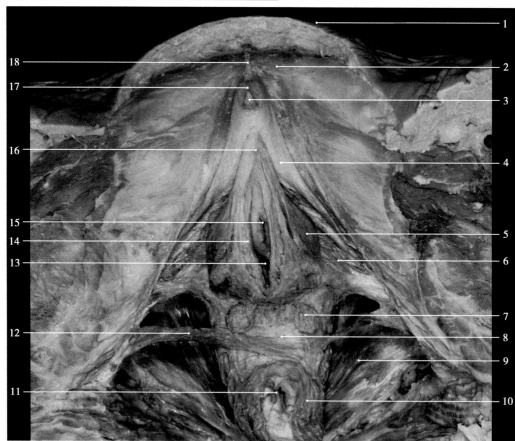

▲ 图 358 **阴蒂、前庭球和前庭大腺**
Clitoris, bulb of vestibule and greater vestibular gland

1. 阴阜 mons pubis
2. 耻骨 pubis
3. 阴蒂头 glans clitoris
4. 阴蒂脚 crus of clitoris
5. 前庭球外侧部 lateral part of bulb of vestibule
6. 尿生殖膈下筋膜 inferior fascia of urogenital diaphragm
7. 前庭大腺 greater vestibular gland
8. 会阴中心腱 perineal central tendon
9. 肛提肌 levator ani

10. 肛门外括约肌 sphincter ani externus
11. 肛门 anus
12. 会阴浅横肌 superficial transverse muscle of perineum
13. 阴道口 vaginal orifice
14. 小阴唇 lesser lip of pudendum
15. 尿道外口 external orifice of urethra
16. 前庭球中间部 intermediate part of bulbs
17. 阴蒂体 body of clitoris
18. 阴蒂悬韧带 suspensory ligament of clitoris

第八章 会阴和腹膜
Perineum and Peritoneum

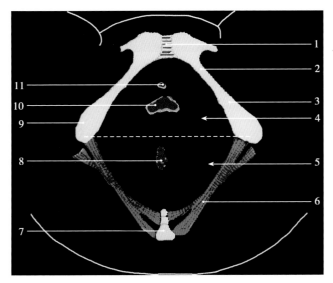

◄ 图 359

会阴的境界和分区 (模式图)
Perineal milien and zonation. Diagram
1. 耻骨联合 pubic symphysis
2. 耻骨下支 inferior ramus of pubis
3. 坐骨支 ramus of ischium
4. 尿生殖区 urogenital region
5. 肛区 anal region
6. 骶结节韧带 sacrotuberous lig.
7. 尾骨 coccyx
8. 肛门 anus
9. 坐骨结节 ischial tuberosity
10. 阴道口 vagina orifice
11. 尿道外口 external orifice of urethra

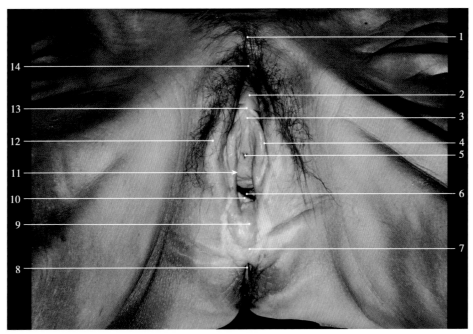

▲ 图 360　**女性外生殖器**
Female external genital organs

1. 阴阜 mons pubis
2. 阴蒂包皮 prepuce of clitoris
3. 阴蒂系带 frenulum of clitoris
4. 小阴唇 lesser lip of pudendum
5. 尿道外口 external orifice of urethra
6. 阴道口 vaginal orifice
7. 唇后连合 posterior labial commissure
8. 肛门 anus
9. 阴唇系带 frenulum of pudendal labia
10. 处女膜痕 carunculae hymenales
11. 阴道前庭 vaginal vestibule
12. 大阴唇 greater lip of pudendum
13. 阴蒂 clitoris
14. 唇前连合 anterior labial commissure

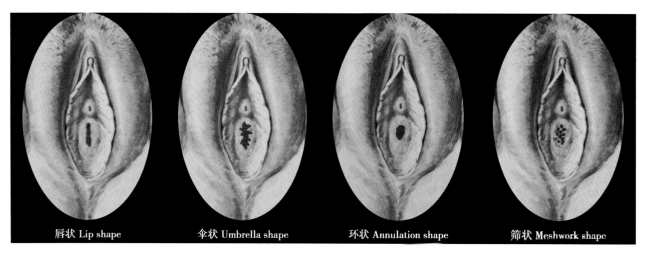

唇状 Lip shape　　　伞状 Umbrella shape　　　环状 Annulation shape　　　筛状 Meshwork shape

▲ 图 361　处女膜的类型
Type of hymen

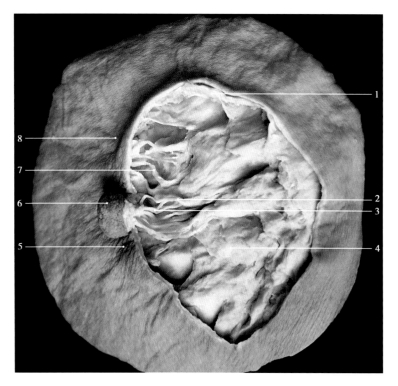

▲ 图 362　女性乳房
Mamma of female

1. 乳房脂肪体 adipose body of mamma
2. 输乳管 lactiferous duct
3. 输乳管窦 lactiferous sinuses
4. 乳腺小叶 lobule of mammary gland
5. 乳晕 areola of breast
6. 乳头 mammary papilla
7. 乳房悬韧带 suspensory ligament of breast
8. 皮肤 skin

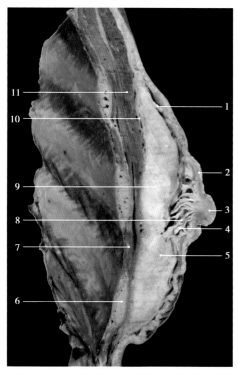

▲ 图 363　女性乳房 (矢状切面)
Mamma of female. Sagittal section

1. 乳房悬韧带 suspensory ligament of breast
2. 乳腺 areolar glands
3. 乳头 mammary papilla
4. 输乳管窦 lactiferous sinuses
5. 乳房脂肪体 adipose body of mamma
6. 肋骨 rib
7. 肋间肌 intercostales
8. 输乳管 lactiferous duct
9. 乳腺小叶 lobule of mammary gland
10. 胸肌筋膜 pectoral fascia
11. 胸大肌 pectoralis major

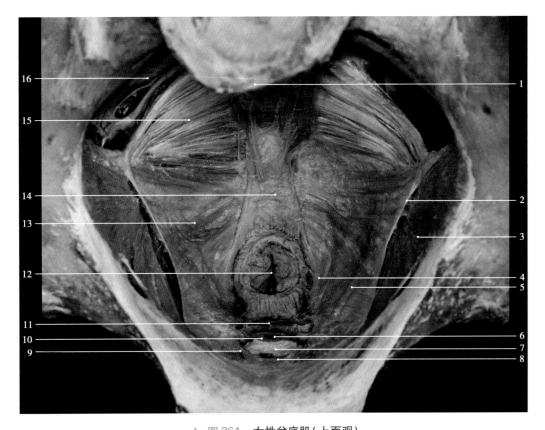

▲ 图 364 **女性盆底肌 (上面观)**
Floor muscles of pelvis in the female. Superior aspect

1. 岬 promontory
2. 肛提肌腱弓 tendinous arch of levator ani
3. 闭孔内肌 obturator internus
4. 耻骨直肠肌 puborectalis
5. 耻尾肌 pubococcygeus
6. 尿道 urethra
7. 尿生殖膈 urogenital diaphragm
8. 耻骨弓状韧带 arcuate pubic lig.
9. 耻骨阴道肌 pubovaginalis
10. 尿道括约肌 sphincter of urethra
11. 阴道 vagina
12. 直肠 rectum
13. 髂尾肌 iliococcygeus
14. 肛尾韧带 anococcygeal lig.
15. 尾骨肌 coccygeus
16. 梨状肌 piriformis

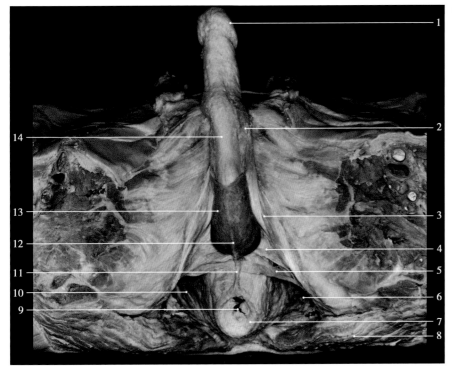

◀ 图 365
男性会阴肌
Muscles of male perineum
1. 阴茎头 glans penis
2. 阴茎海绵体 cavernous body of penis
3. 坐骨海绵体肌 ischiocaverno-sus
4. 尿生殖膈下筋膜 inferior fascia of urogenital diaphragm
5. 会阴浅横肌 superficial transverse muscle of perineum
6. 坐骨肛门窝 ischioanal fossa
7. 肛门外括约肌 sphincter ani externus
8. 臀大肌 gluteus maximus
9. 肛门 anus
10. 肛提肌 levator ani
11. 会阴中心腱 perineal central tendon
12. 尿道球中隔 bulbourethral septum
13. 球海绵体肌 bulbocavernosus
14. 尿道海绵体 cavernous body of urethra

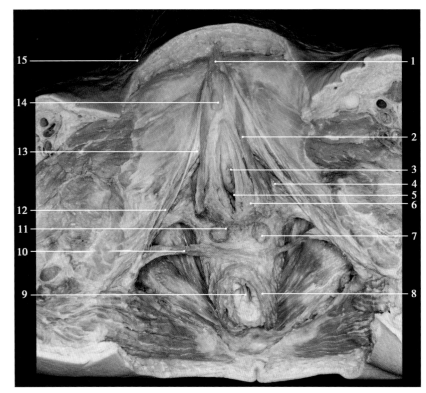

◀ 图 366
女性会阴肌
Muscles of female perineum
1. 阴蒂悬韧带 suspensory ligament of clitoris
2. 球海绵体肌 bulbocavernosus
3. 尿道外口 external orifice of urethra
4. 尿生殖膈下筋膜 inferior fascia of urogenital diaphragm
5. 阴道口 vaginal orifice
6. 前庭球 bulb of vestibule
7. 前庭大腺 greater vestibular gland
8. 肛门外括约肌 sphincter ani externus
9. 肛门 anus
10. 会阴浅横肌 superficial transverse muscle of perineum
11. 前庭大腺小管 canaliculus of greater vestibular gland
12. 坐骨海绵体肌 ischiocavernosus
13. 阴蒂脚 crus of clitoris
14. 阴蒂头 glans of clitoris
15. 阴阜 mons pubis

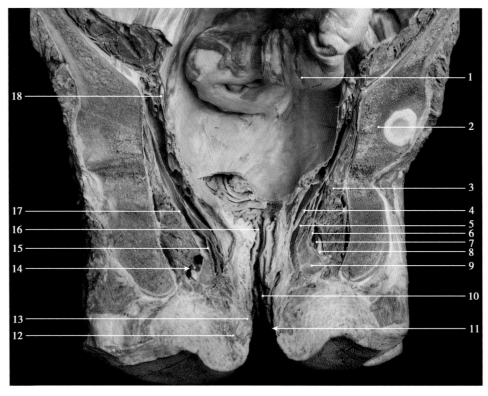

▲ 图 367　男性盆腔冠状切面 (经直肠、肛管)
Coronal section of male pelvic cavity. Through rectum and anal canal

1. 乙状结肠 sigmoid colon
2. 髋骨 hip bone
3. 闭孔内肌 obturator internus
4. 盆膈上筋膜 superior fascia of pelvic diaphragm
5. 肛提肌 levator ani
6. 阴茎背神经 dorsal nerve of penis
7. 阴部内动脉 internal pudendal a.
8. 会阴神经 perineal n.
9. 坐骨肛门窝脂体 adipose body of ischioanal fossa
10. 肛管 anal canal
11. 肛门 anus
12. 肛门外括约肌 sphincter ani externus
13. 肛门内括约肌 sphincter ani internus
14. 阴部管 pudendal canal
15. 盆膈下筋膜 inferior fascia of pelvic diaphragm
16. 直肠 rectum
17. 闭孔筋膜 obturator fascia
18. 输尿管 ureter

图 368 ▶

男性盆腔冠状切面（示尿生殖膈和盆膈）
Coronal section of male pelvic cavity.
Showing urogenital diaphragm and
pelvic diaphragm

1. 膀胱 urinary bladder
2. 闭孔动、静脉 obturator a. and v.
3. 盆膈上筋膜 superior fascia of pelvic diaphragm
4. 肛提肌 levator ani
5. 尿生殖膈上筋膜 superior fascia of urogenital diaphragm
6. 会阴动脉 perineal a.
7. 尿道括约肌 sphincter of urethra
8. 尿道球 bulb of urethra
9. 会阴浅隙 superficial perineal space
10. 会阴深隙 deep perineal space
11. 盆膈下筋膜 inferior fascia of pelvic diaphragm
12. 前列腺 prostate
13. 闭孔内肌 obturator internus
14. 膀胱筋膜 vesical fascia

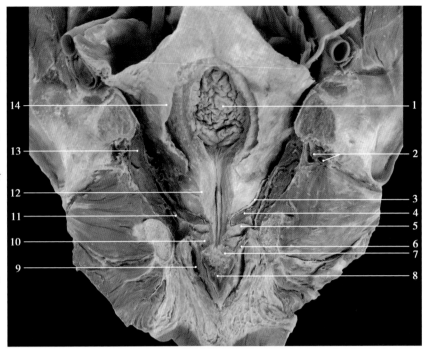

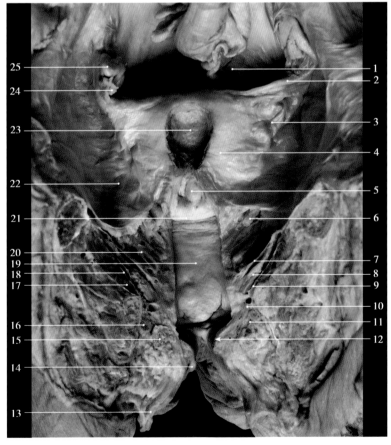

◀ 图 369

女性盆腔冠状切面（通过子宫和阴道）
Coronal section of female pelvis cavity.
Through uterus and vagina

1. 直肠 rectum
2. 输卵管 uterine tube
3. 子宫阔韧带 broad ligament of uterus
4. 子宫 uterus
5. 子宫颈管 canal of cervix of uterus
6. 输尿管 ureter
7. 盆膈上筋膜 superior fascia of pelvic diaphragm
8. 肛提肌 levator ani
9. 盆膈下筋膜 inferior fascia of pelvic diaphragm
10. 会阴深隙 deep perineal space
11. 会阴浅隙 superficial perineal space
12. 阴道口 vaginal orifice
13. 大阴唇 greater lip of pudendum
14. 小阴唇 lesser lip of pudendum
15. 前庭球 bulb of vestibule
16. 阴蒂脚 crus of clitoris
17. 闭孔内肌 obturator internus
18. 闭孔筋膜 obturator fascia
19. 阴道后壁 posterior wall of vagina
20. 阴道静脉丛 vaginal venous plexus
21. 子宫口后唇 posterior lip of orifice of uterus
22. 腹膜 peritoneum
23. 子宫腔 cavity of uterus
24. 输卵管伞 fimbriae of uterine tube
25. 卵巢 ovary

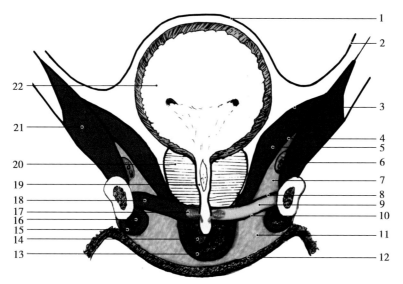

▲ 图370 **男性盆腔冠状切面（模式图）**
Coronal section of male pelvic cavity. Diagram

1. 脏腹膜 visceral peritoneum
2. 壁腹膜 parietal peritoneum
3. 盆膈上筋膜 superior fascia of pelvic diaphragm
4. 盆膈下筋膜 inferior fascia of pelvic diaphragm
5. 肛提肌 levator ani
6. 阴部管 pudendal canal
7. 坐骨肛门窝 ischioanal fossa
8. 尿生殖膈上筋膜 superior fascia of urogenital diaphragm
9. 会阴深隙 deep perineal space
10. 尿生殖膈下筋膜 inferior fascia of urogenital diaphragm
11. 会阴浅隙 superficial perineal space
12. 会阴浅筋膜 superficial fascia of perineum
13. 球海绵体肌 bulbocavernosus
14. 尿道球 bulb of urethra
15. 坐骨海绵体肌 ischiocavernosus
16. 阴茎脚 crus of penis
17. 尿道球腺 bulbourethral gland
18. 会阴深横肌 deep transverse muscle of perineum
19. 尿道 urethra
20. 前列腺 prostate
21. 闭孔内肌 obturator internus
22. 膀胱 urinary bladder

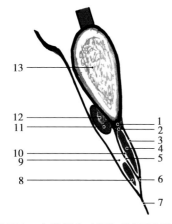

▲ 图371 **右侧尿生殖膈矢状切面（模式图）**
Sagittal section of right urogenital diaphragm. Diagram

1. 耻骨弓状韧带 arcuate pubic lig.
2. 会阴横韧带 transverse ligament of perineum
3. 尿生殖膈上筋膜 superior fascia of urogenital diaphragm
4. 会阴深横肌 deep transverse muscle of perineum
5. 尿生殖膈下筋膜 inferior fascia of urogenital diaphragm
6. 尿生殖膈后缘 posterior border of urogenital diaphragm
7. 盆膈下筋膜 inferior fascia of pelvic diaphragm
8. 会阴浅横肌 superficial transverse muscle of perineum
9. 会阴浅隙 superficial perineal space
10. 会阴深隙 deep perineal space
11. 坐骨海绵体肌 ischiocavernosus
12. 阴茎脚 crus of penis
13. 耻骨 pubis

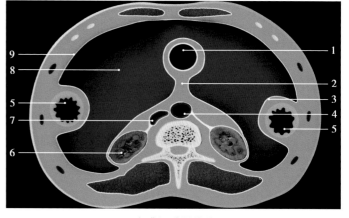

▲ 图372 **腹膜与脏器的关系（下面观）**
Relationship between viscera and peritoneum. Inferior aspect

1. 腹膜内位器官 intraperitoneal viscera
2. 肠系膜 mesentery
3. 脏腹膜 visceral peritoneum
4. 腹主动脉 abdominal aorta
5. 腹膜间位器官 interperitoneal viscera
6. 腹膜后位器官 retoperitoneal viscera
7. 下腔静脉 inferior vena cava
8. 腹膜腔 peritoneal cavity
9. 壁腹膜 parietal peritoneum

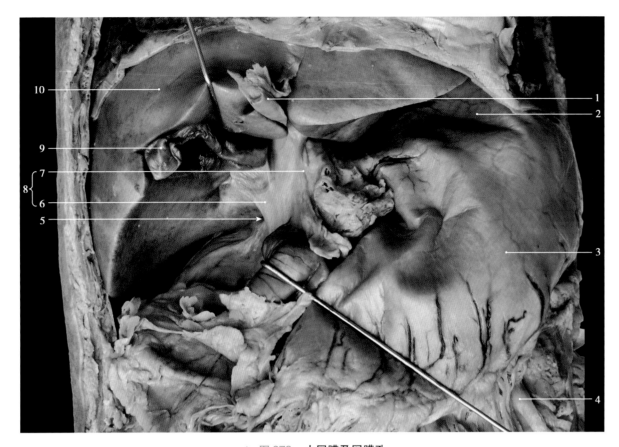

▲ 图 373 **小网膜及网膜孔**
Lesser omentum and omental foramen

1. 肝圆韧带 ligamentum teres hepatis
2. 胃底 fundus of stomach
3. 胃体 body of stomach
4. 大网膜 greater omentum
5. 网膜孔 omental foramen
6. 肝十二指肠韧带 hepatoduodenal lig.
7. 肝胃韧带 hepatogastric lig.
8. 小网膜 less omentum
9. 胆囊 gallbladder
10. 肝 liver

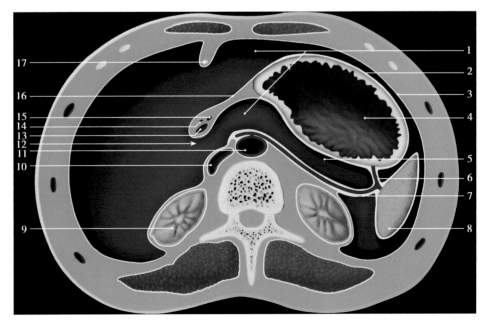

◀ 图 374

网膜囊及网膜孔(下面观)
Omental bursa and omental
foramen. Inferior aspect

1. 腹膜腔 peritoneal cavity
2. 脏腹膜 visceral peritoneum
3. 壁腹膜 parietal peritoneum
4. 胃 stomach
5. 网膜囊 omental bursa
6. 胃脾韧带 gastrosplenic lig.
7. 脾肾韧带 splenorenal lig.
8. 脾 spleen
9. 肾 kidney
10. 下腔静脉 inferior vena
cava
11. 腹主动脉 abdominal
aorta
12. 网膜孔 omental foramen
13. 肝门静脉 hepatic portal v.
14. 胆总管 common bile duct
15. 肝固有动脉 proper
hepatic a.
16. 小网膜 less omentum
17. 肝镰状韧带 falciform
ligament of liver

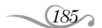

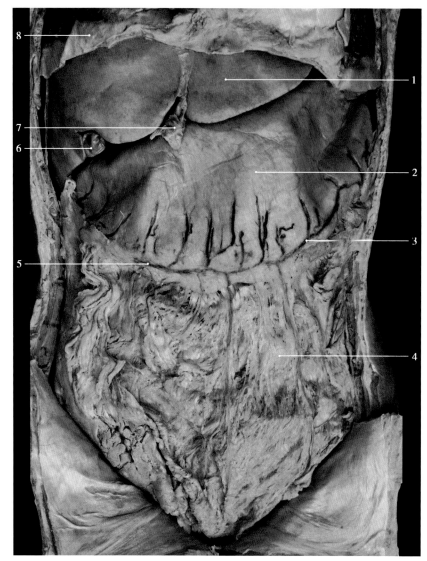

◀ 图 375
大网膜
Greater omentum
1. 肝 liver
2. 胃 stomach
3. 胃网膜左动脉 left gastroomental a.
4. 大网膜 greater omentum
5. 胃网膜右动脉 right gastroomental a.
6. 胆囊 gallbladder
7. 肝圆韧带 ligamentum teres hepatis
8. 膈 diaphragm

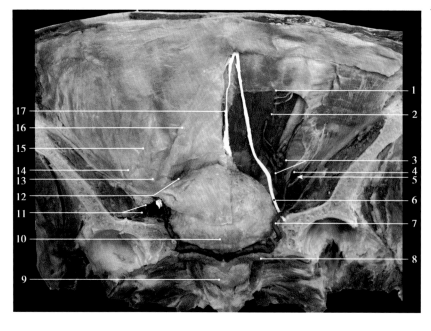

◀ 图 376
腹前壁内面的皱襞和窝
Peritoneal folds and fossa on the inner surface of anterior ventral wall
1. 弓状线 arcuate line
2. 腹直肌 rectus abdominis
3. 腹壁下动、静脉 inferior epigastric a. and v.
4. 睾丸静脉 testicular v.
5. 腹股沟管深环 deep inguinal ring
6. 脐内侧韧带 medial umbilical lig.
7. 输精管 ductus deferens
8. 精囊 seminal vesicle
9. 前列腺 prostate
10. 膀胱 urinary bladder
11. 髂外动、静脉 external iliac a. and v.
12. 膀胱上窝 supravesical fossa
13. 腹股沟内侧窝 medial inguinal fossa
14. 腹股沟外侧窝 lateral inguinal fossa
15. 脐外侧襞 lateral umbilical fold
16. 脐内侧襞 medial umbilical fold
17. 脐尿管索(脐正中襞) chorda urachi

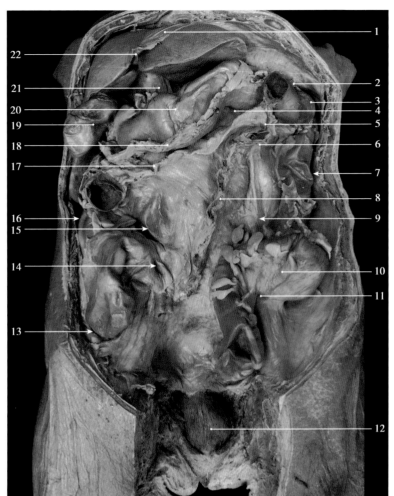

◀ 图 377

腹膜形成的结构
Forming structures of peritoneum
1. 肝镰状韧带 falciform ligament of liver
2. 膈结肠韧带 phrenicocolic lig.
3. 结肠左曲 left colic flexure
4. 胰 pancreas
5. 十二指肠上襞 superior duodenal fold
6. 十二指肠下襞 inferior duodenal fold
7. 左结肠旁沟 left paracolic sulci
8. 肠系膜根 radix of mesentery
9. 左肠系膜窦 left mesenteric sinus
10. 乙状结肠系膜 sigmoid mesocolon
11. 乙状结肠间隐窝 intersigmoid recess
12. 直肠 rectum
13. 盲肠后隐窝 retrocecal recess
14. 回盲上隐窝 superior ileocecal recess
15. 右肠系膜窦 right mesenteric sinus
16. 右结肠旁沟 right paracolic sulci
17. 横结肠系膜 transverse mesocolon
18. 大网膜 greater omentum
19. 胆囊 gallbladder
20. 胃 stomach
21. 小网膜 less omentum
22. 肝圆韧带 ligamentum teres hepatis

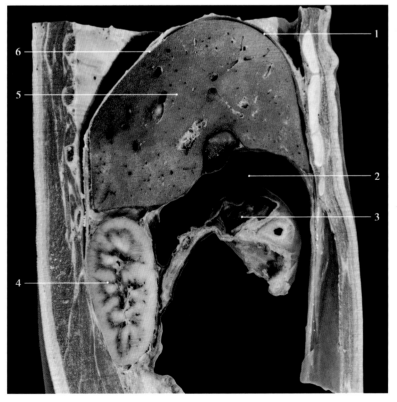

◀ 图 378

结肠上区的间隙
Interspace of superior region of colon
1. 右肝上前间隙 superior anterior interspace of right liver
2. 右肝下间隙 inferior interspace of right liver
3. 横结肠 transverse colon
4. 右肾 right kidney
5. 肝右叶 right lobe of liver
6. 肝裸区 bare area of liver

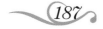

第九章 心血管系统
Cardiovascular System

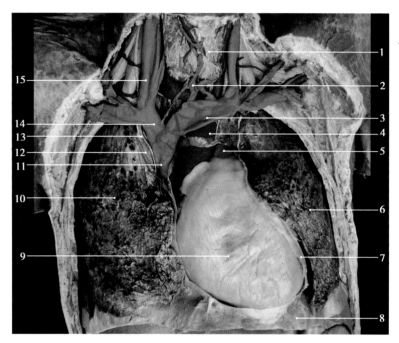

◀ 图 379

心肺的位置
Location of heart and lung

1. 甲状腺 thyroid gland
2. 甲状腺下静脉 inferior thyroid v.
3. 左头臂静脉 left brachiocephalic v.
4. 主动脉弓 aortic arch
5. 肺动脉 pulmonary a.
6. 左肺 left lung
7. 心包 pericardium
8. 膈 diaphragm
9. 心 heart
10. 右肺 right lung
11. 上腔静脉 superior vena cava
12. 纵隔胸膜 mediastinal pleura
13. 膈神经 phrenic n.
14. 右头臂静脉 right brachiocephalic v.
15. 右颈内静脉 right internal jugular v.

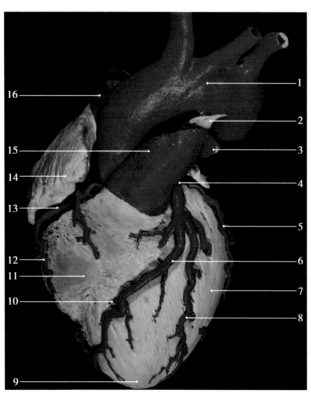

◀ 图 380

冠状动脉（前面观）
Coronary artery. Anterior aspect

1. 主动脉弓 aortic arch
2. 动脉韧带 arterial lig.
3. 左肺动脉 left pulmonary a.
4. 左冠状动脉 left coronary a.
5. 左缘支 left marginal branch
6. 前室间支 anterior interventricular branch
7. 左心室 left ventricle
8. 左室前支 anterior branch of the left ventricle
9. 心尖 cardiac apex
10. 室间隔前支 anterior branch of the interventricular septum
11. 右心室 right ventricle
12. 右缘支 right marginal branch
13. 右冠状动脉 right coronary a.
14. 右心耳 right auricle
15. 肺动脉干 pulmonary trunk
16. 上腔静脉 superior vena cava

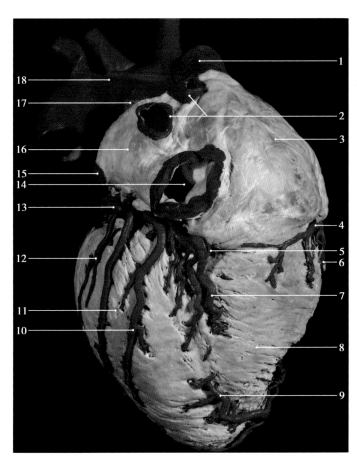

◀ 图 381

冠状动脉（膈面）

Coronary arteries. Diaphragmatic surface

1. 上腔静脉 superior vena cava
2. 右肺静脉 right pulmonary v.
3. 右心房 right atrium
4. 右冠状动脉 right coronary a.
5. 房室结支 branch of atrioventricular node
6. 右缘支 right marginal branch
7. 后室间支 posterior interventricular branch
8. 右心室 right ventricle
9. 前室间支 anterior interventricular branch
10. 左室后支 posterior branch of left ventricle
11. 左心室 left ventricle
12. 左缘支 left marginal branch
13. 旋支 circumflex branch
14. 下腔静脉 inferior vena cava
15. 左肺静脉 left pulmonary v.
16. 左心房 left atrium
17. 动脉韧带 arterial lig.
18. 主动脉弓 aorta arch

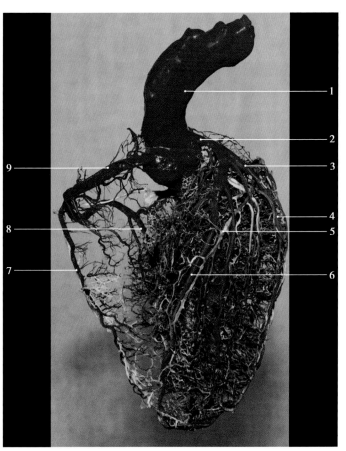

◀ 图 382

冠状动脉铸型

Cast of coronary arteries

1. 升主动脉 ascending aorta
2. 左冠状动脉 left coronary a.
3. 旋支 circumflex branch
4. 左缘支 left marginal branch
5. 心大静脉 great cardiac v.
6. 前室间支 anterior interventricular branch
7. 右缘支 right marginal branch
8. 后室间支 posterior interventricular branch
9. 右冠状动脉 right coronary a.

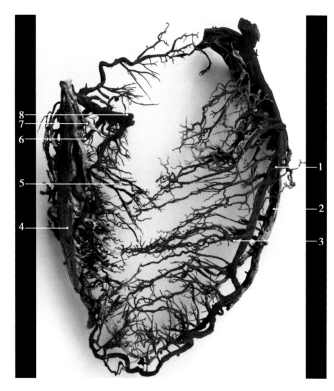

◀ 图 383

室间隔的血管
Blood vessels of interventricular septum
1. 前室间支 anterior interventricular branch
2. 心大静脉 great cardiac v.
3. 室间隔前支 anterior branch of interventricular septum
4. 心中静脉 middle cardiac v.
5. 室间隔后支 posterior branch of interventricular septum
6. 后室间支 posterior interventricular branch
7. 心小静脉 smallest cardiac v.
8. 右冠状动脉 right coronary a.

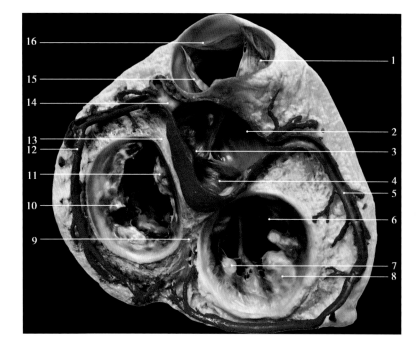

◀ 图 384

心脏的瓣膜（上面观）
Cardiac valves. Superior aspect
1. 肺动脉瓣右半月瓣 right leaflet of pulmonary valve
2. 主动脉瓣右半月瓣 right leaflet of aortic valve
3. 主动脉瓣左半月瓣 left leaflet of aortic valve
4. 主动脉瓣后半月瓣 posterior leaflet of aortic valve
5. 右冠状动脉 right coronary a.
6. 三尖瓣前尖 anterior cusp of tricuspid valve
7. 三尖瓣隔侧尖 septal cusp of tricuspid valve
8. 三尖瓣后尖 posterior cusp of tricuspid valve
9. 右纤维三角 right fibrous trigone
10. 二尖瓣后尖 posterior cusp of mitral valve
11. 二尖瓣前尖 anterior cusp of mitral valve
12. 旋支 circumflex branch
13. 左纤维三角 left fibrous trigone
14. 左冠状动脉 left coronary a.
15. 肺动脉瓣左半月瓣 left leaflet of pulmonary valve
16. 肺动脉瓣前半月瓣 anterior leaflet of pulmonary valve

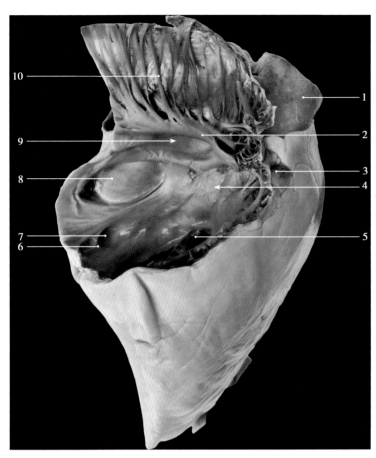

◀ 图 385

右心房
Right atrium

1. 升主动脉 ascending aorta
2. 界嵴 crista terminalis
3. 右心耳 right auricle
4. 主动脉隆凸 aortic carina
5. 三尖瓣隔侧尖 septal cusp of tricuspid valve
6. 冠状窦瓣 valve of coronary sinus
7. 冠状窦口 orifice of coronary sinus
8. 卵圆窝 fossa ovalis
9. 上腔静脉口 orifice of superior vena cava
10. 梳状肌 pectinate m.

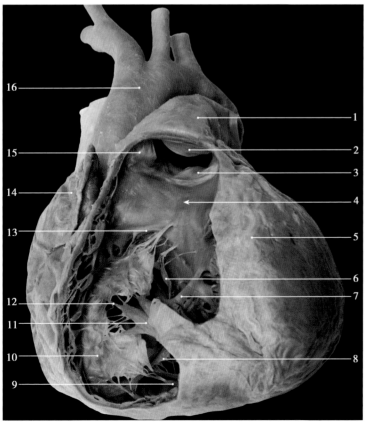

◀ 图 386

右心室
Right ventricle

1. 肺动脉干 pulmonary trunk
2. 肺动脉瓣前半月瓣 anterion leaflet of pulmonary valve
3. 肺动脉瓣左半月瓣 left leaflet of pulmonary valve
4. 动脉圆锥 conus arteriosus
5. 前室间沟 anterior interventricular groove
6. 三尖瓣隔侧尖 septal cusp of tricuspid valve
7. 隔缘肉柱 septomarginal trabecula
8. 三尖瓣后尖 posterior cusp of tricuspid valve
9. 后乳头肌 posterior papillary m.
10. 三尖瓣前尖 anterior cusp of tricuspid valve
11. 前乳头肌 anterior papillary m.
12. 腱索 chorda tendineae
13. 室上嵴 supraventricular crest
14. 右心耳 right auricle
15. 肺动脉瓣右半月瓣 right leaflet of pulmonary valve
16. 主动脉弓 aortic arch

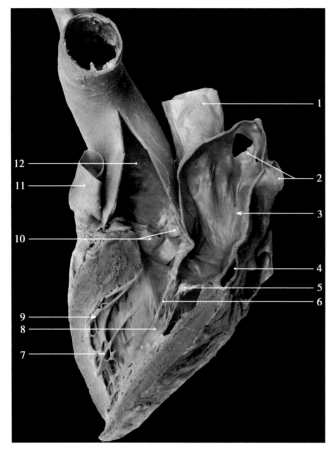

◀ 图 387

左心室和左心房

Left ventricle and atrium

1. 上腔静脉 superior vena cava
2. 右肺静脉 right pulmonary v.
3. 左心房 left atrium
4. 冠状窦 coronary sinus
5. 二尖瓣 mitral valve
6. 腱索 chorda tendineae
7. 肉柱 trabeculae carneae
8. 后乳头肌 posterior papillary m.
9. 左心室 left ventricle
10. 主动脉瓣 aortic valve
11. 肺动脉干 pulmonary trunk
12. 升主动脉 ascending aorta

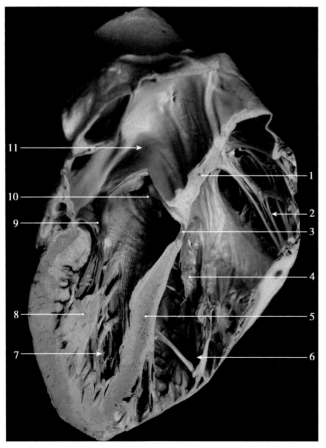

◀ 图 388

室间隔和房间隔

Interventricular septum and interatrial septum

1. 房间隔 interatrial septum
2. 右心房 right atrium
3. 室间隔膜部 membranous part of interventricular septum
4. 三尖瓣隔侧尖 septal cusp
5. 室间隔肌部 muscular part of interventricular septum
6. 右心室 right ventricle
7. 左心室 left ventricle
8. 乳头肌 papillary m.
9. 二尖瓣 mitral valve
10. 主动脉瓣 aortic valve
11. 左心房 left atrium

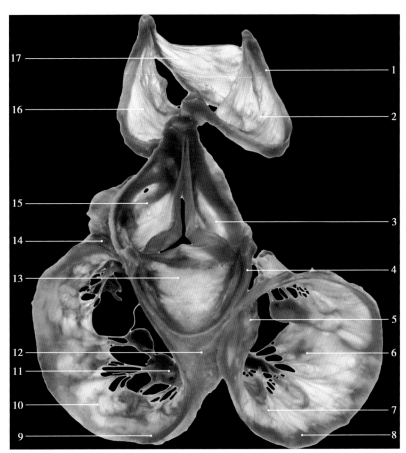

◀ 图 389

心纤维支架（1）
Fibrous framework of the heart（1）

1. 肺动脉瓣环 annulus of pulmonary valve
2. 肺动脉瓣右半月瓣 right leaflet of pulmonary valve
3. 主动脉瓣右半月瓣 right leaflet of aortic valve
4. 主动脉瓣环 annulus of aortic valve
5. 三尖瓣隔侧尖 septal cusp of tricuspid valve
6. 三尖瓣前尖 anterior cusp of tricuspid valve
7. 三尖瓣后尖 posterior cusp of tricuspid valve
8. 三尖瓣环 tricuspid annulus
9. 二尖瓣环 mitral annulus
10. 二尖瓣后尖 posterior cusp
11. 乳头肌 papillary m.
12. 右纤维三角 right fibrous trigone
13. 主动脉瓣后半月瓣 posterior leaflet of aortic valve
14. 左纤维三角 left fibrous trigone
15. 主动脉瓣左半月瓣 left leaflet of aortic valve
16. 肺动脉瓣左半月瓣 left leaflet of pulmonary valve
17. 肺动脉瓣前半月瓣 anterior leaflet of pulmonary valve

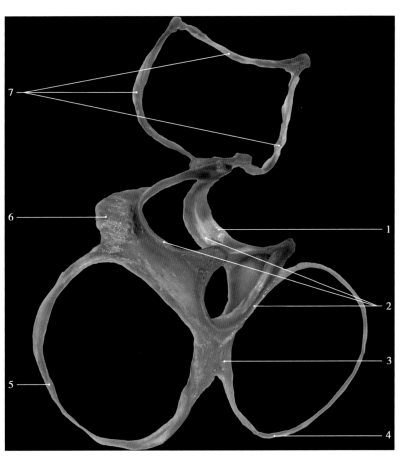

◀ 图 390

心纤维支架（2）
Fibrous framework of the heart（2）

1. 圆锥韧带 conoid lig.
2. 主动脉瓣环 annulus of aortic valve
3. 右纤维三角 right fibrous trigone
4. 三尖瓣环 tricuspid annulus
5. 二尖瓣环 mitral annulus
6. 左纤维三角 left fibrous trigone
7. 肺动脉瓣环 annulus of pulmonary valve

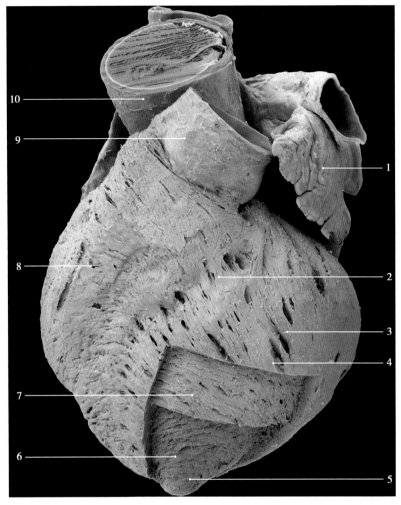

◀ 图 391

心肌

Cardiac muscles

1. 左心耳 left auricle
2. 前室间沟 anterior interventricular groove
3. 左心室 left ventricle
4. 心肌浅层 superficial layer of cardiac m.
5. 心尖 cardiac apex
6. 心肌深层 deep layer of cardiac m.
7. 心肌中层 middle layer of cardiac m.
8. 右心室 right ventricle
9. 肺动脉干 pulmonary trunk
10. 升主动脉 ascending aorta

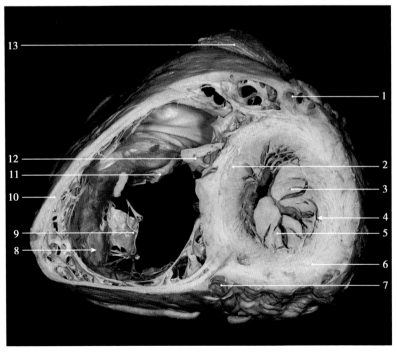

◀ 图 392

心室横切面

Transverse section of ventricles

1. 前室间支 anterior interventricular branch
2. 室间隔肌部 muscular part of interventricular septum
3. 前乳头肌 anterior papillary m.
4. 左心室 left ventricle
5. 后乳头肌 posterior papillary m.
6. 左心室壁 left ventricular wall
7. 心中静脉 middle cardiac v.
8. 右心室 right ventricle
9. 三尖瓣后尖 posterior cusp of tricuspid valve
10. 右心室壁 right ventricular wall
11. 三尖瓣前尖 anterior cusp of tricuspid valve
12. 三尖瓣隔侧尖 septal cusp of tricuspid valve
13. 肺动脉干 pulmonary trunk

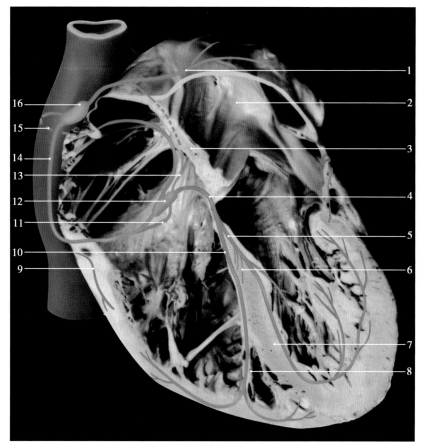

◀ 图 393

心传导系 (1)
Conduction system of the heart (1)
1. 上房间束 superior interatrial tract
2. 左心房 left atrium
3. 房间隔 interatrial septum
4. 房室束 atrioventricular bundle
5. 左束支 left bundle branch
6. Mahaim 纤维 Mahaim fiber
7. 室间隔 interventricular septum
8. 隔缘肉柱 septomarginal trabecula
9. Kent 束 Kent bundle
10. 右束支 right bundle branch
11. James 旁路纤维 alternative pathway fiber of James
12. 房室结 atrioventricular node
13. 前结间束 anterior internodal tract
14. 后结间束 posterior internodal tract
15. 中结间束 middle internodal tract
16. 窦房结 sinuatrial node

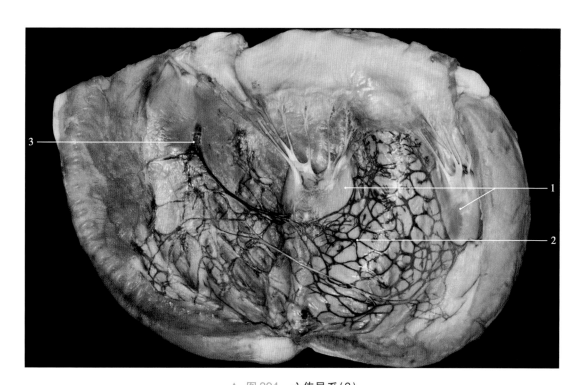

▲ 图 394 **心传导系 (2)**
Conduction system of the heart (2)
1. 乳头肌 papillary m.
2. Purkinje 纤维网 Purkinje fiber web
3. 右束支 right bundle branch

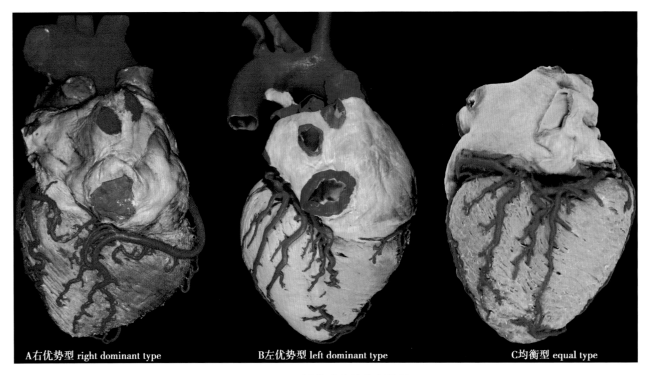

A右优势型 right dominant type B左优势型 left dominant type C均衡型 equal type

▲ 图 395 冠状动脉的分布类型
Distributional type of coronary artery

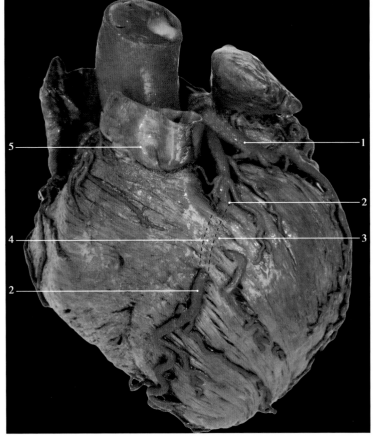

◀ 图 396
壁冠状动脉
Mural coronary artery
1. 旋支 circumflex branch
2. 前室间支 anterior interventricular branch
3. 心肌桥 myocardial bridge
4. 壁冠状动脉 mural coronary a.
5. 肺动脉干 pulmonary trunk

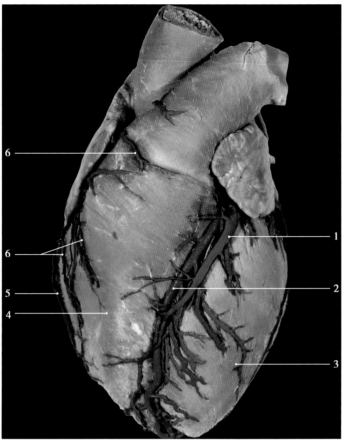

◀ 图 397

心的静脉（前面观）
Cardiac veins. Anterior aspect

1. 心大静脉 great cardiac v.
2. 前室间支 anterior interventricular branch
3. 左心室 left ventricle
4. 右心室 right ventricle
5. 心小静脉 small cardiac v.
6. 心前静脉 anterior cardiac v.

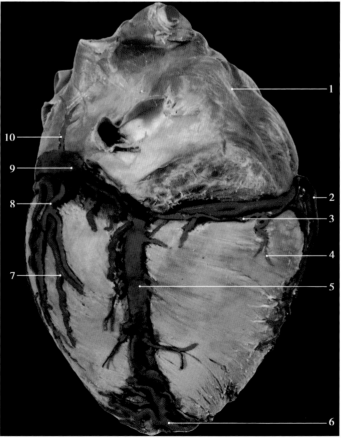

◀ 图 398

心的静脉（膈面）
Cardiac veins. Diaphragmatic surface

1. 右心房 right atrium
2. 右缘静脉 right marginal v.
3. 心小静脉 small cardiac v.
4. 右室后静脉 posterior vein of the right ventricle
5. 心中静脉 middle cardiac v.
6. 前室间支 anterior interventricular branch
7. 左室后支 posterior branch of the left ventricle
8. 左室后静脉 posterior vein of the left ventricle
9. 冠状窦 coronary sinus
10. 左心房斜静脉 oblique vein of the left atrium

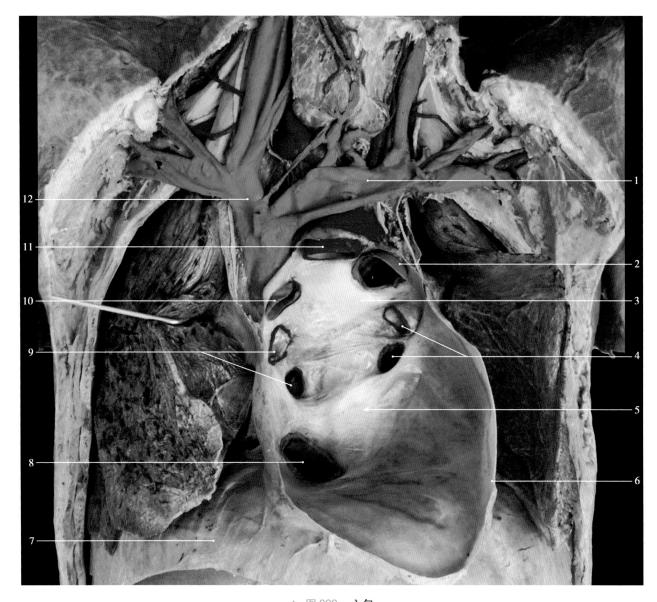

▲ 图 399　心包

Pericardium

1. 左头臂静脉 left brachiocephalic v.　　7. 膈 diaphragm

2. 肺动脉干 pulmonary trunk　　8. 下腔静脉 inferior vena cava

3. 横窦 transverse sinus　　9. 右肺静脉 right pulmonary v.

4. 左肺静脉 left pulmonary v.　　10. 上腔静脉 superior vena cava

5. 斜窦 oblique sinus　　11. 升主动脉 ascending aorta

6. 心包 pericardium　　12. 右头臂静脉 right brachiocephalic v.

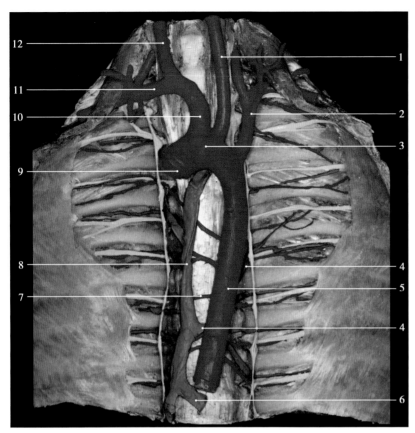

◀ 图 400

主动脉弓和胸主动脉
Aortic arch and thoracic aorta
1. 左颈总动脉 left common carotid a.
2. 左锁骨下动脉 left subclavian a.
3. 主动脉弓 aortic arch
4. 副半奇静脉 accessory hemiazygos v.
5. 胸主动脉 thoracic aorta
6. 半奇静脉 hemiazygos v.
7. 肋间后动脉 posterior intercostal a.
8. 奇静脉 azygos v.
9. 升主动脉 ascending aorta
10. 头臂干 brachiocephalic trunk
11. 右锁骨下动脉 right subclavian a.
12. 右颈总动脉 right common carotid a.

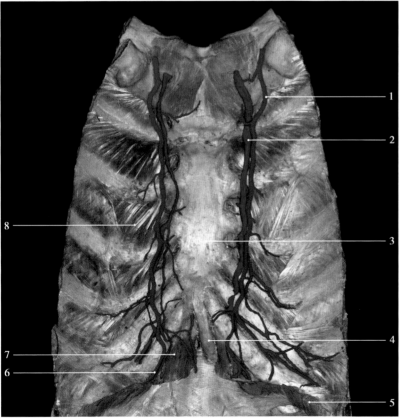

◀ 图 401

胸廓内动脉
Internal thoracic artery
1. 胸廓内动脉 internal thoracic a.
2. 胸廓内静脉 internal thoracic v.
3. 胸骨体 body of sternum
4. 剑突 xiphoid process
5. 膈 diaphragm
6. 腹壁上动脉 superior epigastric a.
7. 腹直肌 rectus abdominis
8. 肋间内肌 intercostales interni

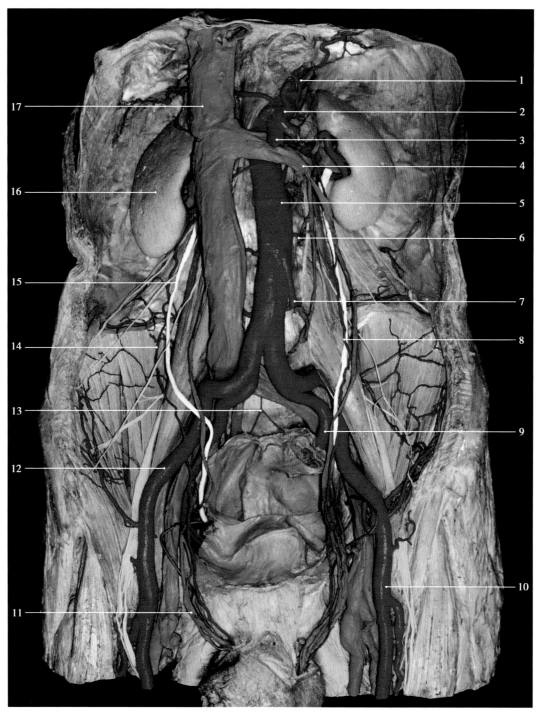

▲ 图402 腹主动脉及其分支
Abdominal aorta and its branches

1. 膈下动脉 inferior phrenic a.
2. 腹腔干 celiac trunk
3. 肠系膜上动脉 superior mesenteric a.
4. 左肾静脉 left renal v.
5. 腹主动脉 abdominal aorta
6. 腰动脉 lumbar a.
7. 肠系膜下动脉 inferior mesenteric a.
8. 左睾丸动脉 left testicular a.
9. 髂内动脉 internal iliac a.

10. 股动脉 femoral a.
11. 蔓状静脉丛 pampiniform plexus
12. 髂外动脉 external iliac a.
13. 骶中动脉 median sacral a.
14. 右睾丸动脉 right testicular a.
15. 输尿管 ureter
16. 右肾 right kidney
17. 下腔静脉 inferior vena cava

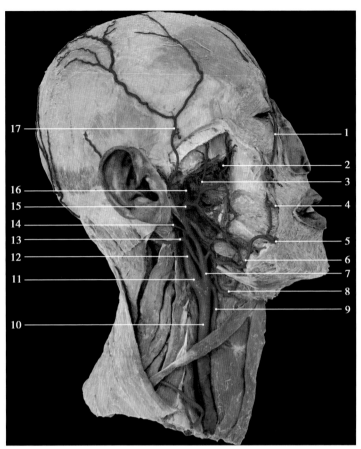

◀ 图 403

颈外动脉及其分支
External carotid artery and its branches

1. 内眦动脉 angular a.
2. 蝶腭动脉 sphenopalatine a.
3. 颞深动脉 deep temporal a.
4. 上唇动脉 superior labial a.
5. 下唇动脉 inferior labial a.
6. 面动脉 facial a.
7. 颈外动脉 external carotid a.
8. 舌动脉 lingual a.
9. 甲状腺上动脉 superior thyroid a.
10. 颈总动脉 common carotid a
11. 颈动脉窦 carotid sinus
12. 颈内动脉 internal carotid a.
13. 枕动脉 occipital a.
14. 耳后动脉 posterior auricular a
15. 上颌动脉 maxillary a.
16. 脑膜中动脉 middle meningeal a.
17. 颞浅动脉 superficial temporal a.

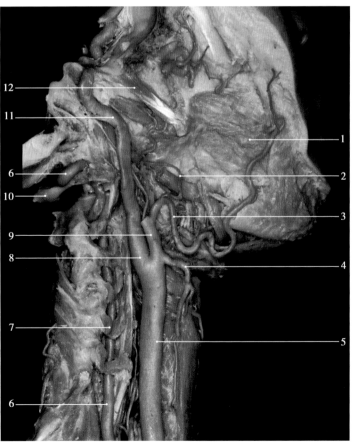

◀ 图 404

颈内动脉和椎动脉
Internal carotid artery and vertebral artery

1. 颊肌 buccinator
2. 腭升动脉 ascending palatine a.
3. 面动脉 facial a.
4. 甲状腺上动脉 superior thyroid a.
5. 颈总动脉 common carotid a.
6. 椎动脉 vertebral a.
7. 横突 transverse process
8. 颈动脉窦 carotid sinus
9. 颈外动脉 external carotid a.
10. 寰椎 atlas
11. 颈内动脉 internal carotid a.
12. 腭帆张肌 tensor veli palati

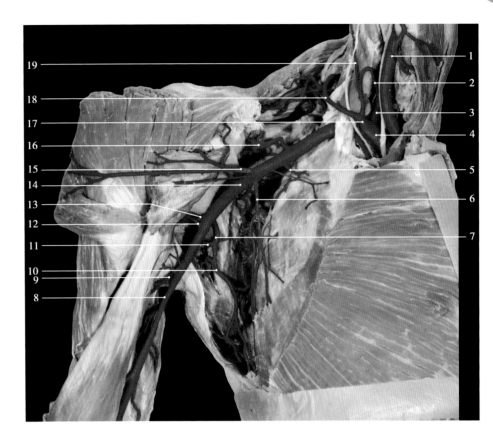

◀ 图 405

锁骨下动脉和腋动脉
Subclavian artery and axillary artery

1. 颈总动脉 common carotid a.
2. 甲状腺下动脉 inferior thyroid a.
3. 椎动脉 vertebral a.
4. 锁骨下动脉 subclavian a.
5. 胸最上动脉 supreme thoracic a.
6. 胸外侧动脉 lateral thoracic a.
7. 肩胛下动脉 subscapular a.
8. 肱动脉 brachial a.
9. 肱深动脉 deep brachial a.
10. 胸背动脉 thoracodorsal a.
11. 旋肩胛动脉 circumflex scapular a.
12. 旋肱前动脉 anterior humeral circumflex a.
13. 旋肱后动脉 posterior humeral circumflex a.
14. 腋动脉 axillary a.
15. 胸肩峰动脉 thoracoacromial a.
16. 肩胛上动脉 suprascapular a.
17. 甲状颈干 thyrocervical trunk
18. 颈横动脉 transverse cervical a.
19. 颈升动脉 ascending cervical a.

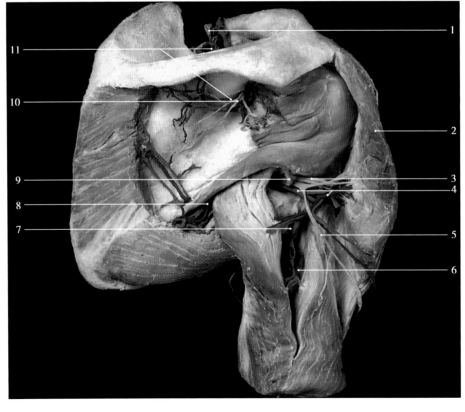

◀ 图 406

肩部的血管和神经 (后面观)
Blood vessels and nerves of the shoulder. Posterior aspect

1. 肩胛上神经 suprascapular n.
2. 三角肌 deltoid
3. 腋神经 axillary n.
4. 旋肱后动、静脉 posterior humeral circumflex a. and v.
5. 臂上外侧皮神经 superior lateral brachial cutaneous n.
6. 肱深动脉 deep brachial a.
7. 旋肱后动脉吻合支 ramus anastomoticus of posterior humeral circumflex a.
8. 旋肩胛动脉 circumflex scapular a.
9. 小圆肌肌支 muscular branch of teres minor
10. 冈下肌肌支 muscular branch of infraspinatus
11. 肩胛上动脉 suprascapular a.

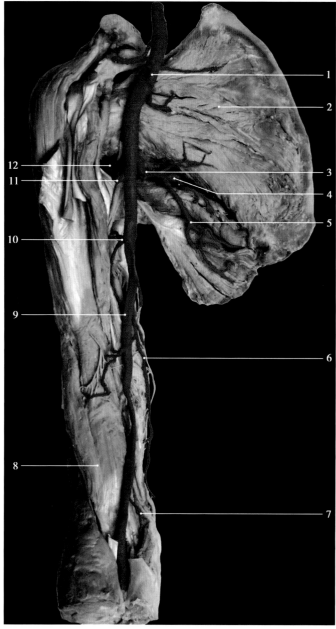

▲ 图 407　臂部的动脉 (前面观)
Arteries of arm. Anterior aspect

1. 腋动脉 axillary a.
2. 肩胛下肌 subscapularis
3. 肩胛下动脉 subscapular a.
4. 旋肩胛动脉 circumflex scapular a.
5. 胸背动脉 thoracodorsal a.
6. 尺侧上副动脉 superior ulnar collateral a.
7. 尺侧下副动脉 inferior ulnar collateral a.
8. 肱肌 brachialis
9. 肱动脉 brachial a.
10. 肱深动脉 deep brachial a.
11. 旋肱前动脉 anterior humeral circumflex a.
12. 旋肱后动脉 posterior humeral circumflex a.

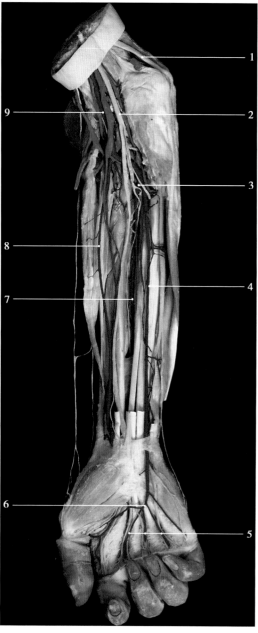

▲ 图 408　前臂的动脉 (前面观)
Arteries of forearm. Anterior aspect

1. 尺神经 ulnar n.
2. 正中神经 median n.
3. 骨间总动脉 common interosseous a.
4. 尺动脉 ulnar a.
5. 指掌侧总动脉 common palmar digital a.
6. 掌浅弓 superficial palmar arch
7. 骨间前动脉 anterior interosseous a.
8. 桡动脉 radial a.
9. 肱动脉 brachial a.

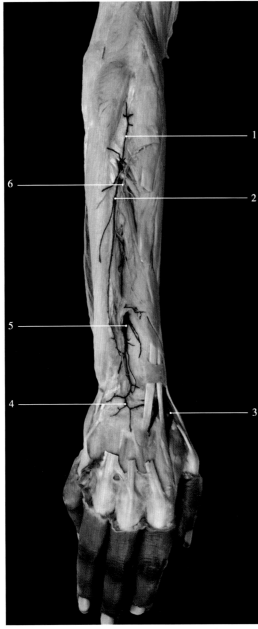

▲ 图409　前臂的动脉（后面观）
Arteries of forearm. Posterior aspect

1. 骨间返动脉 recurrent interosseous a.
2. 骨间后动脉 posterior interosseous a.
3. 桡动脉 radial a.
4. 腕背网 dorsal carpal rete
5. 骨间前动脉背侧支 dorsal branch of anterior
　 interosseous a.
6. 桡神经深支 deep branch of radial n.

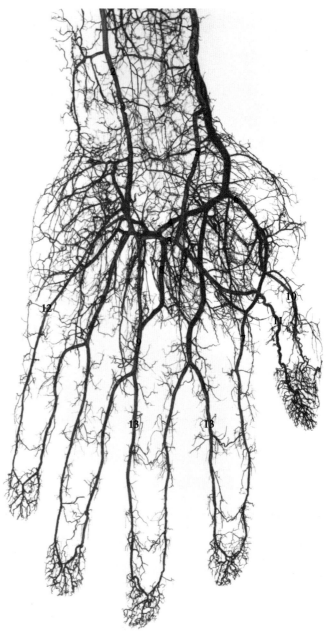

▲ 图410　手动脉铸型
Cast of arteries of hand

1. 桡动脉 radial a.
2. 尺动脉 ulnar a.
3. 掌浅弓 superficial palmar arch
4. 掌深弓 deep palmar arch
5. 掌浅支 superficial palmar branch
6. 拇主要动脉 principal artery of thumb
7. 示指桡侧动脉 radial artery of index
8. 掌心动脉 palmar metacarpal a.
9. 指掌侧总动脉 common palmar digital a.
10. 拇指桡掌侧动脉 radial palmar pollicis a.
11. 拇指尺掌侧动脉 ulnar palmar pollicis a.
12. 小指尺掌侧动脉 ulnar palmar artery of little finger
13. 指掌侧固有动脉 proper palmar digital a.

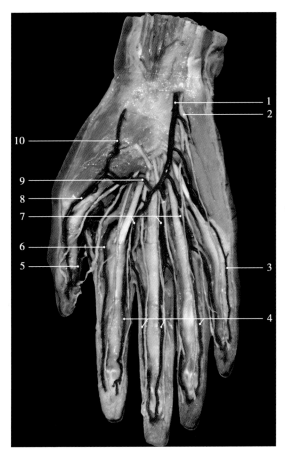

◀ 图 411

手的动脉（前面观 1）
Arteries of hand. Anterior aspect（1）

1. 尺动脉 ulnar a.
2. 尺神经 ulnar n.
3. 小指尺掌侧动脉 ulnar palmar artery of little finger
4. 指掌侧固有动脉 proper palmar digital a.
5. 拇指尺掌侧动脉 ulnar palmar pollicis a.
6. 示指桡侧动脉 radial artery of index
7. 指掌侧总动脉 common palmar digital a.
8. 拇指桡掌侧动脉 radial palmar pollicis a.
9. 掌浅弓 superficial palmar arch
10. 掌浅支 superficial palmar branch

图 412 ▶

手的动脉（前面观 2）
Arteries of hand. Anterior aspect（2）

1. 尺动脉 ulnar a.
2. 掌深支 deep palmar branch
3. 掌心动脉 palmar metacarpal a.
4. 小指尺掌侧动脉 ulnar palmar artery of little finger
5. 指掌侧固有动脉 proper palmar digital a.
6. 示指桡侧动脉 radial artery of index
7. 拇指尺掌侧动脉 ulnar palmar pollicis a.
8. 拇指桡掌侧动脉 radial palmar pollicis a.
9. 拇主要动脉 principal artery of thumb
10. 掌深弓 deep palmar arch
11. 桡动脉 radial a.

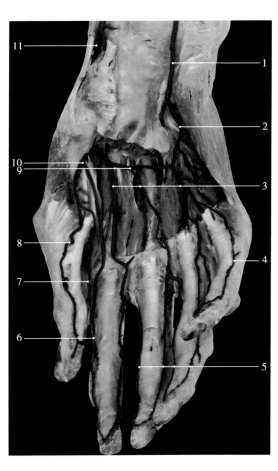

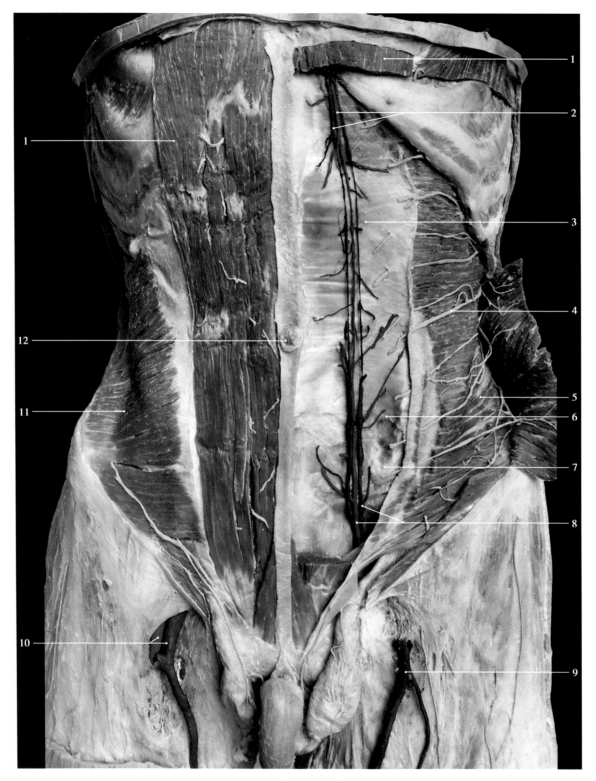

▲ 图 413　腹壁上动脉与腹壁下动脉
Superior epigastric artery and inferior epigastric artery

1. 腹直肌 rectus abdominis
2. 腹壁上动、静脉 superior epigastric a. and v.
3. 腹直肌鞘后层 posterior layer of sheath of rectus abdominis
4. 肋间神经 intercostal n.
5. 腹横肌 transversus abdominis
6. 弓状线 arcuate line

7. 腹横筋膜 transverse fascia
8. 腹壁下动、静脉 inferior epigastric a. and v.
9. 大隐静脉 great saphenous v.
10. 股动、静脉 femoral a. and v.
11. 腹内斜肌 obliquus internus abdominis
12. 脐 umbilicus

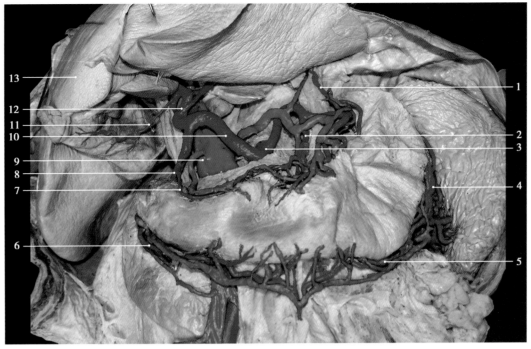

▲ 图 414　腹腔干及其分支（1）
Celiac trunk and its branches（1）

1. 食管支 esophageal branch
2. 胃左动脉 left gastric a.
3. 腹腔干 celiac trunk
4. 胃短动脉 short gastric a.
5. 胃网膜左动脉 left gastroepiploic a.
6. 胃网膜右动脉 right gastroepiploic a.
7. 胃右动脉 right gastric a.
8. 胃十二指肠动脉 gastroduodenal a.
9. 肝门静脉 hepatic portal v.
10. 肝总动脉 common hepatic a.
11. 胆囊动脉 cystic a.
12. 肝固有动脉 proper hepatic a.
13. 肝 liver

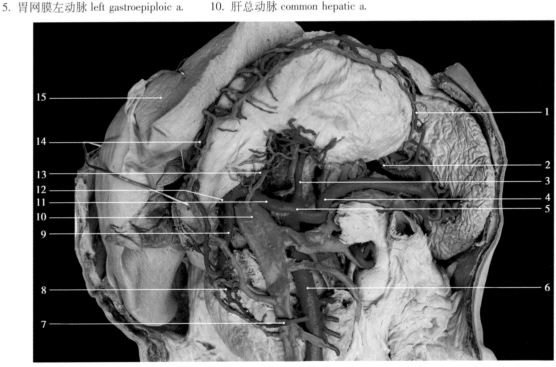

▲ 图 415　腹腔干及其分支（2）
Celiac trunk and its branches（2）

1. 胃网膜左动脉 left gastro-epiploic a.
2. 胃短动脉 short gastric a
3. 胃左动脉 left gastric a.
4. 脾动脉 splenic a.
5. 腹腔干 celiac trunk
6. 肠系膜上动脉 superior mesenteric a.
7. 胰十二指肠下前动脉 anterior inferior pancreaticoduodenal a.
8. 胰十二指肠上前动脉 anterior superior pancreaticoduodenal a
9. 胃十二指肠动脉 gastroduodenal a.
10. 肝门静脉 hepatic portal v.
11. 肝总动脉 common hepatic a.
12. 肝固有动脉 proper hepatic a.
13. 胃右动脉 right gastric a.
14. 胃网膜右动脉 right gastroepiploic a.
15. 肝 liver

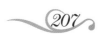

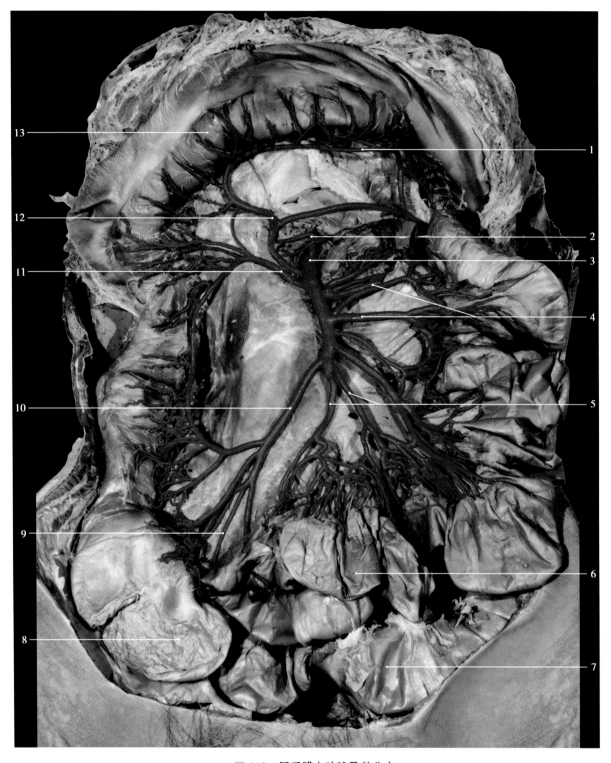

▲ 图 416　肠系膜上动脉及其分支
Superior mesenteric artery and its branches

1. 边缘动脉 marginal a.
2. 胰十二指肠下动脉 inferior pancreaticoduodenal a.
3. 肠系膜上动脉 superior mesenteric a.
4. 空肠动脉 jejunal a.
5. 回肠动脉 ileal a.
6. 回肠 ileum
7. 乙状结肠 sigmoid colon
8. 盲肠 cecum
9. 阑尾动脉 appendicular a.
10. 回结肠动脉 ileocolic a.
11. 右结肠动脉 right colic a.
12. 中结肠动脉 middle colic a.
13. 横结肠 transverse colon

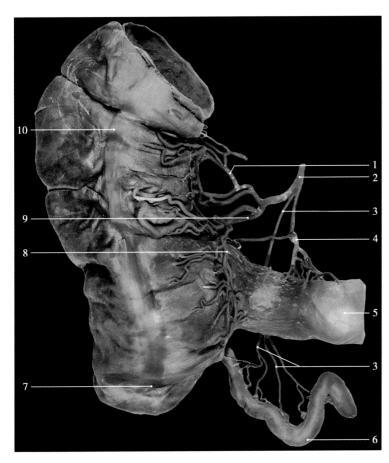

◄ 图 417

回结肠动脉及其分支
Ileocolic artery and its branches

1. 升支 ascending branch
2. 回结肠动脉 ileocolic a.
3. 阑尾动脉 appendicular a.
4. 回肠支 ileal branch
5. 回肠 ileum
6. 阑尾 vermiform appendix
7. 盲肠 cecum
8. 盲肠前动脉 anterior cecal a.
9. 盲肠后动脉 posterior cecal a.
10. 升结肠 ascending colon

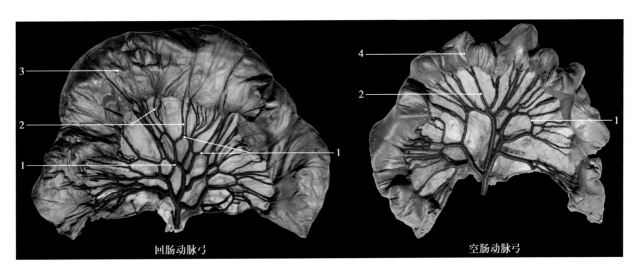

回肠动脉弓　　　　　　　　　空肠动脉弓

▲ 图 418　空、回肠动脉弓
Arterial arcades of ileum and jejunum

1. 动脉弓 arterial arcades　　3. 回肠 ileum
2. 直动脉 straight a.　　　　4. 空肠 jejunum

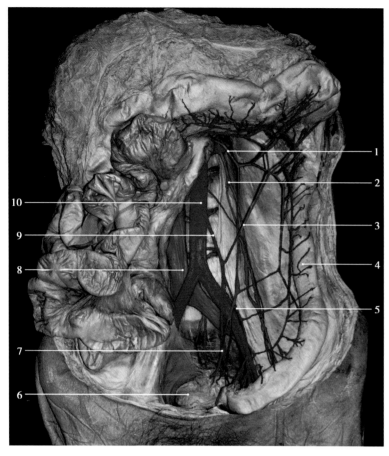

◀ 图 419

肠系膜下动脉及其分支
Inferior mesenteric artery and its branches
1. 肠系膜下静脉 inferior mesenteric v.
2. 睾丸静脉 testicular v.
3. 左结肠动脉 left colic a.
4. 降结肠 descending colon
5. 乙状结肠动脉 sigmoid a.
6. 直肠 rectum
7. 直肠上动脉 superior rectal a.
8. 下腔静脉 inferior vena cava
9. 肠系膜下动脉 inferior mesenteric a.
10. 腹主动脉 abdominal aorta

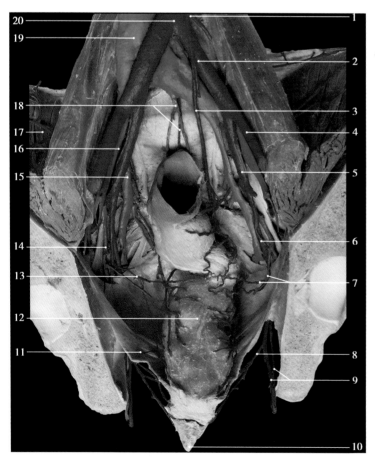

◀ 图 420

直肠和肛管的动脉(前面观)
Arteries of rectum and anal canal. Anterior aspect
1. 肠系膜下动脉 inferior mesenteric a.
2. 髂总动脉 common iliac a
3. 直肠上动脉 superior rectal a.
4. 髂外动脉 external iliac a.
5. 髂内动脉 internal iliac a.
6. 阴部内动脉 internal pudendal a.
7. 直肠下动、静脉 inferior rectal a. and v.
8. 肛动脉 anal a.
9. 阴部内动、静脉 internal pudendal a. and v.
10. 肛门外括约肌 sphincter ani externus
11. 肛提肌 levator ani
12. 直肠 rectum
13. 直肠下动脉 inferior rectal a.
14. 阴部内静脉 internal pudendal v.
15. 髂内静脉 internal iliac v.
16. 髂外静脉 external iliac v.
17. 髂肌 iliacus
18. 骶正中动、静脉 median sacral a. and v.
19. 下腔静脉 inferior vena cava
20. 腹主动脉 abdominal aorta

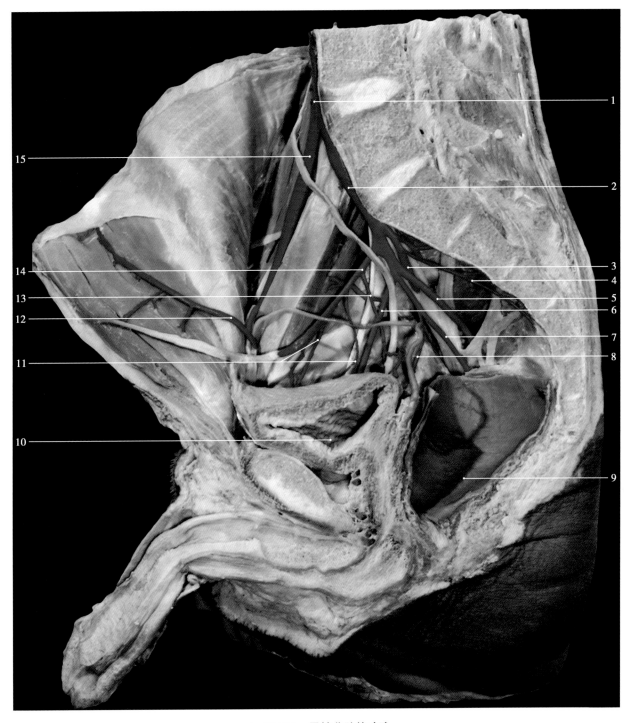

▲ 图 421　**男性盆腔的动脉**
Arteries of the male pelvic cavity

1. 髂总动脉 common iliac a.
2. 髂内动脉 internal iliac a.
3. 臀上动脉 superior gluteal a.
4. 骶外侧动脉 lateral sacral a.
5. 臀下动脉 inferior gluteal a.
6. 闭孔动脉 obturator a.
7. 阴部内动脉 internal pudendal a.
8. 直肠下动脉 inferior rectal a.
9. 直肠 rectum
10. 膀胱 urinary bladder
11. 膀胱上动脉 superior vesical a.
12. 腹壁下动脉 inferior epigastric a.
13. 膀胱下动脉 inferior vesical a.
14. 脐动脉 umbilical a.
15. 髂外动脉 external iliac a.

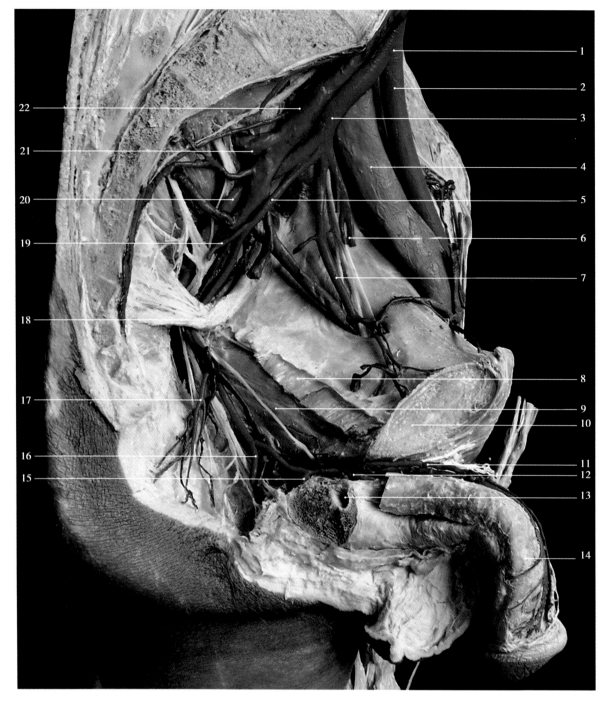

▲ 图 422　阴茎背动脉
Dorsal artery of penis

1. 髂总动脉 common iliac a.
2. 髂外动脉 external iliac a.
3. 髂内动脉 internal iliac a.
4. 髂外静脉 external iliac v.
5. 阴部内动脉 internal pudendal a.
6. 脐动脉 umbilical a.
7. 闭孔动脉 obturator a.
8. 肛提肌 levator ani
9. 闭孔内肌 obturator internus
10. 耻骨联合面 symphysial surface
11. 阴茎背动脉 dorsal artery of penis
12. 阴茎深动脉 deep artery of penis
13. 尿道 urethra
14. 阴茎 penis
15. 尿道球动脉 urethral bulbar a.
16. 阴囊后动脉 posterior scrotal a.
17. 肛动脉 anal a.
18. 坐骨棘 ischial spine
19. 直肠下动脉 inferior rectal a.
20. 臀下动脉 inferior gluteal a.
21. 臀上静脉 superior gluteal v.
22. 髂内静脉 internal iliac v.

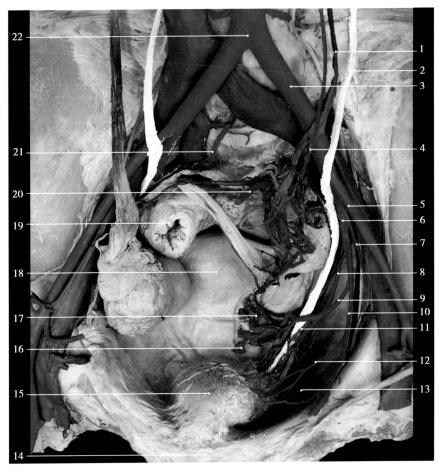

◀ 图 423　**女性盆腔的动脉**
Arteries of the female pelvic cavity
1. 卵巢静脉 ovarian v.
2. 输尿管 ureter
3. 髂总动脉 common iliac a.
4. 卵巢动脉 ovarian a.
5. 髂外动脉 external iliac a.
6. 髂内动脉 internal iliac a.
7. 闭孔动脉 obturator a.
8. 阴道动脉 vaginal a.
9. 子宫动脉 uterine a.
10. 脐动脉 umbilical a.
11. 子宫动脉输尿管支 ureteric branch of uterine a.
12. 膀胱上动脉 superior vesical a.
13. 膀胱下动脉 inferior vesical a.
14. 耻骨 pubis
15. 膀胱 urinary bladder
16. 子宫动脉阴道支 vaginal branch of uterine a.
17. 子宫动脉螺旋支 spiral branch of uterine a.
18. 子宫 uterus
19. 直肠 rectum
20. 直肠上动脉 superior rectal a.
21. 骶正中动脉 median sacral a.
22. 腹主动脉 abdominal aorta

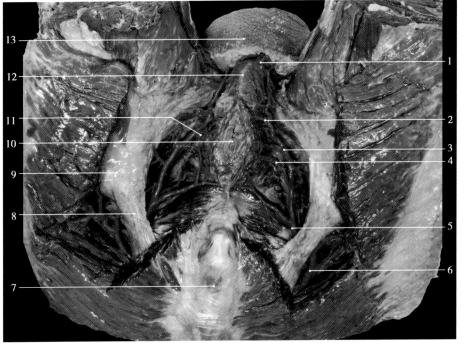

◀ 图 424
会阴部的动脉
Arteries of perineum
1. 阴囊后动脉 posterior scrotal a.
2. 尿道球动脉 urethral bulbar a.
3. 会阴动脉 perineal a.
4. 肛动脉 anal a.
5. 阴部内动脉 internal pudendal a.
6. 臀下动脉 inferior gluteal a.
7. 尾骨 coccyx
8. 骶结节韧带 sacrotuberal lig.
9. 坐骨结节 ischial tuberosity
10. 肛门 anus
11. 阴茎动脉 arteries of penis
12. 球海绵体肌 bulbocaver-nosus
13. 阴囊 scrotum

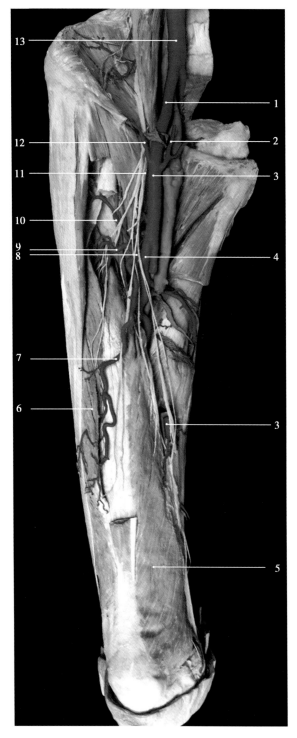

▲ 图425 股部的动脉（前面观）
Arteries of thigh. Anterior aspect

1. 髂外动脉 external iliac a.
2. 腹壁下动脉 inferior epigastric a.
3. 股动脉 femoral a.
4. 股深动脉 deep femoral a.
5. 股内侧肌 vastus medialis
6. 股外侧肌 vastus lateralis
7. 旋股外侧动脉降支 descending branch of lateral femoral circumflex a.
8. 旋股外侧动脉 lateral femoral circumflex a.
9. 旋股外侧动脉横支 transverse branch of lateral femoral circumflex a.
10. 旋股外侧动脉升支 ascending branch of lateral femoral circumflex a.
11. 股神经 femoral n.
12. 旋髂深动脉 deep iliac circumflex a.
13. 髂总动脉 common iliac a.

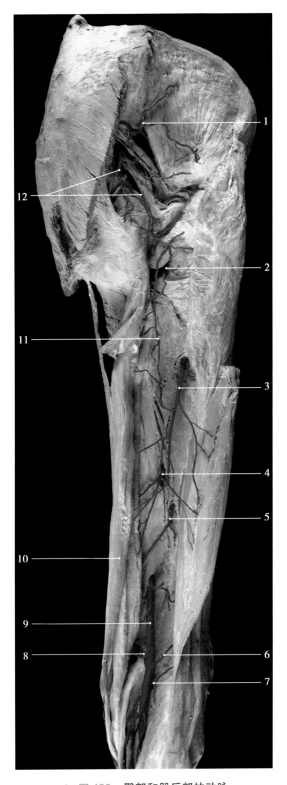

▲ 图 426 **臀部和股后部的动脉**
Arteries of gluteal and posterior femoral regions

1. 臀上动脉 superior gluteal a.
2. 旋股内侧动脉 medial femoral circumflex a.
3. 第 1 穿动脉 1st perforating a.
4. 第 2 穿动脉 2nd perforating a.
5. 第 3 穿动脉 3rd perforating a.
6. 膝上外侧动脉 lateral superior genicular a.
7. 膝中动脉 middle genicular a.
8. 膝上内侧动脉 medial superior genicular a.
9. 腘动脉 popliteal a.
10. 半腱肌 semitendinosus
11. 吻合支 ramus anastomoticus
12. 臀下动脉 inferior gluteal a.

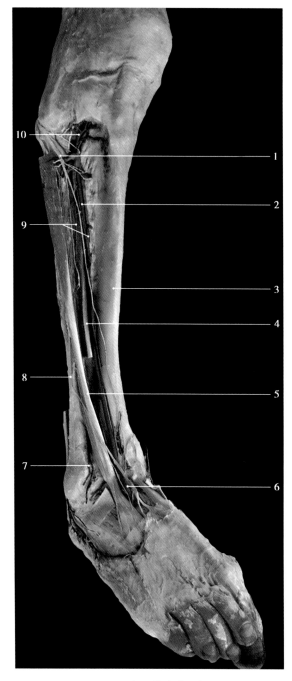

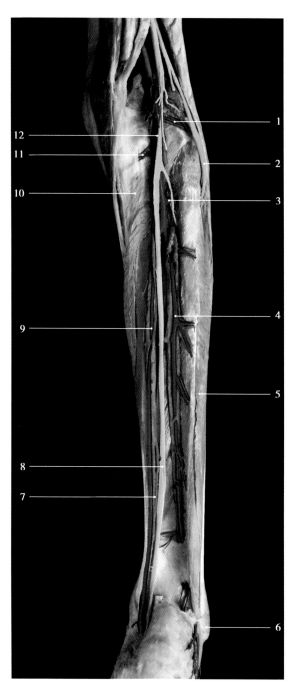

▲ 图 427　小腿的动脉 (前面观)
Arteries of leg. Anterior aspect

1. 腓深神经 deep peroneal n.
2. 胫前动脉 anterior tibial a.
3. 胫骨 tibia
4. 踇长伸肌 extensor hallucis longus
5. 趾长伸肌 extensor digitorum longus
6. 足背动脉 dorsal artery of foot
7. 腓动脉穿支 perforating branch of peroneal a.
8. 腓浅神经 superficial peroneal n.
9. 胫前静脉 anterior tibial v.
10. 胫前返动脉 anterior tibial recurrent a.

▲ 图 428　小腿的动脉 (后面观)
Arteries of leg. Posterior aspect

1. 膝下外侧动脉 lateral inferior genicular a.
2. 腓总神经 common peroneal n.
3. 胫前动脉 anterior tibial a.
4. 腓动脉 fibular a.
5. 腓骨短肌 peroneus brevis
6. 外踝 lateral malleolus
7. 胫后静脉 posterior tibial v.
8. 胫神经 tibial n.
9. 胫后动脉 posterior tibial a.
10. 腘肌 popliteus
11. 膝下内侧动脉 medial inferior genicular a.
12. 腘动脉 popliteal a.

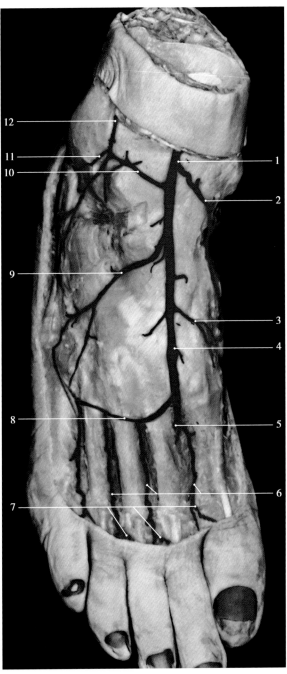

▲ 图 429　足背的动脉
Arteries of the dorsum of foot

1. 胫前动脉 anterior tibial a.
2. 内踝前动脉 medial anterior malleolar a.
3. 跗内侧动脉 medial tarsal a.
4. 足背动脉 dorsal artery of foot
5. 足底深支 deep plantar branch
6. 跖背动脉 dorsal metatarsal a.
7. 趾背动脉 dorsal digital a.
8. 弓状动脉 arcuate a.
9. 跗外侧动脉 lateral tarsal a.
10. 外踝前动脉 lateral anterior malleolar a.
11. 外踝网 lateral malleolar rete
12. 腓动脉穿支 perforating branch of peroneal a.

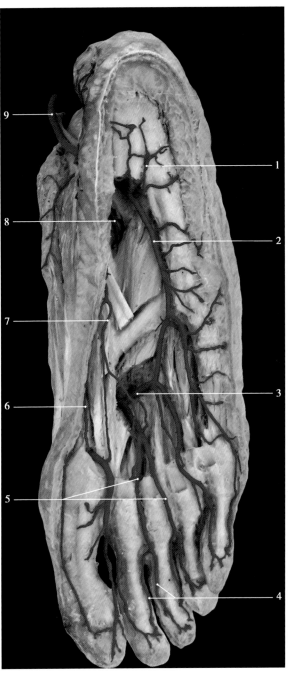

▲ 图 430　足底的动脉
Plantar arteries

1. 跟网 calcaneal rete
2. 足底外侧动脉 lateral plantar a.
3. 足底弓 plantar arch
4. 趾足底固有动脉 proper plantar digital a.
5. 跖足底总动脉 common plantar metatarsal a.
6. 足底内侧动脉浅支 superficial branch of medial plantar a.
7. 足底内侧动脉深支 deep branch of medial plantar a.
8. 足底内侧动脉 medial plantar a.
9. 胫后动脉 posterior tibial a.

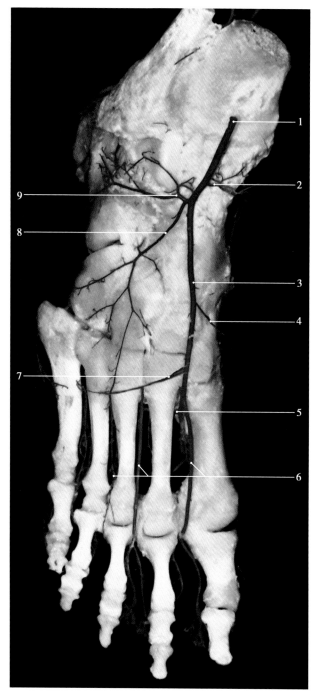

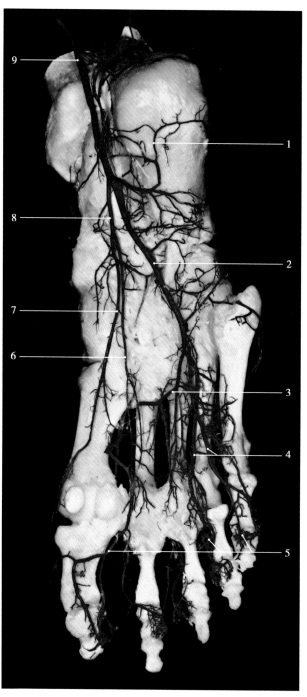

▲ 图 431　足的动脉铸型（上面观）
Cast of arteries of foot. Superior aspect
1. 胫前动脉 anterior tibial a.
2. 内踝前动脉 medial anterior malleolar a.
3. 足背动脉 dorsal artery of foot
4. 跗内侧动脉 medial tarsal a.
5. 足底深支 deep plantar branch
6. 跖背动脉 dorsal metatarsal a.
7. 弓状动脉 arcuate a.
8. 跗外侧动脉 lateral tarsal a.
9. 外踝前动脉 lateral anterior malleolar a.

▲ 图 432　足的动脉铸型（下面观）
Cast of arteries of foot. Inferior aspect
1. 跟网 calcaneal rete
2. 足底外侧动脉 lateral plantar a.
3. 足底弓 plantar arch
4. 跖足底总动脉 common plantar metatarsus a.
5. 趾足底固有动脉 proper plantar digital a.
6. 深支 deep branch
7. 浅支 superficial branch
8. 足底内侧动脉 medial plantar a.
9. 胫后动脉 posterior tibial a.

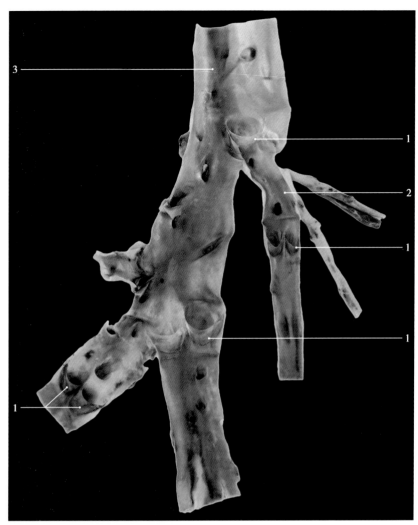

◀ 图 433

静脉瓣
Venous valve

1. 静脉瓣 venous valve
2. 大隐静脉 great saphenous v.
3. 股静脉 femoral v.

图 434 ▶

板障管
Diploic canals

1. 枕板障管 occipital diploic canals
2. 板障 diploë
3. 枕骨大孔 foramen magnum of occipital bone
4. 枕骨 occipital bone

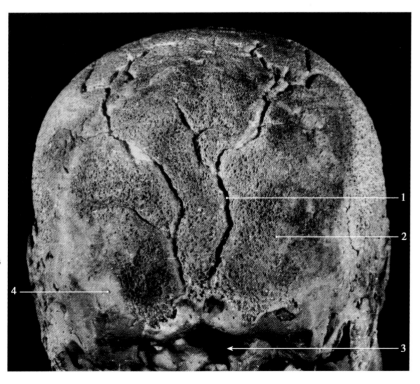

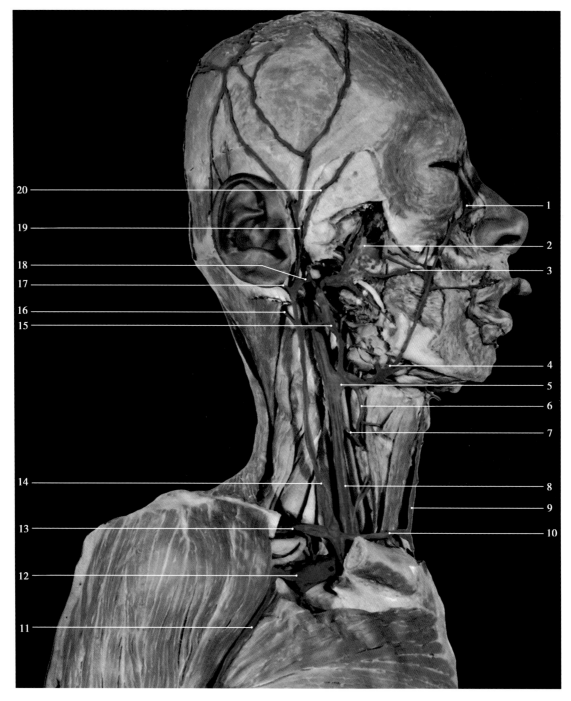

▲ 图 435　头颈部的静脉（侧面观）
Veins of head and neck. Lateral aspect

1. 内眦静脉 angular v.
2. 翼静脉丛 pterygoid venous plexus
3. 面深静脉 deep facial v.
4. 面静脉 facial v.
5. 面总静脉 common facial v.
6. 甲状腺上静脉 superior thyroid v.
7. 甲状腺中静脉 middle thyroid v.
8. 颈内静脉 internal jugular v.
9. 颈前静脉 anterior jugular v.
10. 颈静脉弓 jugular venous arch

11. 头静脉 cephalic v.
12. 锁骨下静脉 subclavian v.
13. 肩胛背静脉 dorsal scapular v.
14. 颈外静脉 external jugular v.
15. 下颌后静脉 retromandibular v.
16. 枕静脉 occipital v.
17. 耳后静脉 posterior auricular v.
18. 上颌静脉 maxillary v.
19. 颞浅静脉 superficial temporal v.
20. 颞中静脉 middle temporal v.

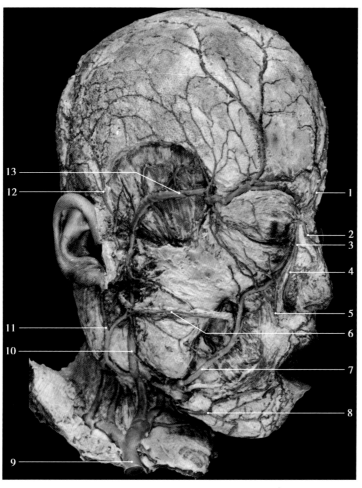

◀ 图 436

面静脉
Facial vein

1. 滑车上静脉 supratrochlear v.
2. 鼻背静脉 dorsal nasal v.
3. 内眦静脉 angular v.
4. 鼻外静脉 external nasal v.
5. 上唇静脉 superior labial v.
6. 面横静脉 facial transverse v.
7. 面静脉 facial v.
8. 下唇静脉 inferior labial v.
9. 颈外静脉 external jugular v.
10. 下颌后静脉 retromandibular v.
11. 耳后静脉 posterior auricular v.
12. 颞浅静脉 superficial temporal v.
13. 颞中静脉 middle temporal v.

图 437 ▶

翼静脉丛
Pterygoid venous plexus

1. 颞中静脉 middle temporal v.
2. 颞深静脉 deep temporal v.
3. 翼静脉丛 pterygoid venous plexus
4. 面深静脉 deep facial v.
5. 面静脉 facial v.
6. 颈外静脉 external jugular v.
7. 下颌后静脉前支 anterior branch of retromandibular
8. 下颌后静脉 retromandibular v.
9. 上颌静脉 maxillary v.
10. 颞浅静脉 superficial temporal v.

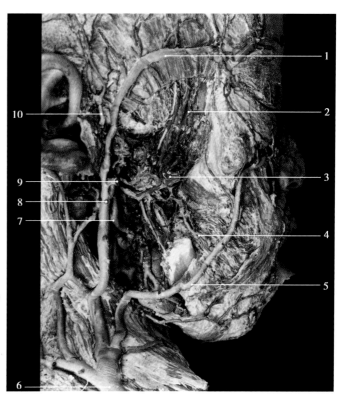

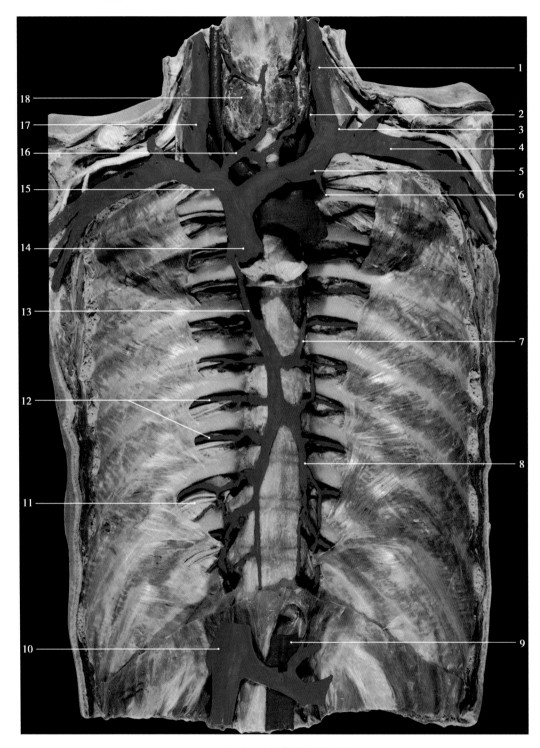

▲ 图 438　上腔静脉及其属支
Superior vena cava and its tributaries

1. 左颈内静脉 left internal jugular v.
2. 椎静脉 vertebral v.
3. 静脉角 venous angle
4. 左锁骨下静脉 left subclavian v.
5. 左头臂静脉 left brachiocephalic v.
6. 肋间最上静脉 highest intercostal v.
7. 副半奇静脉 accessory hemiazygos v.
8. 半奇静脉 hemiazygous v.
9. 腹主动脉 abdominal aorta
10. 下腔静脉 inferior vena cava
11. 肋间神经 intercostal n.
12. 肋间后静脉 posterior intercostal v.
13. 奇静脉 azygos v.
14. 上腔静脉 superior vena cava
15. 右头臂静脉 right brachiocephalic v.
16. 甲状腺下静脉 inferior thyroid v.
17. 右颈内静脉 right internal jugular v.
18. 甲状腺 thyroid gland

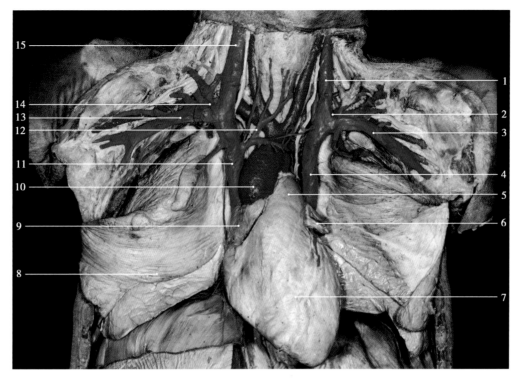

▲ 图 439 双上腔静脉
Double superior vena cave

1. 左颈内静脉 left internal jugular v.
2. 左静脉角 left venous angle
3. 左锁骨下静脉 left subclavian v.
4. 左上腔静脉 left superior vena cava
5. 肺动脉干 pulmonary trunk
6. 左心耳 left auricle
7. 心 heart
8. 右肺 right lung
9. 右心耳 right auricle
10. 升主动脉 ascending aorta
11. 右上腔静脉 right superior vena cava
12. 甲状腺下静脉 inferior thyroid v.
13. 右锁骨下静脉 right subclavian v.
14. 右静脉角 right venous angle
15. 右颈内静脉 right internal jugular v.

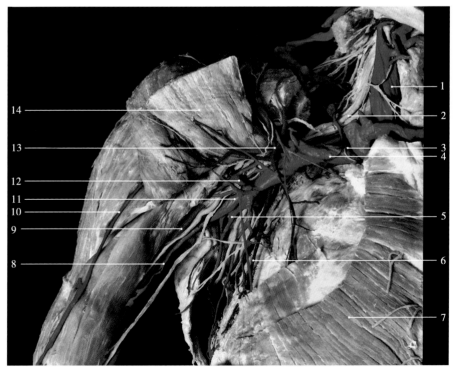

◀ 图 440

锁骨下静脉和腋静脉
Subclavian vein and axillary vein

1. 颈内静脉 internal jugular v.
2. 臂丛 brachial plexus
3. 右淋巴导管 right lymphatic duct
4. 锁骨下静脉 subclavian v.
5. 胸背静脉 thoracodorsal v.
6. 胸外侧动脉 lateral thoracic a.
7. 胸大肌 pectoralis major
8. 肱静脉 brachial v.
9. 肱动脉 brachial a.
10. 头静脉 cephalic v.
11. 腋静脉 axillary v.
12. 旋肱前静脉 anterior humeral circumflex v.
13. 胸肩峰动脉 thoracoacromial a.
14. 胸小肌 pectoralis minor

223

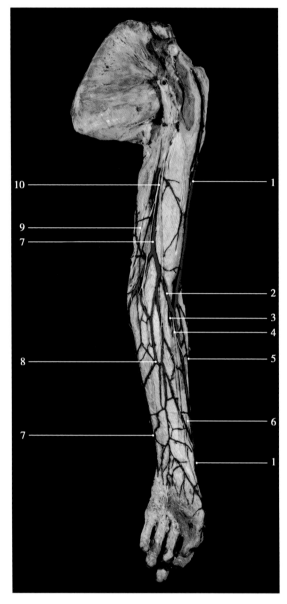

▲ 图 441　上肢浅静脉
Superficial veins of upper limb

1. 头静脉 cephalic v.
2. 肘正中静脉 median cubital v.
3. 深、浅静脉交通支 communicating branch between superficial and deep v.
4. 前臂外侧皮神经 lateral antebrachial cutaneous n.
5. 副头静脉 accessory cephalic v.
6. 桡神经浅支 superficial branch of radial n.
7. 贵要静脉 basilic v.
8. 前臂正中静脉 median antebrachial v.
9. 臂内侧皮神经 medial brachial cutaneous n.
10. 前臂内侧皮神经 medial antebrachial cutaneous n.

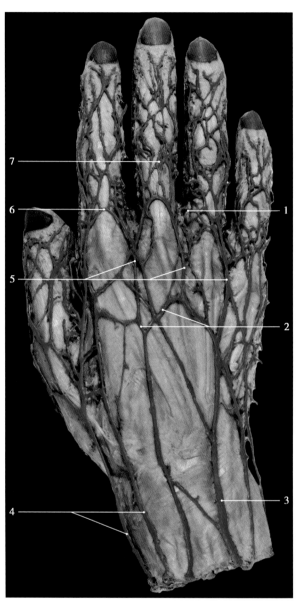

▲ 图 442　手背的浅静脉
Superficial veins of dorsum of hand

1. 掌骨头间静脉 intercapital v.
2. 手背静脉网 dorsal venous rete of hand
3. 贵要静脉 basilic v.
4. 头静脉 cephalic v.
5. 掌背静脉 dorsal metacarpal v.
6. 指静脉弓 digital venous arch
7. 指背静脉 dorsal digital v.

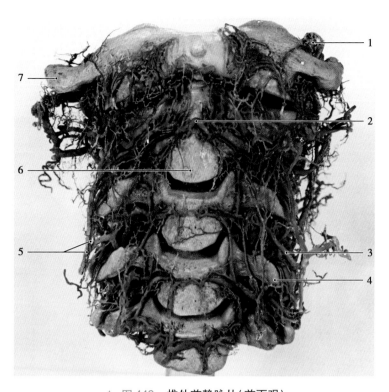

▲ 图 443 **椎外前静脉丛（前面观）**
Anterior external vertebral venous plexus. Anterior aspect

1. 椎静脉 vertebral v.
2. 椎外前静脉丛 anterior external vertebral venous plexus
3. 椎间静脉 intervertebral v.
4. 横突 transverse process
5. 颈升动、静脉 ascending cervical a. and v.
6. 椎体 vertebral body
7. 寰椎横突 transverse process of atlas

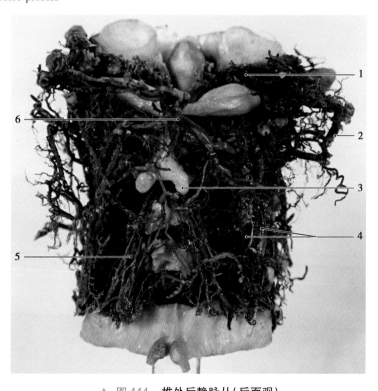

▲ 图 444 **椎外后静脉丛（后面观）**
Posterior external vertebral venous plexus. Posterior aspect

1. 椎动脉旁静脉丛 venous plexus around vertebral a.
2. 枕动脉降支 descending branch of occipital a.
3. 棘突 spinous process
4. 颈深动、静脉 deep cervical a. and v.
5. 椎外后静脉丛 posterior external vertebral venous plexus
6. 枕下静脉丛 suboccipital venous plexus

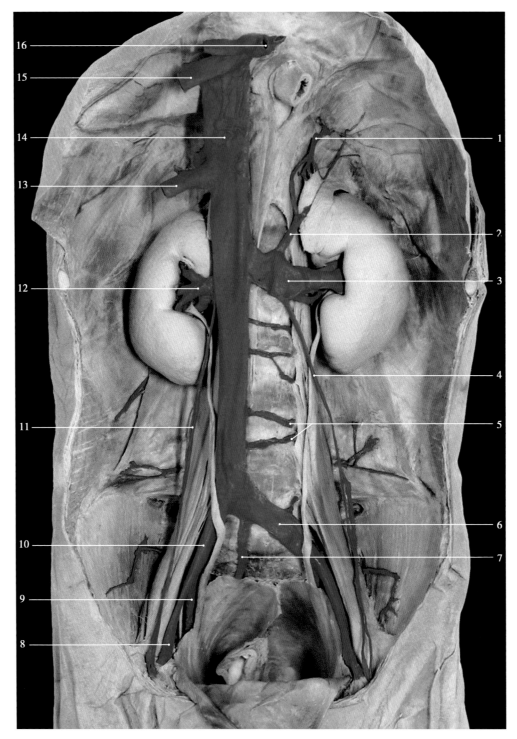

▲ 图445　下腔静脉及其属支
Inferior vena cava and its tributaries

1. 膈下静脉 inferior phrenic v.
2. 左肾上腺静脉 left suprarenal v.
3. 左肾静脉 left renal v.
4. 左睾丸静脉 left testicular v.
5. 腰静脉 lumbar v.
6. 左髂总静脉 left common iliac v.
7. 骶正中静脉 median sacral v.
8. 髂外静脉 external iliac v.

9. 髂内静脉 internal iliac v.
10. 右髂总静脉 right common iliac v.
11. 右睾丸静脉 right testicular v.
12. 右肾静脉 right renal v.
13. 肝右后静脉 right posterior hepatic v.
14. 下腔静脉 inferior vena cava
15. 肝右静脉 right hepatic v.
16. 肝左静脉 left hepatic v.

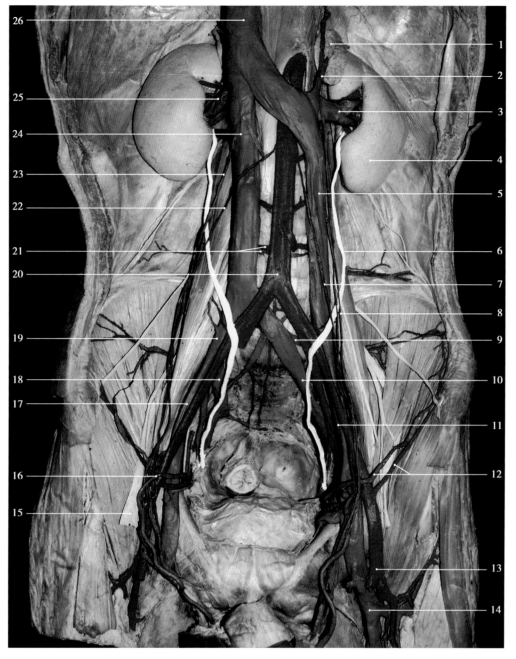

▲ 图 446　双下腔静脉
Double inferior vena cave

1. 左肾上腺 left suprarenal gland
2. 左肾上腺静脉 left suprarenal v.
3. 左肾静脉 left renal v.
4. 左肾 left kidney
5. 左下腔静脉 left inferior vena cava
6. 左输尿管 left ureter
7. 左睾丸动脉 left testicular a.
8. 左睾丸静脉 left testicular v.
9. 吻合支 anastomotic branch
10. 左髂内静脉 left internal iliac v.
11. 左髂外静脉 left external iliac v.
12. 旋髂深动、静脉 deep iliac circumflex a. and v.
13. 股动脉 femoral a.
14. 股静脉 femoral v.
15. 股神经 femoral n.
16. 输精管 ductus deferens
17. 右髂外静脉 right external iliac v.
18. 右髂内静脉 right internal iliac v.
19. 右髂总静脉 right common iliac v.
20. 腹主动脉 abdominal aorta
21. 腰动、静脉 lumbar a. and v.
22. 右睾丸动脉 right testicular a.
23. 右睾丸静脉 right testicular v.
24. 右下腔静脉 right inferior vena cava
25. 右肾静脉 right renal v.
26. 总下腔静脉 common inferior vena cava

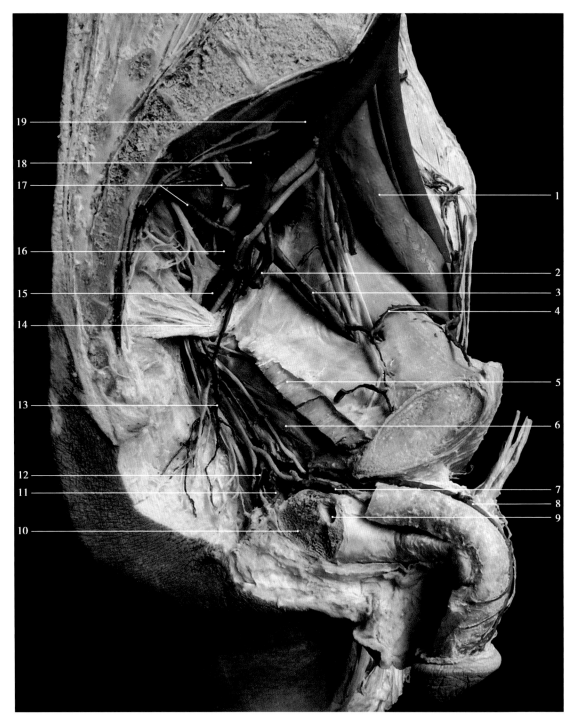

▲ 图 447　盆部的静脉
Veins of pelvis

1. 髂外静脉 external iliac v.
2. 膀胱静脉 vesical v.
3. 闭孔静脉 obturator v.
4. 耻静脉 pubic v.
5. 肛提肌 levator ani
6. 闭孔内肌 obturator internus
7. 阴茎深静脉 deep vein of penis
8. 阴茎背深静脉 deep dorsal vein of penis
9. 尿道 urethra
10. 尿道球 bulb of urethra
11. 尿道球静脉 urethral bulbar v.
12. 阴囊后静脉 posterior scrotal v.
13. 肛静脉 anal v.
14. 坐骨棘 ischial spine
15. 阴部内静脉 interal pudendal v.
16. 臀下静脉 inferior gluteal v.
17. 骶外侧静脉 lateral sacral v.
18. 臀上静脉 superior gluteal v.
19. 髂内静脉 internal iliac v.

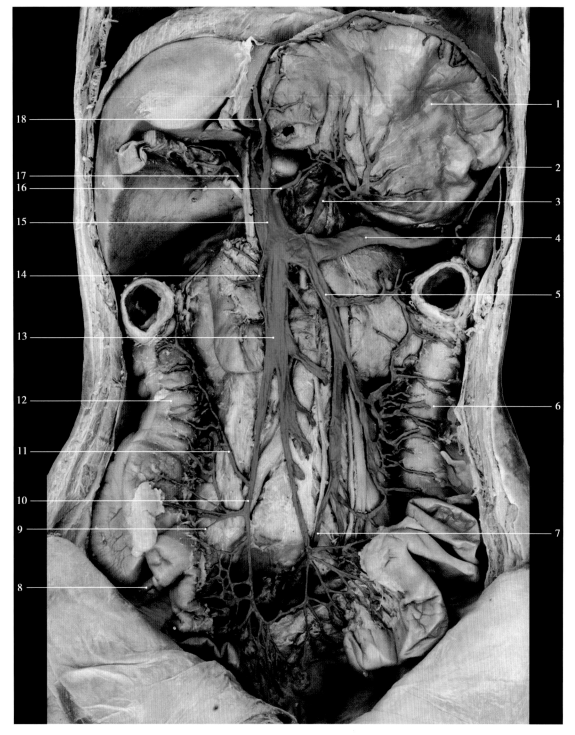

▲ 图 448　肝门静脉及其属支
Hepatic portal vein and its tributaries

1. 胃 stomach
2. 胃网膜左静脉 left gastroepiploic v.
3. 胃左静脉 left gastric v.
4. 脾静脉 splenic v.
5. 肠系膜下静脉 inferior mesenteric v.
6. 降结肠 descending colon
7. 直肠上静脉 superior rectal v.
8. 阑尾 vermiform appendix
9. 阑尾静脉 appendicular v.
10. 回结肠静脉 ileocolic v.
11. 右结肠静脉 right colic v.
12. 升结肠 ascending colon
13. 肠系膜上静脉 superior mesenteric v.
14. 胰十二指肠上前静脉 anterior superior pancreaticoduodenal v.
15. 肝门静脉 hepatic portal v.
16. 胃右静脉 right gastric v.
17. 胆囊静脉 cystic v.
18. 胃网膜右静脉 right gastroepiploic v.

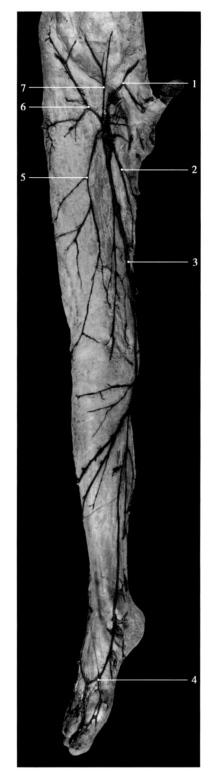

▲ 图 449　大隐静脉及其属支
Great saphenous vein and its tributaries

1. 阴部外静脉 external pudendal v.
2. 股内侧浅静脉 medial femoral superficial v.
3. 大隐静脉 great saphenous v.
4. 足背静脉弓 dorsal venous arch of foot
5. 股外侧浅静脉 lateral femoral superficial v.
6. 旋髂浅静脉 superficial iliac circumflex v.
7. 腹壁浅静脉 superficial epigastric v.

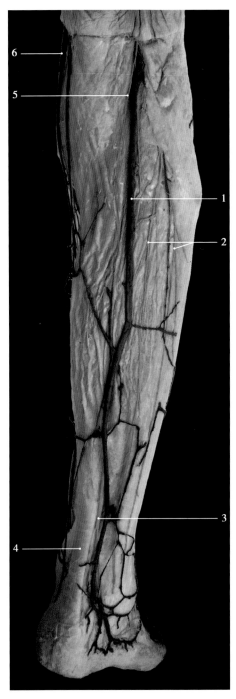

▲ 图 450　小隐静脉
Small saphenous vein

1. 小隐静脉 small saphenous v.
2. 腓肠外侧皮神经 lateral sural cutaneous n.
3. 腓肠神经 sural n.
4. 跟腱 tendo calcaneus
5. 股后皮神经 posterior femoral cutaneous n.
6. 大隐静脉 great saphenous v.

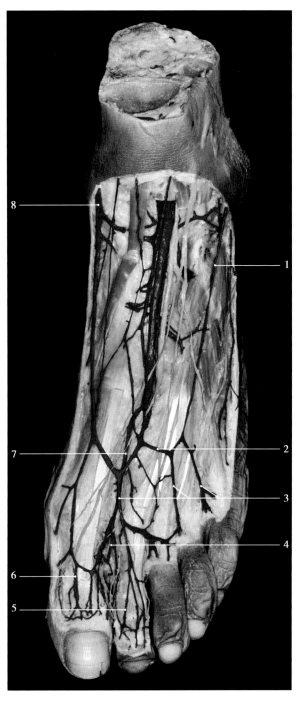

▲ 图 451　足背静脉
Dorsal veins of foot

1. 小隐静脉 small saphenous v.
2. 足背静脉弓 dorsal venous arch of foot
3. 跖背静脉 dorsal metatarsal v.
4. 跖骨头间静脉 intercapital metatarsal v.
5. 趾背静脉 dorsal digital v.
6. 踇趾内侧趾背静脉 dorsal digital vein in medial of hallux
7. 第 1 跖背动脉 1st dorsal metatarsal a.
8. 大隐静脉 great saphenous v.

第十章　淋巴系统
Lymphatic System

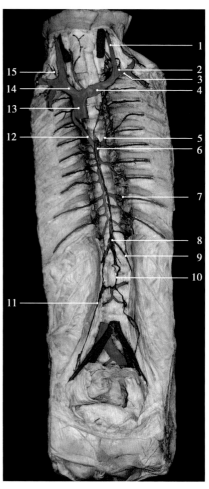

▲ 图 452　淋巴导管
Lymphatic ducts

1. 左颈内静脉 left internal jugular v.
2. 左静脉角 left venous angle
3. 左锁骨下静脉 left subclavian v.
4. 左头臂静脉 left brachiocephalic v.
5. 副半奇静脉 accessory hemiazygos v.
6. 胸导管 thoracic duct
7. 肋间后静脉 posterior intercostal v.
8. 乳糜池 cisterna chyli
9. 肠干 interstinal trunk
10. 左腰干 left lumbar trunk
11. 右腰干 right lumbar trunk
12. 奇静脉 azygos v.
13. 上腔静脉 superior vena cava
14. 右头臂静脉 right brachiocephalic v.
15. 右淋巴导管 right lymphatic duct

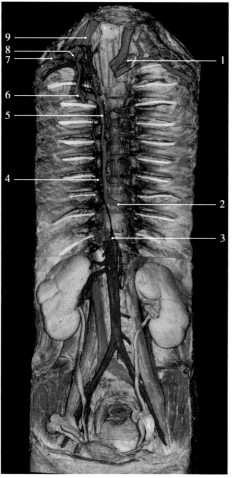

▲ 图 453　右位胸导管
Right thoracic duct(出现率 0. 66%)

1. 左淋巴导管 left lymphatic duct
2. 半奇静脉 hemiazygos v.
3. 乳糜池 cisterna chyli
4. 胸导管 thoracic duct
5. 奇静脉 azygos v.
6. 上腔静脉 superior vena cava
7. 右锁骨下静脉 right subclavian v.
8. 右静脉角 right venous angle
9. 右颈内静脉 right internal jugular v.

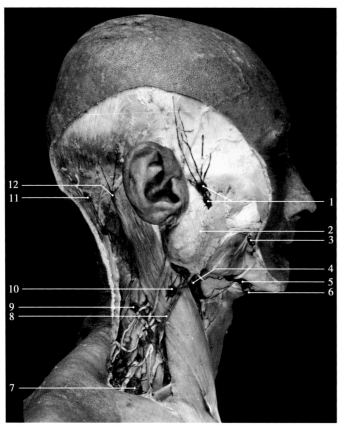

◀ 图 454

颈部的淋巴管和淋巴结(1)
Lymph vessels and nodes of neck（1）

1. 腮腺浅淋巴结 superficial parotid lymph nodes
2. 腮腺 parotid gland
3. 颊肌淋巴结 buccal lymph node
4. 颈内静脉二腹肌淋巴结 jugulodigastric lymph node
5. 下颌下淋巴结 submandibular lymph nodes
6. 颏下淋巴结 submental lymph nodes
7. 锁骨上淋巴结 supraclavicular lymph nodes
8. 颈外静脉 external jugular v.
9. 副神经淋巴结 lymph nodes of accessory n.
10. 颈外侧浅淋巴结 superficial lateral cervical lymph node
11. 枕淋巴结 occipital lymph nodes
12. 乳突淋巴结 mastoid lymph nodes

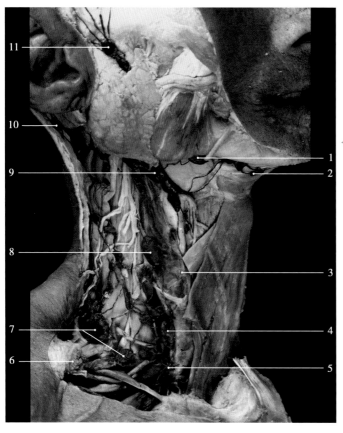

◀ 图 455

颈部的淋巴管和淋巴结(2)
Lymph vessels and nodes of neck(2)

1. 下颌下淋巴结 submandibular lymph nodes
2. 颏下淋巴结 submental lymph nodes
3. 颈内静脉 internal jugular v.
4. 颈外侧下深淋巴结 inferior deep lateral cervical lymph nodes
5. 右淋巴导管 right lymphatic duct
6. 锁骨 clavicle
7. 锁骨上淋巴结 supraclavicular lymph nodes
8. 颈内静脉肩胛舌骨肌淋巴结 juguloomohyoid lymph node
9. 颈内静脉二腹肌淋巴结 jugulodigastric lymph node
10. 乳突淋巴结 mastoid lymph nodes
11. 腮腺浅淋巴结 superficial parotid lymph nodes

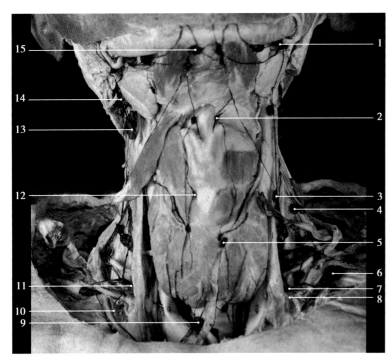

◀ 图 456
颈深部淋巴管和淋巴结 (前面观)
Deep lymph vessels and nodes of neck.
Anterior aspect
1. 下颌下淋巴结 submandibular lymph nodes
2. 舌骨下淋巴结 infrahyoid lymph nodes
3. 颈内静脉外侧淋巴结 lateral jugular lymph nodes
4. 颈内静脉肩胛舌骨肌淋巴结 juguloomohy-oid lymph node
5. 甲状腺淋巴结 thyroid lymph nodes
6. 锁骨上淋巴结 supraclavicular lymph nodes
7. 胸导管 thoracic duct
8. 左静脉角 left venous angle
9. 气管前淋巴结 pretracheal lymph nodes
10. 右支气管纵隔干 right bronchomediastinal trunk
11. 右淋巴导管 right lymphatic duct
12. 喉前淋巴结 prelaryngeal lymph nodes
13. 颈内静脉前淋巴结 anterior jugular lymph node
14. 颈内静脉二腹肌淋巴结 jugulodigastric lymph nodes
15. 颏下淋巴结 submental lymph nodes

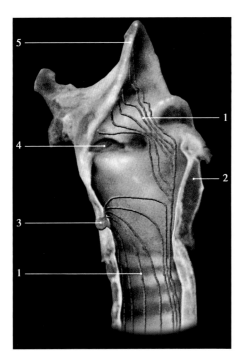

▲ 图 457 喉的淋巴 (矢状切面)
Laryngeal lymph. Sagittal section
1. 淋巴管 lymphatic vessel
2. 甲状软骨 thyroid cartilage
3. 喉前淋巴结 prelaryngeal lymph nodes
4. 喉室 ventricle of larynx
5. 会厌 epiglottis

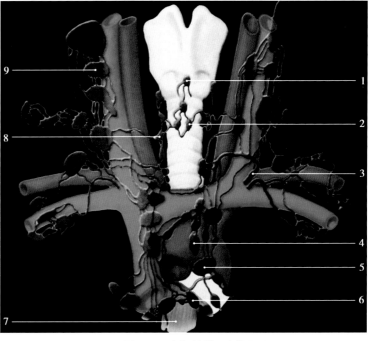

▲ 图 458 喉部的淋巴 (前面观)
Laryngeal lymph. Anterior aspect
1. 喉前淋巴结 prelaryngeal lymph nodes
2. 气管前淋巴结 pretracheal node
3. 胸导管 thoracic duct
4. 纵隔前淋巴结 anterior mediastinal lymph nodes
5. 气管支气管上淋巴结 superior tracheobronchial lymph nodes
6. 气管支气管下淋巴结 inferior tracheobronchial lymph nodes
7. 食管 esophagus
8. 气管旁淋巴结 paratracheal lymph nodes
9. 颈内静脉外侧淋巴结 lateral jugular lymph nodes

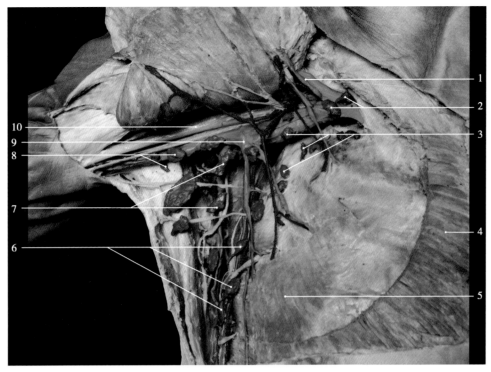

▲ 图 459　腋淋巴结
Axillary lymph nodes

1. 头静脉 cephalic v.
2. 尖淋巴结 apical lymph nodes
3. 中央淋巴结 central lymph nodes
4. 胸大肌 pectoralis major
5. 胸小肌 pectoralis minor
6. 胸肌淋巴结 pectoral lymph nodes
7. 肩胛下淋巴结 subscapular lymph nodes
8. 外侧淋巴结 lateral lymph nodes
9. 腋静脉 axillary v.
10. 正中神经 median n.

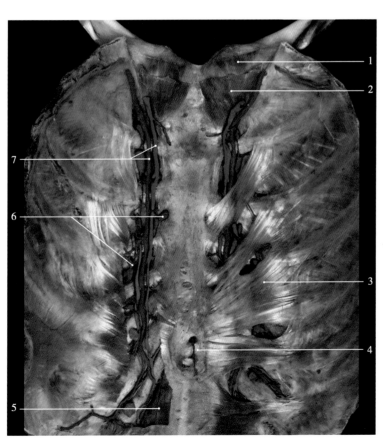

◀ 图 460

胸骨旁淋巴结
Parasternal lymph nodes

1. 胸骨舌骨肌 sternohyoid
2. 胸骨甲状肌 sternothyroid
3. 胸横肌 transversus thoracis
4. 剑突 xiphoid process
5. 腹直肌 rectus abdominis
6. 胸骨旁淋巴结 parasternal lymph nodes
7. 胸廓内动、静脉 internal thoracic a. and v.

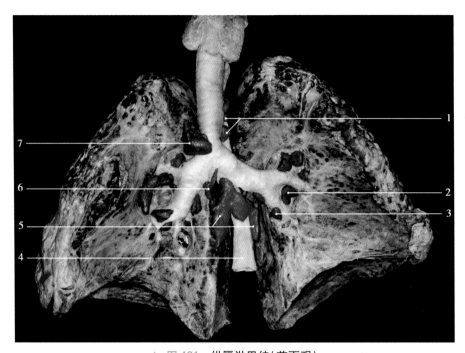

▲ 图 461 纵隔淋巴结(前面观)
Mediastinal lymph nodes. Anterior aspect

1. 气管旁淋巴结 paratracheal lymph nodes
2. 支气管肺淋巴结 bronchopulmonary lymph nodes
3. 肺淋巴结 pulmonary lymph nodes
4. 食管 esophagus
5. 纵隔后淋巴结 posterior mediastinal lymph nodes
6. 气管支气管下淋巴结 inferior tracheobronchial lymph nodes
7. 气管支气管上淋巴结 superior tracheobronchial lymph nodes

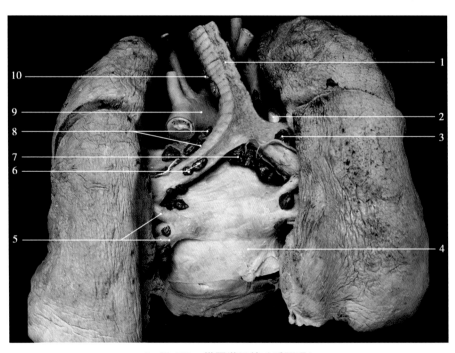

▲ 图 462 纵隔淋巴结（后面观）
Mediastinal lymph nodes. Posterior aspect

1. 气管 trachea
2. 奇静脉 azygos v.
3. 支气管肺淋巴结 bronchopulmonary lymph nodes
4. 心包 pericardium
5. 肺静脉 pulmonary v.
6. 左支气管淋巴结 left bronchial lymph nodes
7. 气管支气管下淋巴结 inferior tracheobronchial lymph nodes
8. 气管支气管上淋巴结 superior tracheobronchial lymph nodes
9. 主动脉弓 aortic arch
10. 气管旁淋巴结 paratracheal lymph nodes

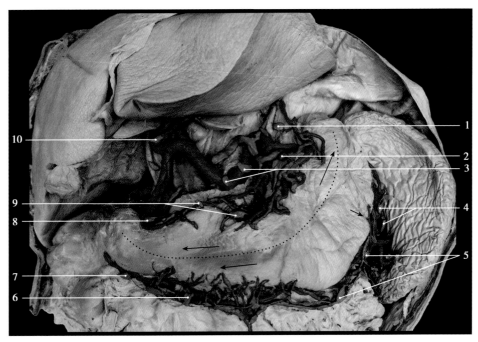

▲ 图463　胃的淋巴管和淋巴结
Lymph vessels and nodes of stomach

1. 贲门淋巴结 cardiac lymph node
2. 胃左淋巴结 left gastric lymph node
3. 腹腔淋巴结 celiac lymph nodes
4. 脾淋巴结 splenic lymph node
5. 胃网膜左淋巴结 left gastroepiploic lymph nodes

6. 胃网膜右淋巴结 right gastroepiploic lymph nodes
7. 幽门下淋巴结 subpyloric lymph node
8. 幽门上淋巴结 suprapyloric lymph node
9. 胃右淋巴结 right gastric lymph nodes
10. 肝淋巴结 hepatic lymph nodes

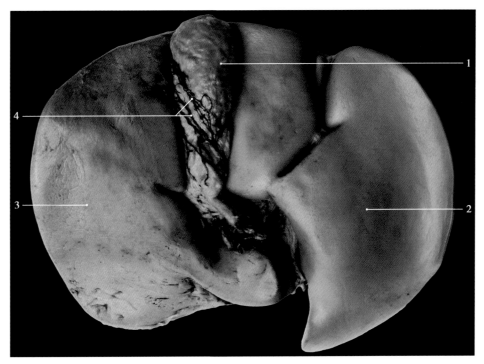

▲ 图464　胆囊的淋巴管
Lymph vessels of gallbladder

1. 胆囊 gallbladder
2. 肝左叶 left lobe of liver
3. 肝右叶 right lobe of live
4. 胆囊淋巴管 lymph vessel of gallbladder

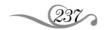

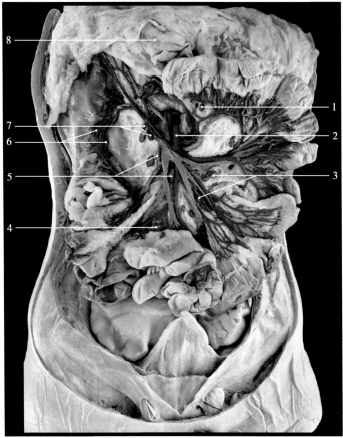

◀ 图 465

肠系膜上淋巴结
Superior mesenteric lymph nodes
1. 肠淋巴结 intestinal lymph node
2. 肠系膜上动脉 superior mesenteric a.
3. 肠系膜淋巴结 mesenteric lymph nodes
4. 回结肠淋巴结 ileocolic lymph nodes
5. 肠系膜上淋巴结 superior mesenteric lymph nodes
6. 右结肠淋巴结 right colic lymph nodes
7. 中结肠淋巴结 middle colic lymph nodes
8. 横结肠 transverse colon

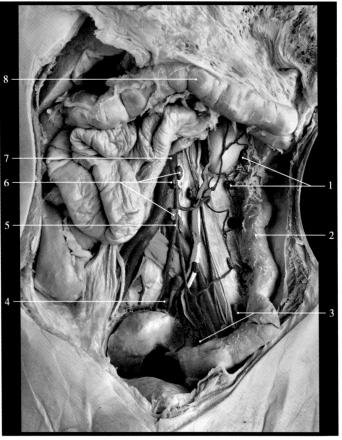

◀ 图 466

肠系膜下淋巴结
Inferior mesenteric lymph nodes
1. 左结肠淋巴结 left colic lymph nodes
2. 降结肠 descending colon
3. 乙状结肠淋巴结 sigmoid lymph nodes
4. 直肠上淋巴结 superior rectal lymph nodes
5. 肠系膜下动脉 inferior mesenteric a.
6. 肠系膜下淋巴结 inferior mesenteric lymph nodes
7. 腹主动脉 abdominal aorta
8. 横结肠 transverse colon

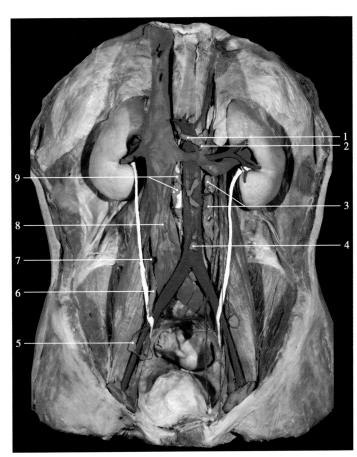

◀ 图 467

腹膜后间隙的淋巴结
Lymph nodes of retroperitoneal space

1. 腹腔淋巴结 celiac lymph nodes
2. 肠系膜上淋巴结 superior mesenteric lymph nodes
3. 主动脉外侧淋巴结 lateral aortic nodes
4. 肠系膜下淋巴结 inferior mesenteric lymph nodes
5. 髂外淋巴结 lateral iliac lymph nodes
6. 髂总淋巴结 common iliac lymph nodes
7. 腔静脉外侧淋巴结 lateral caval lymph nodes
8. 腔静脉前淋巴结 precaval lymph nodes
9. 中间腰淋巴结 intermediate lumbar lymph nodes

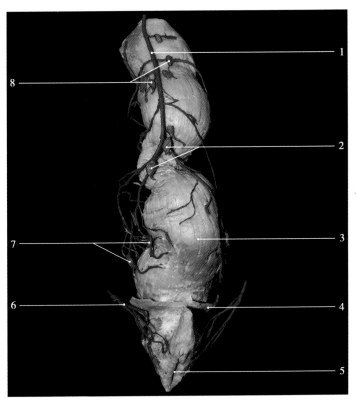

◀ 图 468

直肠旁淋巴结(后面观)
Lymph nodes beside rectum. Posterior aspect

1. 直肠上动脉 superior rectal a.
2. 直肠后淋巴结 posterior rectal lymph nodes
3. 直肠骶曲 sacral flexure of rectum
4. 肛提肌 levator ani
5. 肛门 anus
6. 肛动脉 anal a.
7. 直肠下淋巴结 inferior rectal lymph nodes
8. 直肠上淋巴结 superior rectal lymph nodes

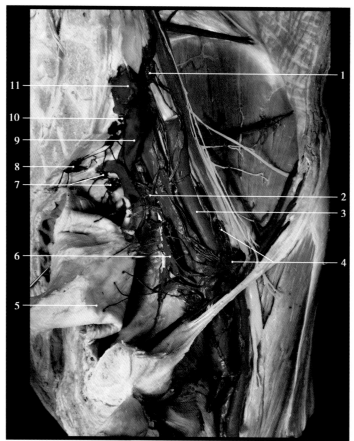

◀ 图 469

男性盆腔淋巴管及淋巴结
Lymph vessels and nodes of male pelvic cavity
1. 髂总淋巴结 common iliac lymph nodes
2. 髂内淋巴结 medial iliac lymph nodes
3. 髂外动脉 external iliac a.
4. 髂外淋巴结 external iliac lymph nodes
5. 膀胱 urinary bladder
6. 闭孔淋巴结 obturator lymph nodes
7. 骶外侧淋巴结 lateral sacral lymph nodes
8. 骶淋巴结 sacral lymph nodes
9. 髂内静脉 internal iliac v.
10. 主动脉下淋巴结 subaortic lymph nodes
11. 髂总静脉 common iliac v.

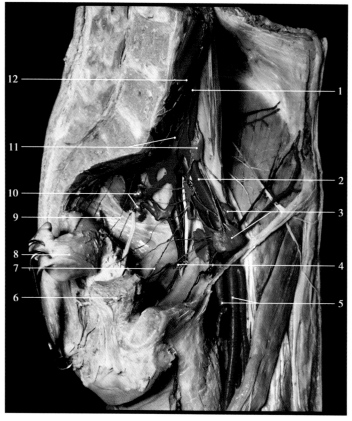

◀ 图 470

女性盆腔淋巴管及淋巴结
Lymph vessels and nodes of female pelvic cavity
1. 髂总动脉 common iliac a.
2. 髂外动脉 external iliac a.
3. 髂外淋巴结 external iliac lymph node
4. 闭孔淋巴结 obturator lymph node
5. 股动、静脉 femoral a. and v.
6. 膀胱 urinary bladder
7. 膀胱淋巴管 lymphatic vessel of urinary bladder
8. 子宫 uterus
9. 子宫淋巴管 lymphatic vessel of uterus
10. 髂内淋巴结 medial iliac lymph nodes
11. 髂总淋巴结 common iliac lymph nodes
12. 主动脉下淋巴结 subaortic lymph nodes

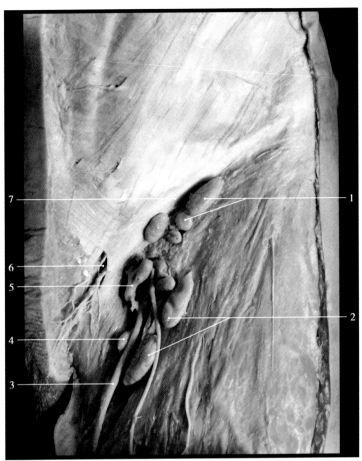

◀ 图 471

腹股沟浅淋巴结
Superficial inguinal lymph nodes

1. 腹股沟上外侧浅淋巴结 superolateral superficial inguinal lymph nodes
2. 腹股沟下外侧浅淋巴结 inferior lateral superficial inguinal lymph nodes
3. 大隐静脉 great saphenous v.
4. 腹股沟下内侧浅淋巴结 inferior medial superficial inguinal lymph nodes
5. 腹股沟上内侧浅淋巴结 superomedial superficial inguinal lymph nodes
6. 腹股沟管浅环 superficial inguinal ring
7. 腹股沟韧带 inguinal lig.

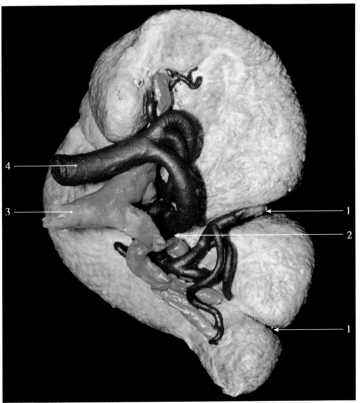

◀ 图 472

脾
Spleen

1. 脾切迹 splenic notch
2. 脾门 hilum of spleen
3. 脾静脉 splenic v.
4. 脾动脉 splenic a.

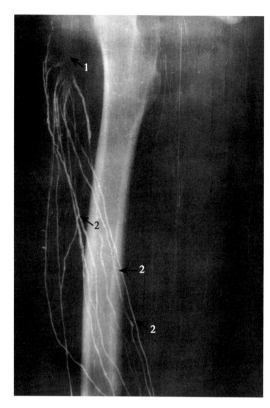

◀ 图 473

下肢淋巴管造影
Lymphangiography of lower limb
1. 淋巴结 lymphatic nodes
2. 淋巴管 lymphatic vessels

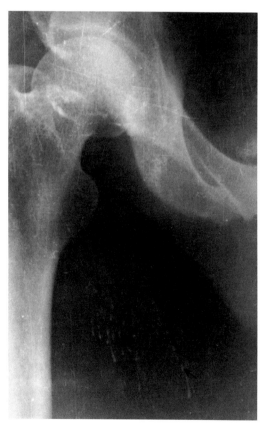

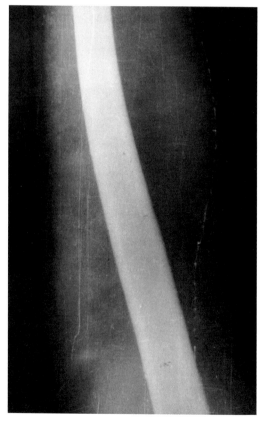

▲ 图 474 **淋巴管瓣膜造影**
Visualization of lymphatic valve
箭头示:淋巴管瓣膜 lymphatic valve

第十一章 视器 Visual Organ

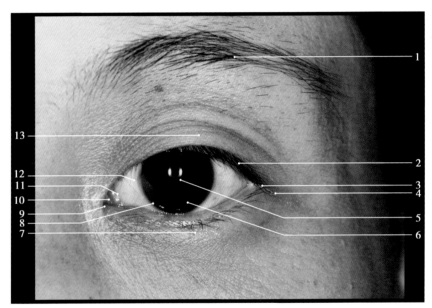

◀ 图 475
左眼(前面观)
Left eye. Anterior aspect
1. 眉毛 eyebrow
2. 睫毛 eyelashes
3. 外眦 lateral angle of eye
4. 睑外侧连合 lateral palpebral commissure
5. 瞳孔 pupil
6. 角膜 cornea
7. 下睑 lower eyelid
8. 角膜缘 limbus corneae
9. 睑内侧连合 medial palpebral commissure
10. 泪阜 lacrimal caruncle
11. 结膜半月襞 conjunctival semilunar fold
12. 球结膜 bulbar conjunctiva
13. 上睑 upper eyelid

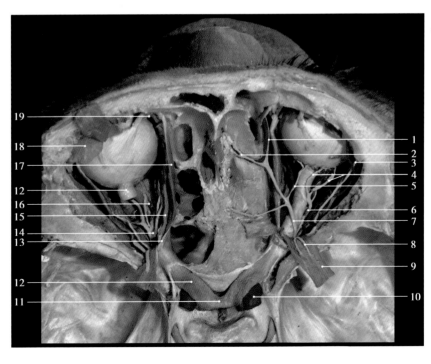

◀ 图 476
眶壁、眼球、视神经和视交叉
Orbital wall, eyeball, optic nerve and optic chiasma
1. 滑车下神经 infratrochlear n.
2. 筛前神经 anterior ethmoidal n.
3. 泪腺神经 lacrimal n.
4. 睫状短神经 short ciliary n.
5. 睫状长神经 long ciliary n.
6. 睫状神经节 ciliary ganglion
7. 鼻睫神经 nasociliary n.
8. 上直肌支 muscular branch of superior rectus
9. 上直肌 superior rectus
10. 颈内动脉 internal carotid a.
11. 视交叉 optic chiasma
12. 视神经 optic n.
13. 滑车神经 trochlear n.
14. 动眼神经 oculomotor n.
15. 内直肌 medial rectus
16. 下直肌 inferior rectus
17. 上斜肌 superior obliquus
18. 泪腺 lacrimal gland
19. 滑车 trochlea

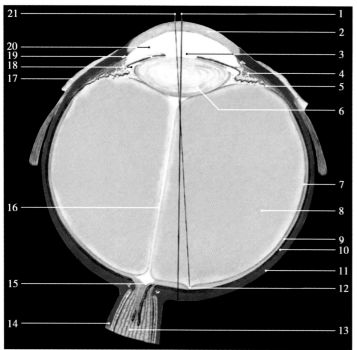

◀ 图477

眼球水平切面
Horizontal section of the eyeball

1. 眼轴 ophthalmic axis
2. 角膜 cornea
3. 瞳孔 pupil
4. 睫状体 ciliary body
5. 视网膜睫状体部 ciliary part of the retina
6. 晶状体 lens
7. 玻璃体膜 vitreous membrane
8. 玻璃体 vitreous body
9. 视网膜 retina
10. 脉络膜 choroid
11. 巩膜 sclera
12. 中央凹 fovea centralis
13. 视神经 optic n.
14. 视神经硬膜鞘 dural sheath of optic n.
15. 视神经盘 optic disc
16. 玻璃体管 hyaloid canal
17. 球结膜 bulbar conjunctiva
18. 眼球后房 posterior chamber of eyeball
19. 虹膜 iris
20. 眼球前房 anterior chamber of eyeball
21. 视轴 optic axis

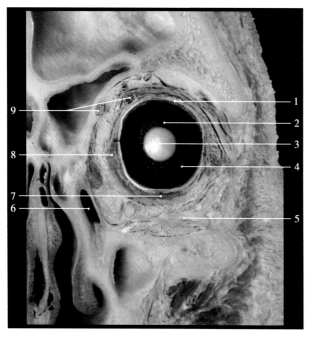

▲ 图478 眶及眼球的冠状切面(后面观1)
Coronal section of orbit and eyeball.
Posterior aspect (1)

1. 巩膜 sclera
2. 睫状突 ciliary processes
3. 晶状体 lens
4. 睫状环 ciliary ring
5. 眶脂体 adipose body of orbit
6. 鼻泪管 nasolacrimal duct
7. 下直肌 inferior rectus
8. 内直肌 medial rectus
9. 上斜肌腱 superior oblique tendon

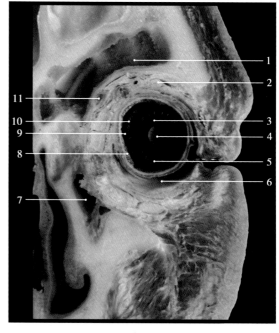

▲ 图479 眶及眼球的冠状切面(后面观2)
Coronal section of orbit and eyeball. Posterior aspect(2)

1. 额窦 frontal sinus
2. 眶脂体 adipose body of orbit
3. 虹膜 iris
4. 瞳孔 pupil
5. 睫状突 ciliary processes
6. 结膜下穹 inferior conjunctival fornix
7. 鼻泪管 nasolacrimal duct
8. 巩膜 sclera
9. 脉络膜 choroid
10. 视网膜 retina
11. 上斜肌腱 superior oblique tendon

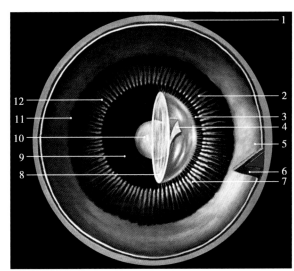

◀ 图 480

虹膜和睫状体（后面观）
Iris and ciliary body. Posterior aspect

1. 巩膜 sclera
2. 睫状突 ciliary process
3. 睫状小带 ciliary zonule
4. 晶状体囊 lens capsule
5. 视网膜 retina
6. 脉络膜 choroid
7. 睫状襞 ciliary folds
8. 晶状体 lens
9. 虹膜 iris
10. 瞳孔 pupil
11. 锯状缘 ora serrata
12. 睫状环 ciliary ring

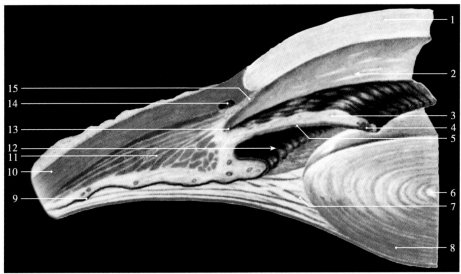

▲ 图 481　**角膜缘结构**
Structures of limbus corneae

1. 角膜 cornea
2. 眼球前房 anterior chamber of eyeball
3. 虹膜 iris
4. 瞳孔括约肌 sphincter pupillae
5. 瞳孔开大肌 dilator pupillae
6. 晶状体核 lens nucleus
7. 睫状小带 ciliary zonule
8. 晶状体皮质 cortex of lens
9. 脉络膜 choroid
10. 巩膜 sclera
11. 睫状肌 ciliary muscle
12. 眼球后房 posterior chamber of eyeball
13. 虹膜角膜角 iridocorneal angle
14. 巩膜静脉窦 sinus venosus sclerae
15. 小梁网 trabecular reticulum

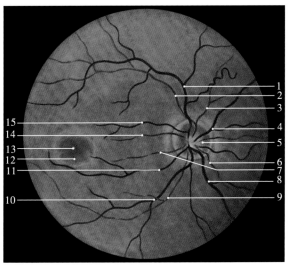

◀ 图 482

视网膜血管
Blood vessels of retina

1. 视网膜颞侧上小静脉 superior temporal venule of retina
2. 视网膜颞侧上小动脉 superior temporal arteriole of retina
3. 视网膜鼻侧上小动脉 superior nasal arteriole of retina
4. 视网膜鼻侧上小静脉 superior nasal venule of retina
5. 视神经盘 optic disc
6. 视网膜鼻侧下小动脉 inferior nasal arteriole of retina
7. 黄斑下小动脉 inferior macular arteriole
8. 视网膜鼻侧下小静脉 inferior nasal venule of retina
9. 视网膜颞侧下小动脉 inferior temporal arteriole of retina
10. 视网膜颞侧下小静脉 inferior temporal venule of retina
11. 黄斑下小静脉 inferior macular venule
12. 黄斑 macula lutea
13. 中央凹 fovea centralis
14. 黄斑上小动脉 superior macular arteriole
15. 黄斑上小静脉 superior macular venule

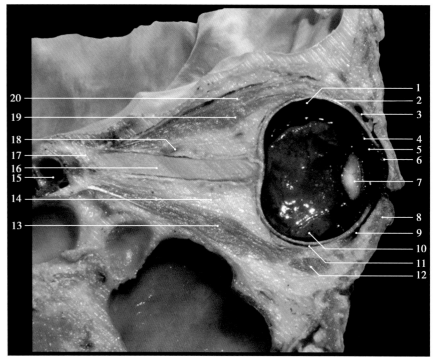

◀ 图 483

眶及眼球的矢状切面
Sagittal section of orbit and eyeball

1. 脉络膜 choroid
2. 巩膜 sclera
3. 结膜上穹 superior conjunctival fornix
4. 虹膜 iris
5. 前房 anterior chamber
6. 角膜 cornea
7. 晶状体 lens
8. 眼轮匝肌 orbicularis oculi
9. 结膜下穹 inferior conjunctival fornix
10. 视网膜 retina
11. 巩膜外隙 episcleral space
12. 下斜肌 inferior obliquus
13. 下直肌 inferior rectus
14. 眶脂体 adipose body of orbit
15. 颈内动脉 internal carotid a.
16. 视神经 optic n.
17. 总腱环 common tendinous ring
18. 眼动脉 ophthalmic a.
19. 上直肌 superior rectus
20. 上睑提肌 levator palpebrae superioris

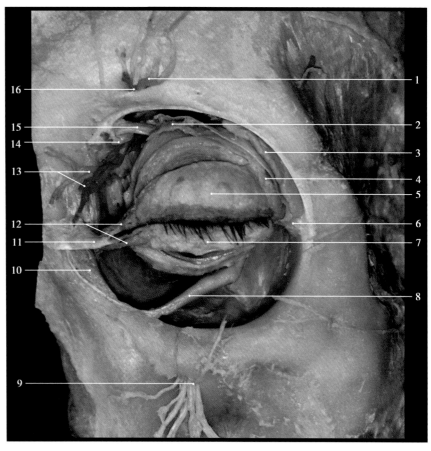

◀ 图 484

眶周围结构
Peripheral structures of orbit

1. 眶上神经 supraorbital n.
2. 上睑提肌 levator palpebrae superioris
3. 泪腺眶部 orbital part of lacrimal gland
4. 泪腺睑部 palpebral part of lacrimal gland
5. 上睑板 superior tarsus
6. 睑外侧韧带 lateral palpebral lig.
7. 下睑板 inferior tarsus
8. 下斜肌 inferior obliquus
9. 眶下神经 infraorbital n.
10. 泪囊 lacrimal sac
11. 睑内侧韧带 medial palpebral lig.
12. 泪小管 lacrimal ductule
13. 鼻背动、静脉 dorsal nasal a. and v.
14. 滑车 trochlea
15. 上斜肌腱 tendon of superior obliquus
16. 眶上孔 supraorbital foramen

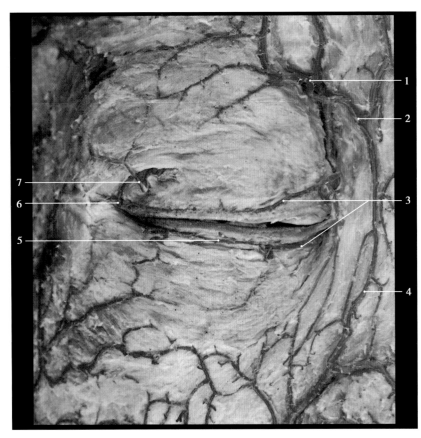

◀ 图 485

眼睑部的动脉
Arteries of eyelids
1. 眶上动脉 supraorbital a.
2. 鼻背动脉 dorsal nasal a.
3. 睑内侧动脉 medial palpebral a.
4. 内眦动脉 angular a.
5. 下睑缘弓 arterial arch of infrapalpebral margin
6. 睑外侧动脉 lateral palpebral a.
7. 泪腺动脉 lacrimal a.

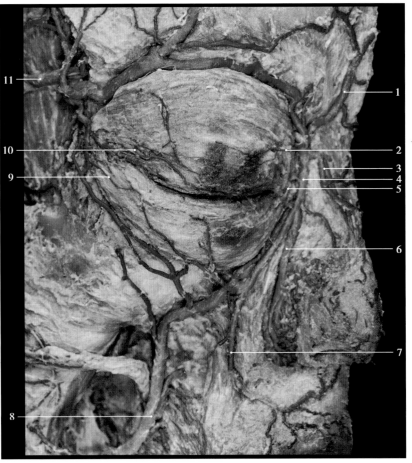

◀ 图 486

眼睑部的静脉
Veins of eyelids
1. 滑车上静脉 supratrochlear v.
2. 上睑内侧静脉 medial superior palpebral v.
3. 鼻背静脉 dorsal nasal v.
4. 内眦静脉 angular v.
5. 下睑内侧静脉 medial inferior palpebral v.
6. 鼻翼静脉 ala nasal v.
7. 上唇静脉 superior labial v.
8. 面静脉 facial v.
9. 下睑外侧静脉 lateral inferior palpebral v.
10. 上睑外侧静脉 lateral superior palpebral v.
11. 颞中静脉 middle temporal v.

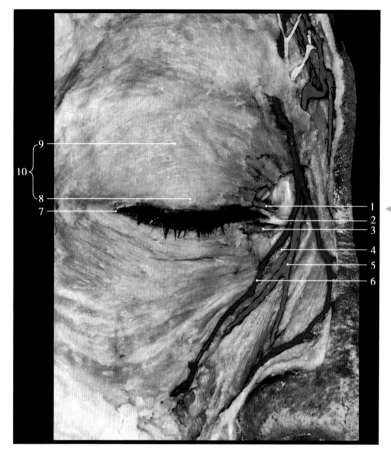

◀ 图 487

泪器(1)
Lacrimal apparatus(1)
1. 上泪小管 superior canaliculus
2. 睑内侧韧带 medial palpebral lig.
3. 下泪小管 inferior lacrimal ductule
4. 泪囊 lacrimal sac
5. 内眦静脉 angular v.
6. 内眦动脉 angular a.
7. 外眦 lateral angle of eye
8. 睑部 palpebral part
9. 眶部 orbital part
10. 眼轮匝肌 orbicularis oculi

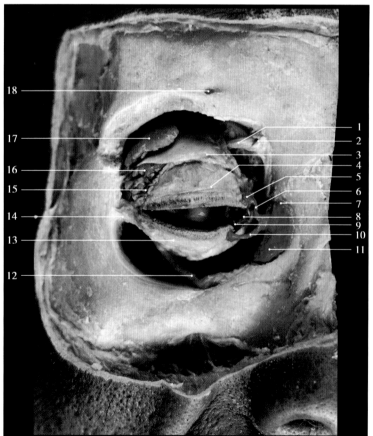

◀ 图 488

泪器(2)
Lacrimal apparatus(2)
1. 上斜肌腱 tendon of superion obliquus
2. 滑车 trochlea
3. 上睑提肌筋膜 fascia of levator palpebrae
   superioris
4. 上睑板 superior tarsus
5. 泪小管壶腹 ampulla of lacrimal ductule
6. 上泪小管 superior lacrimal ductule
7. 泪囊穹 fornix of lacrimal sac
8. 泪阜 lacrimal caruncle
9. 泪湖 lacrimal lacus
10. 下泪小管 inferior lacrimal ductule
11. 泪囊 lacrimal sac
12. 下斜肌 inferior obliquus
13. 下睑板 inferior tarsus
14. 睑外侧韧带 lateral palpebral lig.
15. 泪腺排泄小管 excretory ductules of
    lacrimal gland
16. 泪腺睑部 palpebral part of lacrimal gland
17. 泪腺眶部 orbital part of lacrimal gland
18. 眶上孔 supraorbital foramen

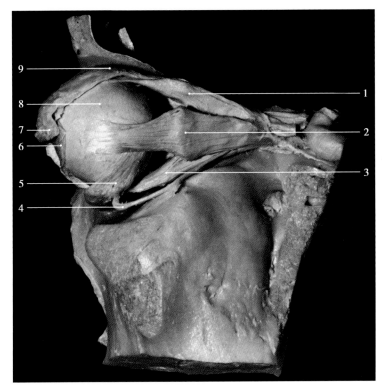

◀ 图 489

眼外肌(外侧面观)

Extraocular muscles. Lateral aspect

1. 上直肌 superior rectus
2. 外直肌 lateral rectus
3. 下直肌 inferior rectus
4. 下斜肌神经 nerve to inferior obliquus
5. 下斜肌 inferior obliquus
6. 角膜 cornea
7. 上睑板 superior tarsus
8. 眼球 eyeball
9. 上睑提肌 levator palpebrae superioris

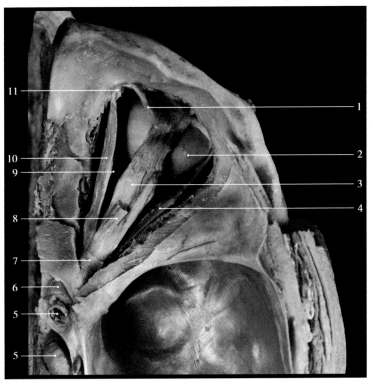

◀ 图 490

眼外肌(上面观)

Extraocular muscles. Superior aspect

1. 上斜肌腱 tendon of superior obliquus
2. 眼球 eyeball
3. 上直肌 superior rectus
4. 外直肌 lateral rectus
5. 颈内动脉 internal carotid a.
6. 视神经 optic n.
7. 总腱环 common tendinous ring
8. 上睑提肌 levator palpebrae superioris
9. 内直肌 medial rectus
10. 上斜肌 superior obliquus
11. 滑车 trochlea

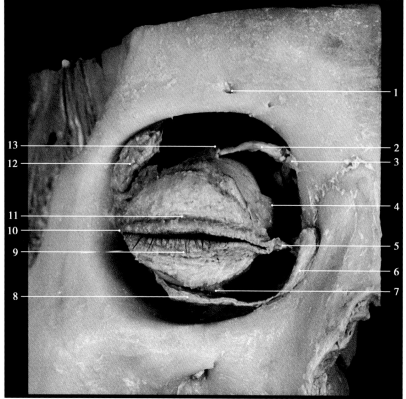

◀ 图 491

眼外肌 (前面观)

Extraocular muscles. Anterior aspect

1. 眶上孔 supraorbital foramen
2. 上斜肌腱 tendon of superior obliquus
3. 滑车 trochlea
4. 内直肌 medial rectus
5. 睑内侧韧带 medial palpebral lig.
6. 泪囊 lacrimal sac
7. 下直肌 inferior rectus
8. 下斜肌 inferior obliquus
9. 下睑板 inferior tarsus
10. 睑外侧韧带 lateral palpebral lig.
11. 上睑板 superior tarsus
12. 泪腺 lacrimal gland
13. 上直肌 superior rectus

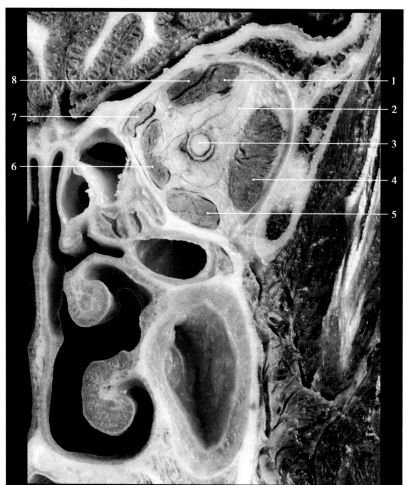

◀ 图 492

眶腔的冠状切面

Coronal section of orbital cavity

1. 上直肌 superior rectus
2. 眶脂体 adipose body of orbit
3. 视神经 optic n.
4. 外直肌 lateral rectus
5. 下直肌 inferior rectus
6. 内直肌 medial rectus
7. 上斜肌 superior obliquus
8. 上睑提肌 levator palpebrae superioris

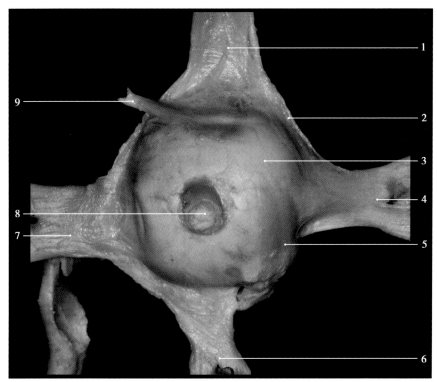

◀ 图 493
眼球筋膜鞘（后面观 1）
Sheath of eyeball. Posterior aspect
(1)
1. 上直肌 superior rectus
2. 肌间膜 intermuscular membrane
3. 眼球筋膜鞘 sheath of eyeball
4. 外直肌 lateral rectus
5. 下斜肌 inferior obliquus
6. 下直肌 inferior rectus
7. 内直肌 medial rectus
8. 视神经 optic n.
9. 上斜肌腱 tendon of superior
   obliquus

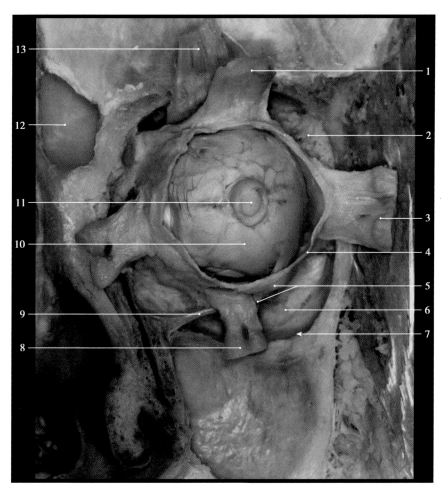

◀ 图 494
眼球筋膜鞘（后面观 2）
Sheath of eyeball. Posterior aspect
(2)
1. 上直肌 superior rectus
2. 泪腺 lachrymal gland
3. 外直肌 lateral rectus
4. 眼球筋膜鞘 sheath of eyeball
5. 下支持带 inferior check lig.
6. 眶脂体 adipose body of orbit
7. 眶 orbit
8. 下直肌 inferior rectus
9. 下斜肌 inferior obliquus
10. 眼球 eyeball
11. 视神经 optic n.
12. 额窦 frontal sinus
13. 上睑提肌 levator palpebrae
    superioris

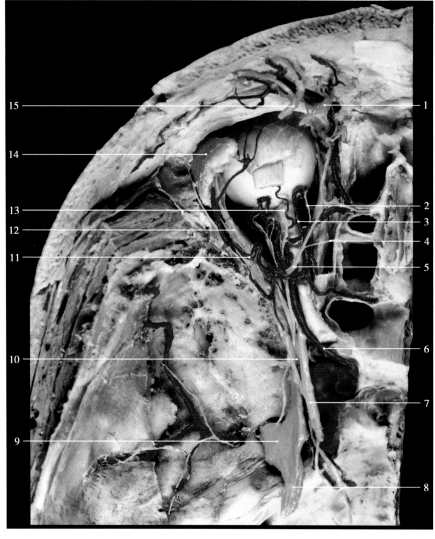

◀ 图 495

睚腔内的血管和神经(上面观)
Blood vessels and nerves in the orbital cavity. Superior aspect

1. 滑车上神经 supratrochlear n.
2. 睫状长神经 long ciliary n.
3. 睫后长动脉 long posterior ciliary a.
4. 筛后神经 posterior ethmoidal n.
5. 鼻睫神经 nasociliary n.
6. 眼动脉 ophthalmic a.
7. 动眼神经 oculomotor n.
8. 三叉神经 trigeminal n.
9. 三叉神经节 trigeminal ganglion
10. 眼神经 ophthalmic n.
11. 泪腺动脉 lacrimal a.
12. 泪腺神经 lacrimal n.
13. 睫状短神经 short ciliary n.
14. 泪腺 lachrymal gland
15. 睚上神经 supraorbital n.

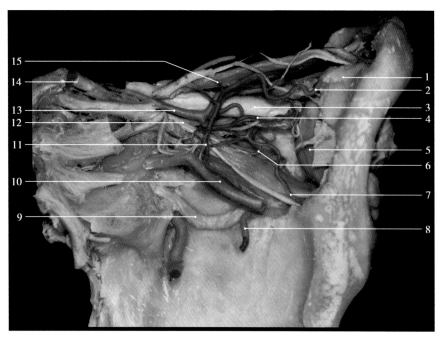

◀ 图 496

眼动脉及其分支(外侧面观)
Ophthalmic artery and its branches. Lateral aspect

1. 泪腺 lacrimal gland
2. 泪腺动脉 lacrimal gland a.
3. 视神经 optic n.
4. 睫后长动脉 long posterior ciliary a.
5. 下斜肌 inferior obliquus
6. 下直肌动脉 artery of inferior rectus
7. 下斜肌动脉 artery of inferior obliquus
8. 睚下动脉 infraorbital a.
9. 上颌神经 maxillary n.
10. 外直肌 lateral rectus
11. 外直肌动脉 artery of lateral rectus
12. 动眼神经 oculomotor n.
13. 眼动脉 ophthalmic a.
14. 颈内动脉 internal carotid a.
15. 上直肌动脉 artery of superior rectus

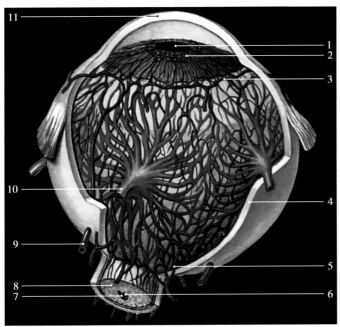

◀ 图 497

虹膜的动脉和涡静脉
Arteries of iris and vorticose veins

1. 瞳孔 pupil
2. 虹膜动脉小环 lesser arterial circle of iris
3. 虹膜动脉大环 greater arterial circle of iris
4. 巩膜 sclera
5. 睫后短动脉 short posterior ciliary a.
6. 视网膜中央动脉 central artery of retina
7. 视网膜中央静脉 central vein of retina
8. 视神经 optic n.
9. 睫后长动脉 long posterior ciliary a.
10. 涡静脉 vorticose v.
11. 角膜 cornea

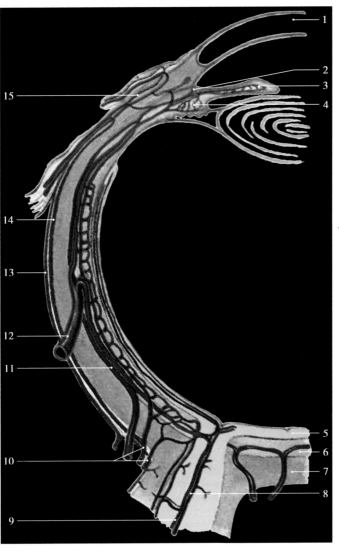

◀ 图 498

眼球的血管
Blood vessels of eyeball

1. 角膜 cornea
2. 虹膜动脉大环 greater arterial circle of iris
3. 虹膜动脉小环 lesser arterial circle of iris
4. 睫状突血管 blood vessels of ciliary process
5. 视网膜 retina
6. 脉络膜 choroid
7. 巩膜 sclera
8. 视网膜中央静脉 central vein of retina
9. 视网膜中央动脉 central artery of retina
10. 睫后短动脉 short posterior ciliary a.
11. 睫后长动脉 long posterior ciliary a.
12. 涡静脉 vorticose v.
13. 巩膜外静脉 episcleral v.
14. 巩膜外动脉 episcleral a.
15. 睫状前动脉 anterior ciliary a.

第十二章 前庭蜗器
Vestibulocochlear Organ

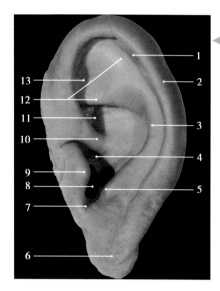

◀ 图 499
耳廓
Auricle
1. 耳舟 scapha
2. 耳轮 helix
3. 对耳轮 antihelix
4. 耳甲腔 cavity of auricular concha
5. 对耳屏 antitragus
6. 耳垂 auricular lobule
7. 耳屏间切迹 intertragic notch
8. 外耳门 external acoustic pore
9. 耳屏 tragus
10. 耳轮脚 crus of helix
11. 耳甲艇 cymba of auricular concha
12. 对耳轮脚 crura of antihelix
13. 三角窝 triangular fossa

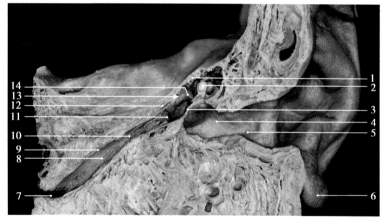

◀ 图 500
咽鼓管和外耳道
Auditory tube and the external acoustic meatus
1. 鼓室盖 tegmen tympani
2. 听小骨 auditory ossicles
3. 鼓膜 tympanic membrane
4. 外耳道骨性部 bony part of external acoustic meatus
5. 外耳道软骨部 cartilaginous part of external acoustic meatus
6. 耳垂 auricular lobule
7. 咽鼓管咽口 pharyngeal opening of auditory tube
8. 咽鼓管软骨部 cartilaginous part of auditory tube
9. 咽鼓管软骨 cartilage of auditory tube
10. 咽鼓管骨部 bony part of auditory tube
11. 咽鼓管鼓室口 tympanic opening of auditory tube
12. 鼓膜张肌 tensor tympani
13. 中耳 middle ear
14. 匙突 cochleariform process

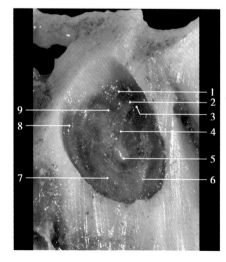

◀ 图 501
鼓膜 (外侧面观)
Tympanic membrane. Lateral aspect
1. 松弛部 flaccid part
2. 锤凸 malleolar prominence
3. 锤骨前襞 anterior malleolar fold
4. 锤纹 malleolar stria
5. 鼓膜脐 umbo of tympanic membrane
6. 光锥 cone of light
7. 紧张部 tense part
8. 纤维软骨环 fibrocartilaginous ring
9. 锤骨后襞 posterior malleolar fold

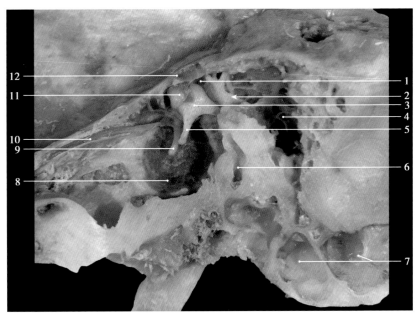

◀ 图 502

鼓室鼓膜壁（内侧面观）
Membranous wall of tympanic cavity.
Medial aspect

1. 鼓室上隐窝 epitympanic recess
2. 乳突窦入口 entrance to mastoid antrum
3. 砧骨 incus
4. 乳突窦 mastoid antrum
5. 砧骨长脚 long crus of incus
6. 面神经管 canal for facial n.
7. 乳突小房 mastoid cells
8. 鼓膜 tympanic membrane
9. 锤骨柄 manubrium of malleus
10. 鼓膜张肌 tensor tympani
11. 锤骨头 head of malleus
12. 盖壁 tegmental wall

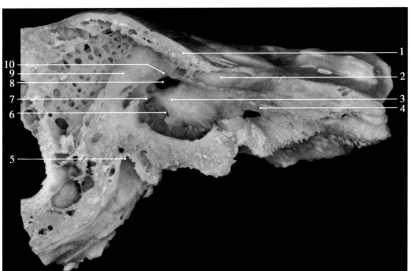

◀ 图 503

鼓室迷路壁（外侧面观）
Labyrinthine wall of tympanic cavity.
Lateral aspect

1. 鼓室盖 tegmen tympani
2. 鼓膜张肌半管 semicanal for tensor tympani
3. 岬 promontory
4. 咽鼓管半管 semicanal for auditory tube
5. 茎乳孔 stylomastoid foramen
6. 蜗窗 fenestra cochleae
7. 锥隆起 pyramidal eminence
8. 前庭窗 fenestra vestibuli
9. 外半规管凸 prominence of lateral semi-circular canal
10. 面神经管凸 prominence of facial canal

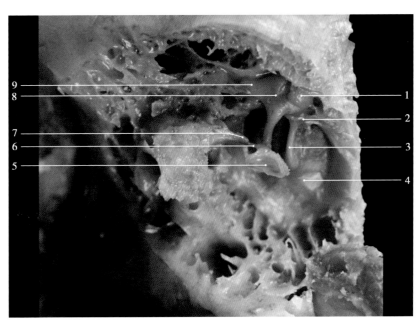

◀ 图 504

鼓室（内侧面观）
Tympanic cavity. Medial aspect

1. 锤骨头 head of malleus
2. 鼓索 chorda tympani
3. 锤骨柄 manubrium of malleus
4. 鼓膜 tympanic membrane
5. 镫骨底 base of stapes
6. 镫骨肌腱 tendon of stapedius
7. 锥隆起 pyramidal eminence
8. 砧骨 incus
9. 砧骨短脚 short crus of incus

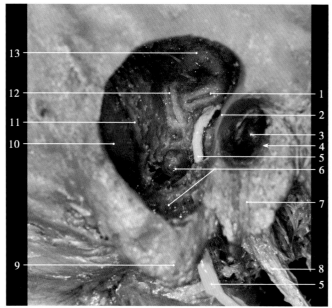

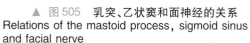

▲ 图505　乳突、乙状窦和面神经的关系
Relations of the mastoid process, sigmoid sinus
and facial nerve
1. 外骨半规管 lateral semicircular duct
2. 外耳道后壁 posterior wall of external acoustic meatus
3. 鼓膜 tympanic membrane
4. 外耳道 external acoustic meatus
5. 面神经 facial n.
6. 乳突小房 mastoid cells
7. 鼓部 tympanic part
8. 茎突 styloid process
9. 乳突 mastoid process
10. 乙状窦 sigmoid sinus
11. 乙状窦前壁 anterior wall of sigmoid sinus
12. 后骨半规管 posterior semicircular duct
13. 前骨半规管 anterior semicircular duct

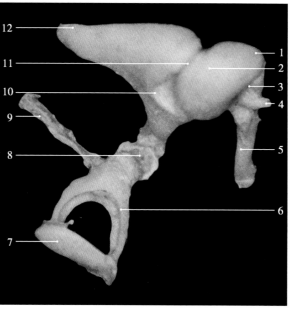

▲ 图506　听骨链
Chain of auditory ossicles
1. 锤骨 malleus
2. 锤骨头 head of malleus
3. 锤骨颈 neck of malleus
4. 前突（长突）anterior process
5. 锤骨柄 manubrium of malleus
6. 镫骨 stapes
7. 镫骨底 base of stapes
8. 砧镫关节 incudostapedial join
9. 镫骨肌 stapedius
10. 砧骨 incus
11. 砧锤关节 incudomalleolar joint
12. 砧骨短脚 short crus of incus

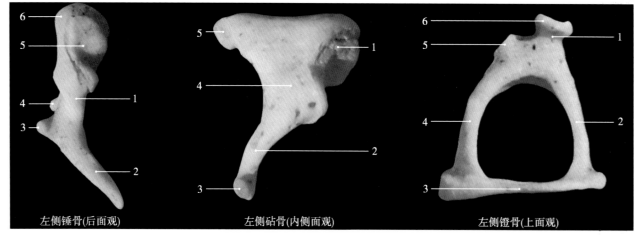

左侧锤骨(后面观)　　　　左侧砧骨(内侧面观)　　　　左侧镫骨(上面观)

▲ 图507　听小骨
Auditory ossicles

1. 锤骨颈 neck of malleus
2. 锤骨柄 manubrium of malleus
3. 外侧突（短突）lateral process
4. 前突（长突）anterior process
5. 砧锤关节面 incudomalleolar articular surface
6. 锤骨头 head of malleus

1. 砧锤关节面 incudomalleolar articular surface
2. 长脚 long crus
3. 豆状突 lenticular process
4. 砧骨体 body of incus
5. 短脚 short crus

1. 镫骨颈 neck of stapes
2. 前脚 anterior crus
3. 镫骨底 base of stapes
4. 后脚 posterior crus
5. 镫骨肌止点 insertion of stapedius
6. 镫骨头 head of stapes

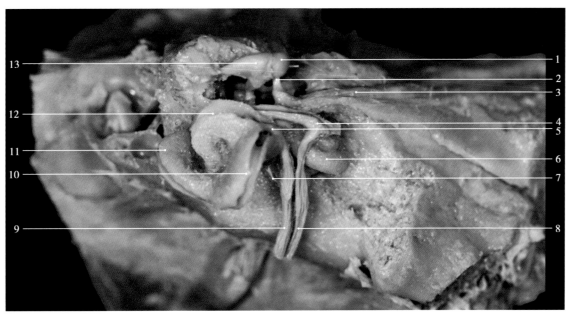

▲ 图 508　**前庭蜗器**
Vestibulocochlear organ

1. 锤骨头 head of malleus
2. 鼓膜张肌腱 tendon tensor tympani
3. 鼓膜张肌 tensor tympani
4. 膝神经节 geniculate ganglion
5. 外壶腹神经 lateral ampullary n.
6. 耳蜗 cochlea
7. 后壶腹神经 posterior ampullary n.
8. 面神经 facial n.
9. 前庭蜗神经 vestibulocochlear n.
10. 前骨半规管 anterior semicircular canal
11. 后骨半规管 posterior semicircular canal
12. 外骨半规管 lateral semicircular canal
13. 砧骨体 body of incus

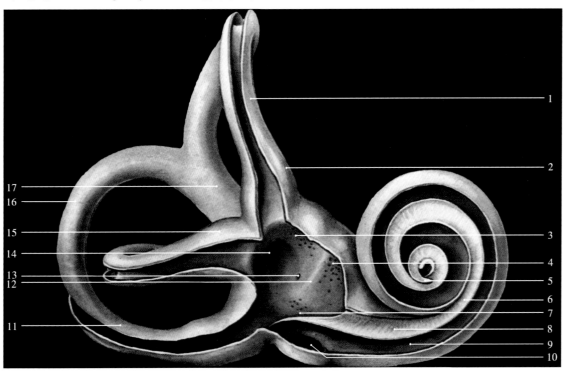

▲ 图 509　**骨迷路**
Bony labyrinth

1. 前骨半规管 anterior semicircular canal
2. 前骨壶腹 anterior bony ampulla
3. 椭圆囊隐窝 elliptical recess
4. 球囊隐窝 spherical recess
5. 螺旋板钩 hamulus of spiral lamina
6. 骨螺旋板 osseous spiral lamina
7. 蜗管隐窝 cochlear recess
8. 前庭阶 scala vestibuli
9. 鼓阶 scala tympani
10. 蜗窗 fenestra cochleae
11. 后骨半规管 posterior semicircular canal
12. 前庭嵴 vestibular crest
13. 前庭管内口 internal aperture of vestibular aqueduct
14. 总骨脚开口 opening of common bony crus
15. 外骨壶腹 lateral bony ampulla
16. 后骨半规管 posterior semicircular canal
17. 总骨脚 common bony crus

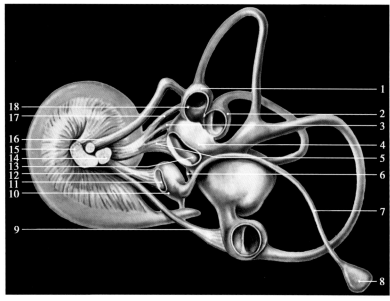

◀ 图 510
膜迷路
Membranous labyrinth
1. 前膜壶腹 anterior membranous ampulla
2. 外膜壶腹 lateral membranous ampulla
3. 外壶腹神经 lateral ampullary n.
4. 椭圆囊 utricle
5. 椭圆囊神经 utricular n.
6. 椭圆球囊管 utriculosaccular duct
7. 内淋巴管 endolymphatic duct
8. 内淋巴囊 endolymphatic sac
9. 后壶腹神经 posterior ampullary n.
10. 球囊 saccule
11. 球囊斑 macula sacculi
12. 球囊神经 saccular n.
13. 椭圆囊斑 macula utriculi
14. 前庭神经 vestibular n.
15. 蜗神经 cochlear n.
16. 面神经 facial n.
17. 前壶腹神经 anterior ampullary n.
18. 壶腹嵴 crista ampullaris

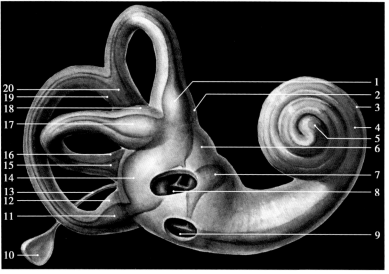

◀ 图 511
骨迷路和膜迷路
Bony labyrinth and membranous labyrinth
1. 前膜壶腹 anterior membranous ampulla
2. 前骨壶腹 anterior bony ampulla
3. 耳蜗 cochlea
4. 蜗管 cochlear duct
5. 蜗顶 cupula of cochlea
6. 前庭 vestibule
7. 球囊 saccule
8. 前庭窗 fenestra vestibuli
9. 蜗窗 fenestra cochleae
10. 内淋巴囊 endolymphatic sac
11. 后膜壶腹 posterior membranous ampulla
12. 后骨壶腹 posterior bony ampulla
13. 内淋巴管 endolymphatic duct
14. 椭圆囊 utricle
15. 单膜脚 simple membranous crus
16. 单骨脚 simple bony crus
17. 外膜壶腹 lateral membranous ampulla
18. 外骨壶腹 lateral bony ampulla
19. 总骨脚 common bony crus
20. 总膜脚 common membranous crus

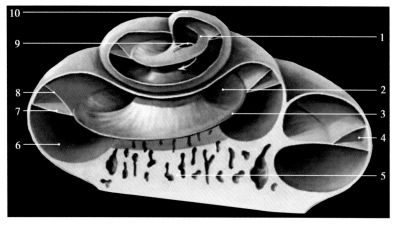

◀ 图 512
耳蜗（剖面1）
Cochlea. Section（1）
1. 螺旋板钩 hamulus of spiral lamina
2. 前庭阶 scala vestibuli
3. 骨螺旋板 osseous spiral lamina
4. 蜗管 cochlear duct
5. 蜗轴 cochlear axis
6. 鼓阶 scala tympani
7. 螺旋膜 spiral membrani
8. 前庭膜 vestibule membrani
9. 蜗孔 helicotrema
10. 蜗顶 cupula of cochlea

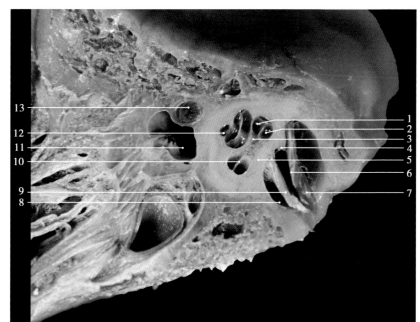

◀ 图 513

耳蜗（剖面 2）
Cochlea. Section（2）

1. 前庭阶 scala vestibuli
2. 鼓阶 scala tympani
3. 蜗轴 cochlear axis
4. 横嵴 transverse crest
5. 蜗底 base of cochlea
6. 面神经 facial n.
7. 前庭神经 vestibular n.
8. 内耳道 internal acoustic meatus
9. 蜗神经 cochlear n.
10. 骨螺旋板 osseous spiral lamina
11. 咽鼓管 auditory tube
12. 蜗孔 helicotrema
13. 鼓膜张肌 tensor tympani

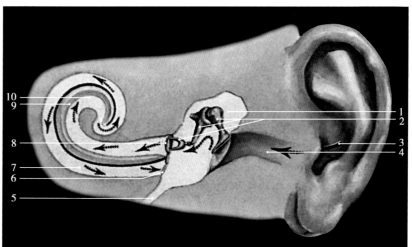

◀ 图 514

声波的传导途径
Conducting pathway of sound wave

1. 鼓室 tympanic cavity
2. 听小骨 auditory ossicles
3. 声波 sound wave
4. 外耳道 external acoustic meatus
5. 咽鼓管 auditory tube
6. 蜗窗 fenestra cochleae
7. 鼓阶 scala tympani
8. 前庭窗 fenestra vestibuli
9. 蜗管 cochlear duct
10. 前庭阶 scala vestibuli

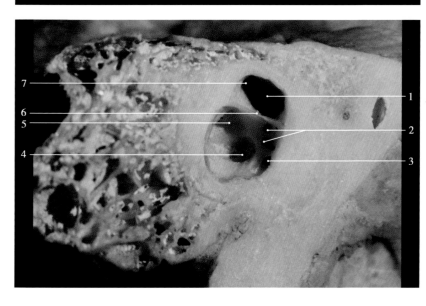

◀ 图 515

内耳道底
Fundus of internal acoustic meatus

1. 前庭上区 superior vestibular area
2. 前庭下区 inferior vestibular area
3. 单孔 single foramen
4. 螺旋孔裂 foraminous spiral tract
5. 蜗区 cochlear area
6. 横嵴 transverse crest
7. 面神经区 area of facial n.

第十三章　中枢神经系统
Central Nervous System

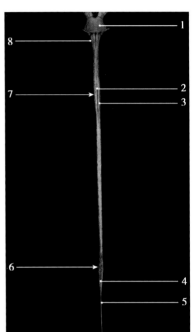
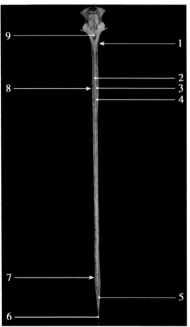

◀ 图 516

脊髓外形
Shape of spinal cord
前面观 Anterior aspect
1. 脑桥 pons
2. 前正中裂 anterior median fissure
3. 前外侧沟 anteriolateral sulcus
4. 脊髓圆锥 conus medullaris
5. 终丝 filum terminale
6. 腰骶膨大 lumbosacral enlargement
7. 颈膨大 cervical enlargement
8. 延髓 spinal cord
后面观 Posterior aspect
1. 延髓 spinal cord
2. 后正中沟 posterior median sulcus
3. 后根丝 posterior rootlets
4. 后外侧沟 posterolateral sulcus
5. 脊髓圆锥 conus medullaris
6. 终丝 filum terminale
7. 腰骶膨大 lumbosacral enlargement
8. 颈膨大 cervical enlargement
9. 菱形窝 rhomboid fossa

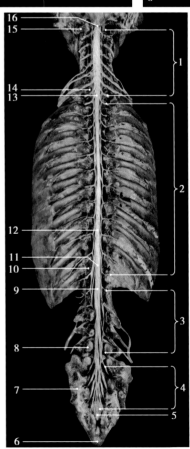

◀ 图 517

脊髓节段和脊神经与椎骨的关系
Relation of segment of spinal cord and spinal nerve to the vertebrae
1. 颈神经 cervical n.
2. 胸神经 thoracic n.
3. 腰神经 lumbar n.
4. 骶神经 sacral plexus
5. 尾神经 coccygeal n.
6. 尾骨 coccyx
7. 骶骨 sacrum
8. 第 5 腰椎 5th lumbar vertebra
9. 尾段 coccygeal segments
10. 第 12 胸椎 12th thoracic vertebra
11. 第 1 骶段 1st sacral segment (S_1)
12. 第 1 腰段 1st lumbar segment (L_1)
13. 第 1 胸段 1st thoracic segment (T_1)
14. 第 7 颈椎 7th cervical vertebra
15. 寰椎 atlas
16. 第 1 颈段 1st cervical segment (C_1)

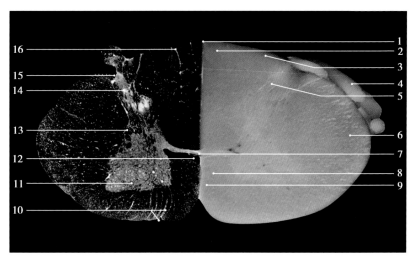

◀ 图 518

脊髓的颈段 (横切面)
Cervical segment of spinal cord. Cross section

1. 后正中沟 posterior median sulcus
2. 薄束 fasciculus gracilis
3. 楔束 fasciculus cuneatus
4. 后根 posterior root
5. 后角 posterior horn
6. 脊髓丘脑侧束 lateral spinothalamic tract
7. 中央管 central canal
8. 内侧纵束 medial longitudinal fasciculus
9. 皮质脊髓前束 anterior corticospinal tract
10. 前根 anterior root
11. 前角 anterior horn
12. 白质前连合 anterior white commissure
13. 网状结构 reticular formation
14. 胶状质 substantia gelatinosa
15. 后外侧沟 posterolateral sulcus
16. 后中间沟 posterior intermediate sulcus

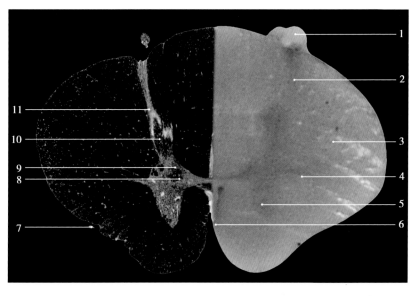

◀ 图 519

脊髓的胸段 (横切面)
Thoracic segment of spinal cord. Cross section

1. 后根 posterior root
2. 后角 posterior horn
3. 皮质脊髓侧束 lateral corticospinal tract
4. 侧角 lateral horn
5. 前角 anterior horn
6. 皮质脊髓前束 anterior corticospinal tract
7. 前根 anterior root
8. 中间内侧核 intermediomedial nucleus
9. 胸核 thoracic nucleus
10. 后角固有核 nucleus proprius
11. 胶状质 substantia gelatinosa

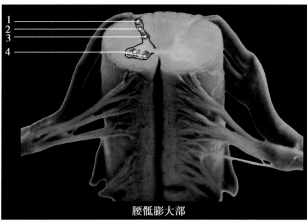

腰骶膨大部

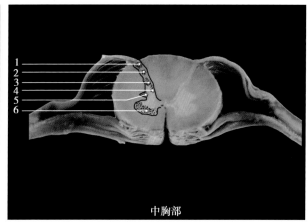

中胸部

▲ 图 520　**脊髓灰质主要核团**
Principal gray nucleus

1. 后角边缘层 marginal layer of posterior horn
2. 胶状质 substantia gelatinosa
3. 后角固有核 nucleus proprius
4. 前角运动核 motor nucleus of anterior horn

1. 后角边缘层 marginal layer of posterior horn
2. 胶状质 substantia gelatinosa
3. 后角固有核 nucleus proprius
4. 胸核 thoracic nucleus
5. 中间外侧核 intermediolateral nucleus
6. 前角运动核 motor nucleus of anterior horn

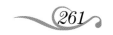

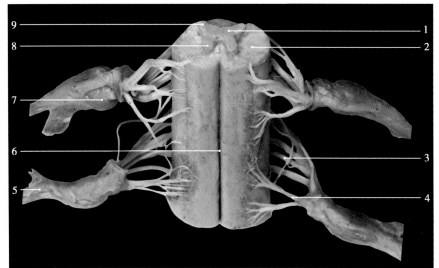

◄ 图 521

脊髓与脊神经根
Spinal cord and roots of spinal nerves
1. 灰质 gray matter
2. 白质 white matter
3. 后根 posterior root
4. 前根 anterior root
5. 脊神经 spinal n.
6. 前正中裂 anterior median fissure
7. 脊神经节 spinal ganglia
8. 前角 anterior horn
9. 后角 posterior horn

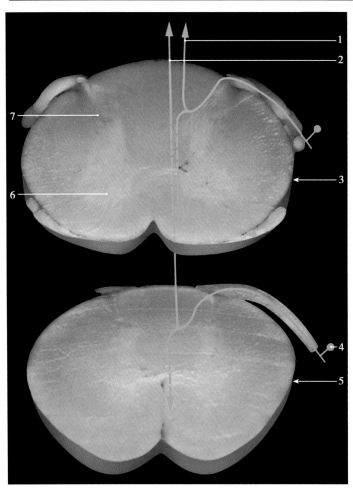

▲ 图 522 薄束和楔束
Fasciculus gracilis and fasciculus cuneatus
1. 楔束 fasciculus cuneatus
2. 薄束 fasciculus gracilis
3. 颈段 cervical segments
4. 脊神经节 spinal ganglia
5. 腰段 lumbar segments
6. 前角 anterior horn
7. 后角 posterior horn

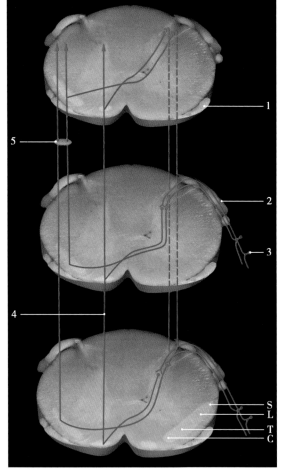

▲ 图 523 脊髓丘脑侧束和前束
Lateral spinothalamic tract and anterior spinothalamic tract
1. 前根 anterior root
2. 后根 posterior root
3. 脊神经节 spinal ganglia
4. 脊髓丘脑前束 anterior spinothalamic tract
5. 脊髓丘脑侧束 lateral spinothalamic tract

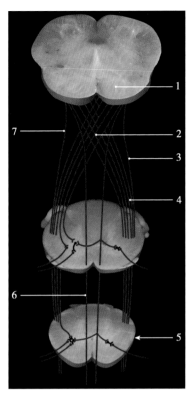

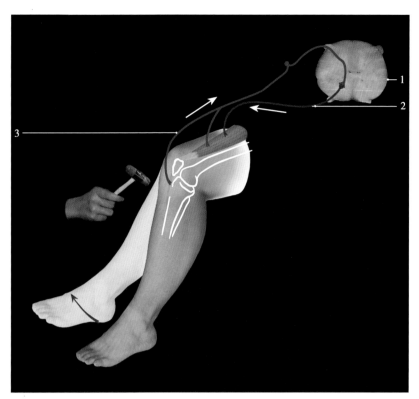

▲ 图 524　皮质脊髓前束和侧束
Anterior corticospinal tract
and lateral corticospinal tract

1. 延髓锥体 pyramid of medulla oblongata
2. 锥体交叉 decussation of pyramid
3. 皮质脊髓前外侧束 antero-lateral corticospinal tract
4. 皮质脊髓侧束 lateral cortico-spinal tract
5. 脊髓 spinal cord
6. 皮质脊髓前束 anterior cortico-spinal tract
7. 未交叉纤维 fiber of non-decus-sation

▲ 图 525　牵张反射（模式图）
Stretch reflex. Diagram
1. 脊髓 spinal cord
2. 传出纤维 efferent fiber
3. 传入纤维 afferent fiber

图 526 ▶
屈曲反射（模式图）
Flexion reflex. Diagram
1. 脊髓 spinal cord
2. 传出纤维 efferent fiber
3. 传入纤维 afferent fiber

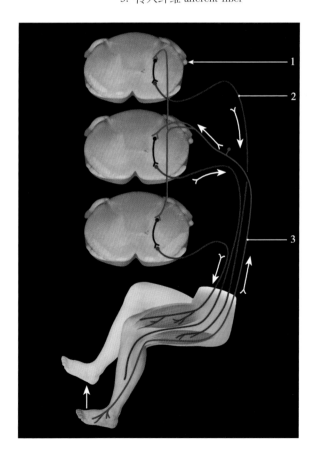

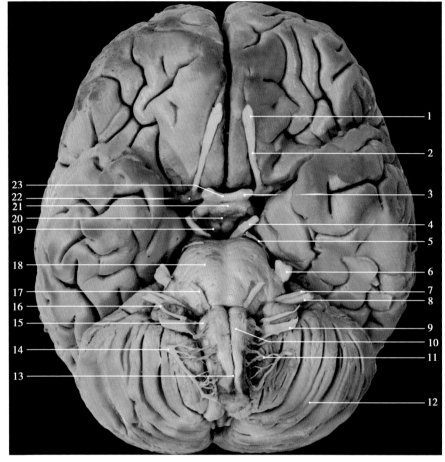

◀ 图 527
脑的底面
Basal surface of brain
1. 嗅球 olfactory bulb
2. 嗅束 olfactory tract
3. 视神经 optic n.
4. 动眼神经 oculomotor n.
5. 滑车神经 trochlear n.
6. 三叉神经 trigeminal n.
7. 面神经 facial n.
8. 前庭蜗神经 vestibulocochlear n.
9. 迷走神经 vagus n.
10. 锥体 pyramid
11. 舌下神经 hypoglossal n.
12. 小脑 cerebellum
13. 锥体交叉 decussation of pyramid
14. 副神经 accessory n.
15. 橄榄 olive
16. 舌咽神经 glossopharyngeal n.
17. 展神经 abducent n.
18. 脑桥 pons
19. 乳头体 mamillary body
20. 灰结节 tuber cinereum
21. 垂体 hypophysis
22. 嗅三角 olfactory trigone
23. 视交叉 optic chiasma

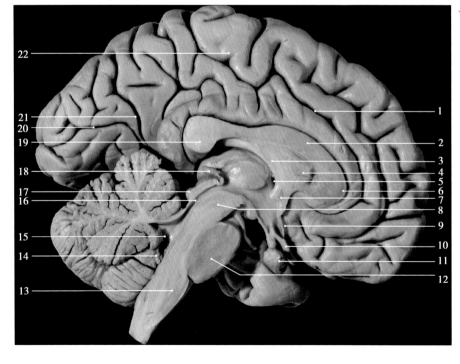

◀ 图 528
脑内侧面
Medial surface of brain
1. 扣带沟 cingulate sulcus
2. 胼胝体干 trunk of corpus callosum
3. 穹隆 fornix
4. 透明隔 septum pellucidum
5. 室间孔 interventricular foramen
6. 胼胝体膝 genu of corpus callosum
7. 前连合 anterior commissure
8. 大脑脚 cerebral peduncle
9. 终板 lamina terminalis
10. 视交叉 optic chiasm
11. 垂体 hypophysis
12. 脑桥 pons
13. 延髓 medulla oblongata
14. 第四脑室脉络丛 choroid plexus of fourth ventricle
15. 第四脑室 fourth ventricle
16. 中脑水管 mesencephalic aqueduct
17. 下丘 inferior colliculus
18. 松果体 pineal body
19. 胼胝体压部 splenium of corpus callosum
20. 距状沟 calcarine sulcus
21. 顶枕沟 parietooccipital sulcus
22. 中央旁小叶 paracentral lobule

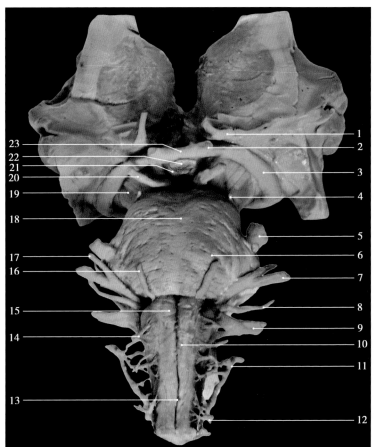

◀ 图 529
脑干 (腹面观)
Brain stem. Ventral aspect
1. 嗅三角 olfactory triangle
2. 视神经 optic n.
3. 视束 optic tract
4. 滑车神经 trochlear n.
5. 三叉神经 trigeminal n.
6. 脑桥 pons
7. 前庭蜗神经 vestibulocochlear n.
8. 舌咽神经 glossopharyngeal n.
9. 迷走神经 vagus n.
10. 延髓 medulla oblongata
11. 副神经 accessory n.
12. 第 1 脊神经 the 1st spinal n.
13. 锥体交叉 decussation of pyramid
14. 舌下神经 hypoglossal n.
15. 锥体 pyramid
16. 展神经 abducent n.
17. 面神经 facial n.
18. 基底沟 basilar sulcus
19. 大脑脚 cerebral peduncle
20. 动眼神经 oculomotor n.
21. 乳头体 mamillary body
22. 垂体 hypophysis
23. 视交叉 optic chiasma

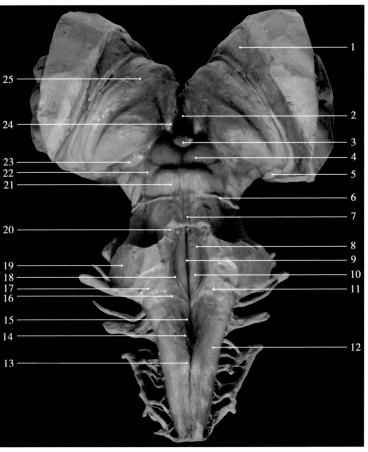

◀ 图 530
脑干 (背面观)
Brain stem. Dorsal aspect
1. 尾状核 caudate nucleus
2. 第三脑室 third ventricle
3. 松果体 pineal body
4. 上丘 superior colliculus
5. 外侧膝状体 lateral geniculate body
6. 滑车神经 trochlear n.
7. 上髓帆 superior medullary velum
8. 蓝斑 locus ceruleus
9. 正中沟 median sulcus
10. 面神经丘 facial colliculus
11. 前庭区 vestibular area
12. 延髓 medulla oblongata
13. 薄束结节 gracile tubercle
14. 迷走神经三角 vagal triangle
15. 舌下神经三角 hypoglossal triangle
16. 髓纹 striae medullares
17. 小脑下脚 inferior cerebellar peduncle
18. 界沟 sulcus limitans
19. 小脑中脚 middle cerebellar peduncle
20. 小脑上脚 superior cerebellar peduncle
21. 下丘 inferior colliculus
22. 下丘臂 brachium of inferior colliculus
23. 内侧膝状体 medial geniculate body
24. 缰三角 haberular trigone
25. 背侧丘脑 dorsal thalamus

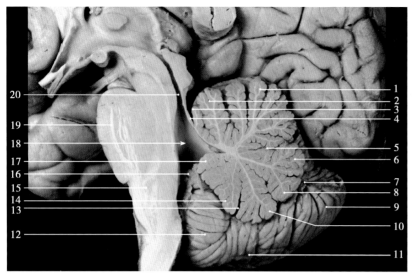

◀ 图 531

脑干、小脑和第四脑室正中切面
Median section of brain stem, cerebellum and the fourth ventricle
1. 山顶 culmen
2. 中央小叶 central lobule
3. 小脑小舌 lingula of cerebellum
4. 上髓帆 superior medullary velum
5. 原裂 primary fissure
6. 山坡 declive
7. 水平裂 horizontal fissure
8. 蚓结节 tuber of vermis
9. 下半月小叶 inferior semilunar lobule
10. 蚓锥体 pyramid of vermis
11. 二腹小叶 biventral lobule
12. 小脑扁桃体 tonsil of cerebellum
13. 次裂 secondary fissure
14. 蚓垂 uvula of vermis
15. 延髓 medulla oblongata
16. 第四脑室脉络丛 choroid plexus of the fourth ventricle
17. 小结 nodule
18. 第四脑室 fourth ventricle
19. 脑桥 pons
20. 中脑水管 mesencephalic aqueduct

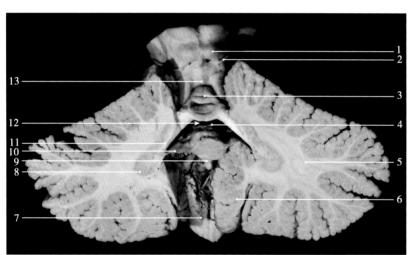

◀ 图 532

小脑冠状切面
Coronal section of cerebellum
1. 下丘 inferior colliculus
2. 滑车神经 trochlear n.
3. 中央小叶 central lobule
4. 第四脑室脉络丛 choroid plexus of the fourth ventricle
5. 髓质 medulla
6. 小脑扁桃体 tonsil of cerebellum
7. 延髓 medulla oblongata
8. 齿状核 dentate nucleus
9. 小结 nodule
10. 下髓帆 inferior medullary velum
11. 齿状核门 hilum of dentate nucleus
12. 第四脑室 fourth ventricle
13. 上髓帆 superior medullary velum

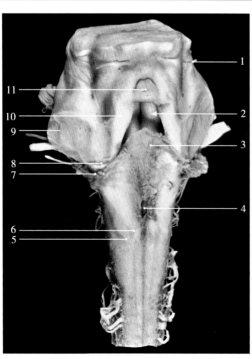

◀ 图 533

第四脑室脉络组织
Tela choroidea of the fourth ventricle
1. 滑车神经 trochlear n.
2. 第四脑室 fourth ventricle
3. 第四脑室脉络组织 tela choroidea of the fourth ventricle
4. 第四脑室正中孔 median aperture of the fourth ventricle
5. 楔束结节 cuneate tubercle
6. 薄束结节 gracile tubercle
7. 第四脑室外侧孔 lateral aperture of the fourth ventricle
8. 小脑下脚 inferior cerebellar peduncle
9. 小脑中脚 middle cerebellar peduncle
10. 小脑上脚 superior cerebellar peduncle
11. 小舌 lingula of cerebellum

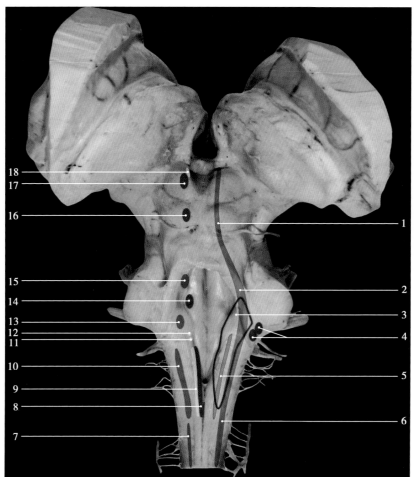

◀ 图 534

脑神经核在脑干的投影 (背面观)
Projection of nuclei of cranial nerves in the brain stem. Dorsal aspect

1. 三叉神经中脑核 mesencephalic nucleus of trigeminal n.
2. 三叉神经脑桥核 pontine nucleus of trigeminal n.
3. 前庭神经核 vestibular nuclei
4. 蜗神经核 cochlear nuclei
5. 孤束核 nucleus of solitary tract
6. 三叉神经脊束核 spinal nucleus of trigeminal n.
7. 副神经核 accessory nucleus
8. 舌下神经核 nucleus of hypoglossal n.
9. 迷走神经背核 dorsal nucleus of vagus n.
10. 疑核 nucleus ambiguus
11. 下泌涎核 inferior salivatory nucleus
12. 上泌涎核 superior salivatory nucleus
13. 面神经核 nucleus of facial n.
14. 展神经核 nucleus of abducent n.
15. 三叉神经运动核 motor nucleus of trigeminal n.
16. 滑车神经核 nucleus of trochlear n.
17. 动眼神经核 nucleus of oculomotor n.
18. 动眼神经副核 accessory nucleus of oculomotor n.

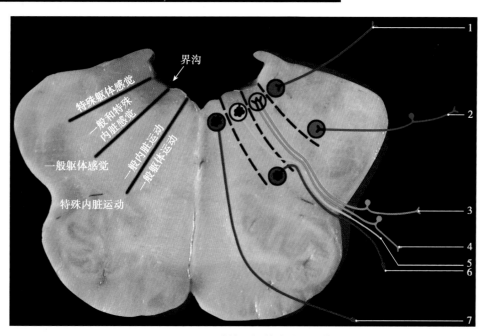

▲ 图 535 脑神经核基本排列规律
Fundamental arrangement of nuclei of cranial nerves

1. 特殊躯体感觉 special somatesthesia
2. 一般躯体感觉 general somatesthesia
3. 一般内脏感觉 general visceral sensation
4. 特殊内脏感觉 special visceral sensation
5. 一般内脏运动 general visceral movement
6. 特殊内脏运动 special visceral movement
7. 一般躯体运动 general body movement

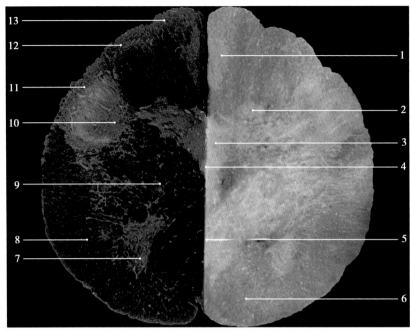

▲ 图 536　延髓横切面（经锥体交叉）
Transverse section of medulla oblongata. Through the decussation of pyramid

1. 薄束核 gracile nucleus
2. 楔束核 cuneate nucleus
3. 中央灰质 central gray matter
4. 中央管 central canal
5. 锥体交叉 decussation of pyramid
6. 锥体束 pyramidal tract
7. 第 1 颈神经运动核 motor nucleus of the 1st cervical n.
8. 脊髓丘脑束 spinothalamic tract
9. 皮质脊髓侧束 lateral corticospinal tract
10. 三叉神经脊束核 spinal nucleus of trigeminal n.
11. 三叉神经脊束 spinal tract of trigeminal n.
12. 楔束 fasciculus cuneatus
13. 薄束 fasciculus gracilis

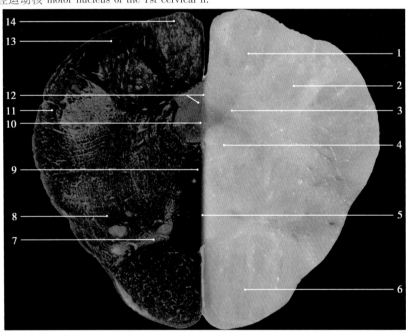

▲ 图 537　延髓横切面（经内侧丘系交叉）
Transverse section of medulla oblongata. Through the decussation of medial lemniscus

1. 薄束核 gracile nucleus
2. 楔束核 cuneate nucleus
3. 孤束核 nucleus of solitary tract
4. 舌下神经核 nucleus of hypoglossal n.
5. 内侧丘系交叉 decussation of medial lemniscus
6. 锥体束 pyramidal tract
7. 内侧副橄榄核 medial accessory olivary nucleus
8. 脊髓丘脑束 spinothalamic tract
9. 内侧纵束 medial longitudinal fasciculus
10. 中央管 central canal
11. 三叉神经脊束 spinal tract of trigeminal n.
12. 中央灰质 central gray
13. 楔束 fasciculus cuneatus
14. 薄束 fasciculus gracilis

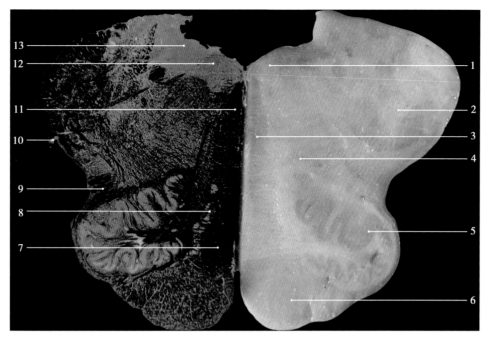

▲ 图 538　延髓横切面 (经橄榄中部)
Transverse section of medulla oblongata. Through the middle portion of olive

1. 舌下神经核 nucleus of hypoglossal n.
2. 三叉神经脊束核 spinal nucleus of trigeminal n.
3. 顶盖脊髓束 tectospinal tract
4. 背侧副橄榄核 dorsal accessory olivary nucleus
5. 下橄榄主核 inferior olivary nucleus
6. 锥体束 pyramidal tract
7. 内侧丘系 medial lemniscus
8. 内侧副橄榄核 medial accessory olivary nucleus
9. 脊髓丘脑束 spinothalamic tract
10. 迷走神经根 root of vagus n.
11. 内侧纵束 medial longitudinal fasciculus
12. 迷走神经背核 dorsal nucleus of vagus n.
13. 前庭内侧核 medial vestibular nucleus

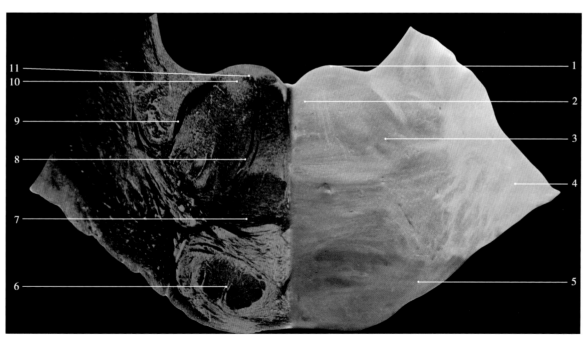

▲ 图 539　脑桥横切面 (经面神经丘)
Transverse section of pons. Through the facial colliculus

1. 面神经丘 facial colliculus
2. 内侧纵束 medial longitudinal fasciculus
3. 面神经核 nucleus of facial n.
4. 小脑中脚 middle cerebellar peduncle
5. 脑桥浅横纤维 superficial horizontal fibers of pons
6. 锥体束 pyramidal tract
7. 斜方体及内侧丘系 trapezoid body and medial lemniscus
8. 展神经根 root of abducens n.
9. 面神经根 root of facial n.
10. 展神经核 nucleus of abducent n.
11. 面神经膝 genu of facial n.

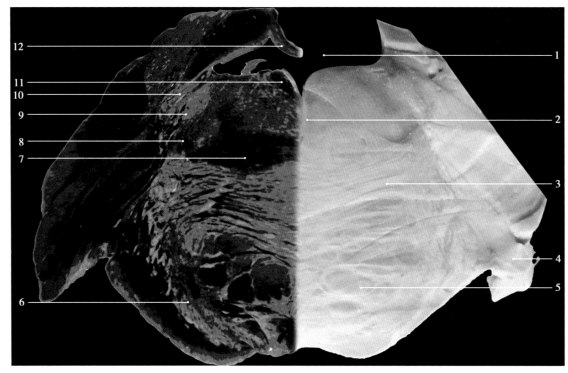

▲ 图 540　脑桥横切面（经三叉神经根）
Transverse section of pons. Through the root of trigeminal nerve

1. 第四脑室 fourth ventricle
2. 内侧纵束 medial longitudinal fasciculus
3. 脑桥深横纤维 deep transverse fibers of pons
4. 三叉神经根 root of trigeminal n.
5. 锥体束与皮质脑桥束 pyramidal tract and corticopontine tracts
6. 脑桥核 pontine nucleus
7. 斜方体及内侧丘系 trapezoid body and medial lemniscus
8. 外侧丘系 lateral lemniscus
9. 三叉神经运动核 motor nucleus of trigeminal n.
10. 三叉神经脑桥核 pontine nucleus of trigeminal n.
11. 背侧纵束 dorsal longitudinal fasciculus
12. 上髓帆 superior medullary velum

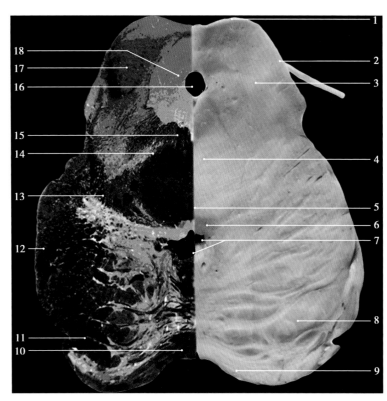

◀ 图 541

中脑横切面（经下丘）
Transverse section of midbrain. Through the inferior colliculus

1. 下丘 inferior colliculus
2. 下丘臂 brachium of inferior colliculus
3. 外侧丘系 lateral lemniscus
4. 内侧纵束 medial longitudinal fasciculus
5. 小脑上脚交叉 decussation of superior cerebellar peduncle
6. 脚间核 interpeduncular nucleus
7. 脚间窝 interpeduncular fossa
8. 锥体束 pyramidal tract
9. 脑桥基底部 basilar part of pons
10. 脑桥横行纤维 transverse fibers of pons
11. 额桥束 frontopontile tract
12. 顶枕颞桥束 parietooccipitotemporopontine tract
13. 三叉丘系及内侧丘系 trigeminal lemniscus and medial lemniscus
14. 顶盖脊髓束 tectospinal tract
15. 滑车神经核 nucleus of trochlear n.
16. 中脑水管 mesencephalic aqueduct
17. 下丘核 nucleus of inferior colliculus
18. 导水管周围灰质 periaoueductal gray matter

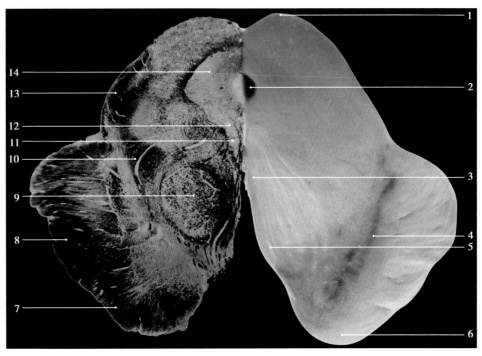

▲ 图 542 **中脑横切面(经上丘)**
Transverse section of midbrain. Through the superior colliculus

1. 上丘 superior colliculus
2. 中脑水管 mesencephalic aqueduct
3. 内侧纵束 medial longitudinal fasciculus
4. 黑质 substantia nigra
5. 动眼神经根 oculomotor root
6. 额桥束 frontopontine tract
7. 皮质核束 corticonuclear tract
8. 皮质脊髓束 corticospinal tract
9. 红核 red nucleus
10. 三叉丘系及内侧丘系 lemniscus trigeminalis and medial lemniscus
11. 动眼神经核 nucleus of oculomotor n.
12. 动眼神经副核 accessory nucleus of oculomotor n.
13. 内侧膝状体 medial geniculate body
14. 导水管周围灰质 periaoueductal gray matter

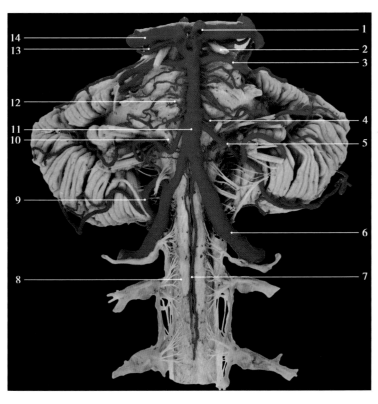

◄ 图 543
脑干的动脉
Arteries of brain stem
1. 后交通动脉 posterior communicating a.
2. 动眼神经 oculomotor n.
3. 小脑上动脉 superior cerebellar a.
4. 迷路动脉 labyrinthine a.
5. 小脑下前动脉 anterior inferior cerebellar a.
6. 椎动脉 vertebral a.
7. 脊髓前动脉 anterior spinal a.
8. 脊髓 spinal cord
9. 小脑下后动脉 posterior inferior cerebellar a.
10. 展神经 abducent n.
11. 基底动脉 basilar a.
12. 脑桥动脉 pontine a.
13. 脉络丛后内侧支 posterior medial choroidal branch
14. 大脑后动脉 posterior cerebral a.

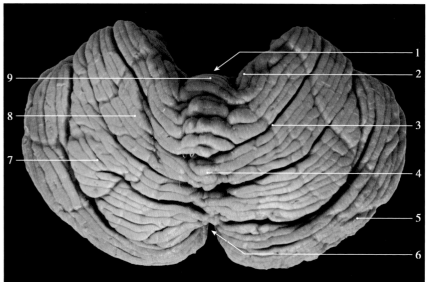

◀ 图 544

小脑（上面观）
Cerebellum. Superior aspect

1. 小脑前切迹 anterior cerebellar notch
2. 中央小叶翼 ala of central lobule
3. 原裂 primary fissure
4. 小脑蚓 vermis
5. 水平裂 horizontal fissure
6. 小脑后切迹 posterior cerebellar notch
7. 方形小叶后部 posterior quadrangular lobule
8. 方形小叶前部 anterior quadrangular lobule
9. 中央小叶 central lobule

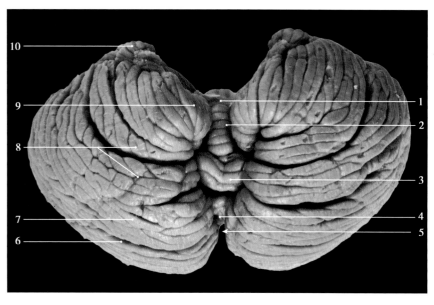

◀ 图 545

小脑（下面观）
Cerebellum. Inferior aspect

1. 小结 nodule
2. 蚓垂 uvula of vermis
3. 蚓锥体 pyramid of vermis
4. 蚓结节 tuber of vermis
5. 小脑后切迹 posterior cerebellar notch
6. 水平裂 horizontal fissure
7. 下半月小叶 inferior semilunar lobule
8. 二腹小叶 biventral lobule
9. 小脑扁桃体 tonsil of cerebellum
10. 绒球 flocculus

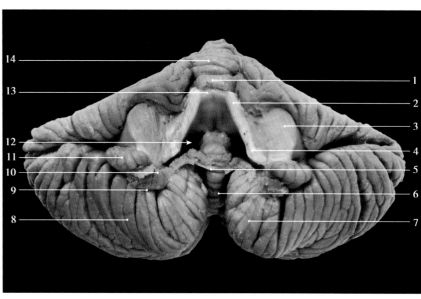

◀ 图 546

小脑（前面观）
Cerebellum. Anterior aspect

1. 小脑小舌 lingula of cerebellum
2. 小脑上脚 superior cerebellar peduncle
3. 小脑中脚 middle cerebellar peduncle
4. 小脑下脚 inferior cerebellar peduncle
5. 下髓帆 inferior medullary velum
6. 蚓垂 uvula of vermis
7. 小脑扁桃体 tonsil of cerebellum
8. 二腹小叶 biventral lobule
9. 后外侧裂 posterolateral fissure
10. 第四脑室脉络丛 choroid plexus of the fourth ventricle
11. 绒球 flocculus
12. 第四脑室 fourth ventricle
13. 上髓帆 superior medullary velum
14. 中央小叶 central lobule

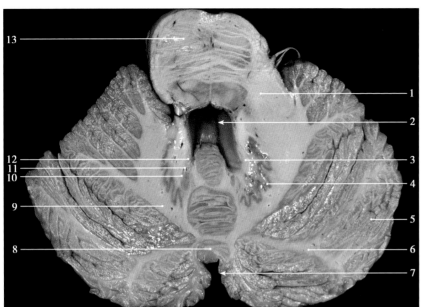

◀ 图 547

小脑水平切面
Horizontal section of cerebellum

1. 小脑中脚 middle cerebellar peduncle
2. 第四脑室 fourth ventricle
3. 齿状核门 hilum of dentate nucleus
4. 齿状核 dentate nucleus
5. 小脑皮质 cerebellar cortex
6. 髓板 medullary plate
7. 小脑后切迹 posterior cerebellar notch
8. 小脑蚓 vermis
9. 小脑髓质 cerebellar medulla
10. 栓状核 emboliform nucleus
11. 球状核 globose nucleus
12. 顶核 fastigial nucleus
13. 脑桥 pons

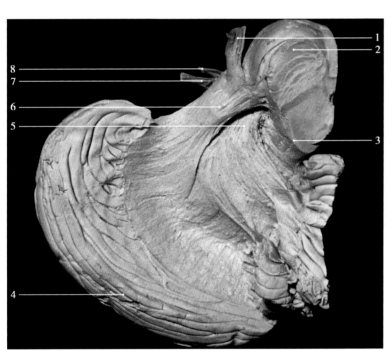

▲ 图 548　小脑脚（1）
Peduncles of cerebellum（1）

1. 三叉神经 trigeminal n.
2. 脑桥 pons
3. 小脑上脚 superior cerebellar peduncle
4. 小脑半球 cerebellar hemisphere
5. 小脑下脚 inferior cerebellar peduncle
6. 小脑中脚 middle cerebellar peduncle
7. 前庭蜗神经 vestibulocochlear n.
8. 面神经 facial n.

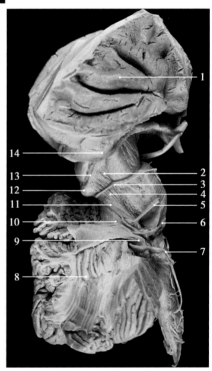

▲ 图 549　小脑脚（2）
Peduncles of cerebellum（2）

1. 岛叶 insular lobe
2. 内侧丘系 medial lemniscus
3. 滑车神经 trochlear n.
4. 外侧丘系 lateral lemniscus
5. 三叉神经 trigeminal n.
6. 面神经 facial n.
7. 前庭蜗神经 vestibulocochlear n.
8. 齿状核 dentate nucleus
9. 小脑下脚 inferior cerebellar peduncle
10. 小脑上脚 superior cerebellar peduncle
11. 脊髓小脑前束 anterior spinocerebellar tract
12. 下丘 inferior colliculus
13. 下丘臂 brachium of inferior colliculus
14. 外侧膝状体 lateral geniculate body

 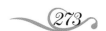

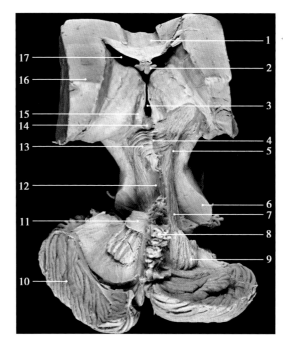

◀ 图 550
小脑齿状核和小脑脚
Dentate nucleus and peduncles of cerebellum
1. 胼胝体 corpus callosum
2. 穹隆体 body of fornix
3. 第三脑室 third ventricle
4. 小脑上脚交叉 decussation of superior cerebellar peduncle
5. 小脑上脚不交叉纤维 not-decussation fibers of superior cerebellar peduncle
6. 小脑中脚 middle cerebellar peduncle
7. 小脑上脚 superior cerebellar peduncle
8. 小脑蚓 vermis
9. 齿状核 dentate nucleus
10. 小脑半球 cerebellar hemisphere
11. 小脑下脚 inferior cerebellar peduncle
12. 上髓帆 superior medullary velum
13. 小脑上脚交叉纤维 decussation fibers of superior cerebellar peduncle
14. 松果体 pineal body
15. 缰三角 habenular trigone
16. 内囊 internal capsule
17. 侧脑室 lateral ventricle

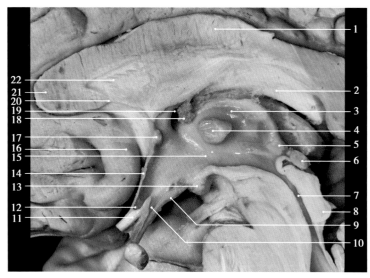

◀ 图 551
间脑内侧面
Medial surface of diencephalon
1. 胼胝体 corpus callosum
2. 穹隆体 body of fornix
3. 背侧丘脑 dorsal thalamus
4. 丘脑间黏合 interthalamic adhesion
5. 缰连合 habenular commissure
6. 松果体 pineal body
7. 中脑水管 mesencephalic aqueduct
8. 下丘 inferior colliculus
9. 灰结节 tuber cinereum
10. 漏斗隐窝 infundibular recess
11. 视交叉 optic chiasma
12. 视隐窝 optic recess
13. 乳头体 mamillary body
14. 终板 lamina terminalis
15. 下丘脑沟 hypothalamic sulcus
16. 胼胝体下区 subcallosal area
17. 前连合 anterior commissure
18. 第三脑室脉络丛 choroid plexus of the third ventricle
19. 室间孔 interventricular foramen
20. 胼胝体嘴 rostrum of corpus callosum
21. 胼胝体膝 genu of corpus callosum
22. 透明隔 septum pellucidum

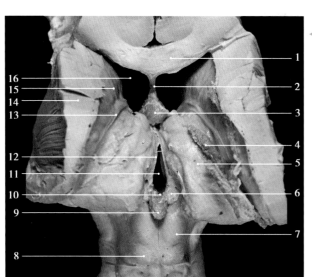

◀ 图 552
间脑的背面
Dorsal surface of diencephalon
1. 胼胝体 corpus callosum
2. 透明隔 septum pellucidum
3. 穹隆 fornix
4. 侧脑室脉络丛 choroid plexus of lateral ventricle
5. 背侧丘脑 dorsal thalamus
6. 缰三角 habenular trigone
7. 上丘 superior colliculus
8. 下丘 inferior colliculus
9. 松果体 pineal body
10. 缰连合 habenular commissure
11. 第三脑室 third ventricle
12. 丘脑髓纹 thalamic medullary stria
13. 终纹 terminal stria
14. 内囊 internal capsule
15. 尾状核头 head of caudate nucleus
16. 侧脑室前角 anterior horn of lateral ventricle

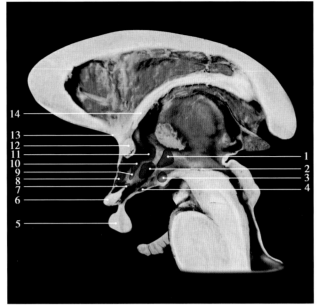

▲ 图 553　下丘脑的主要核团（矢状切面）
Hypothalamic main nuclei. Sagittal section
1. 后核 posterior nucleus
2. 腹内侧核 ventromedial nucleus
3. 乳头体核 mamillary body nucleus
4. 漏斗核 infundibular nucleus
5. 垂体 hypophysis
6. 视交叉 optic chiasma
7. 视上核 supraoptic nucleus
8. 视前核 anterior nucleus
9. 前核 anterior nucleus
10. 室旁核 paraventricular nucleus
11. 背内侧核 dorsomedial nucleus
12. 前连合 anterior commissure
13. 终板 lamina terminalis
14. 穹隆 fornix

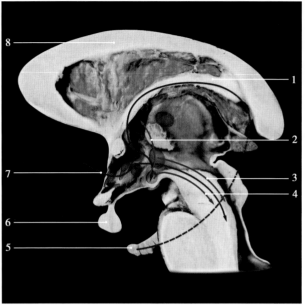

▲ 图 554　下丘脑的纤维联系（矢状切面）
Hypothalamic fiber connection. Sagittal section
1. 穹隆 fornix
2. 乳头丘脑束 mamillothalamic tract
3. 背侧纵束 dorsal longitudinal fasciculus
4. 乳头被盖束 mamillotegmental tract
5. 海马 hippocampus
6. 垂体 hypophysis
7. 前脑内侧束 medial forebrain bundle
8. 胼胝体 corpus callosum

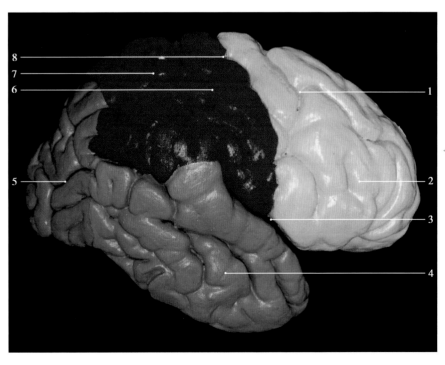

◀ 图 555

脑外侧面（1）
Lateral surface of brain（1）
1. 中央前沟 precentral sulcus
2. 额叶 frontal lobe
3. 外侧沟 lateral sulcus
4. 颞叶 temporal lobe
5. 枕叶 occipital lobe
6. 中央后沟 postcentral sulcus
7. 顶叶 parietal lobe
8. 中央沟 central sulcus

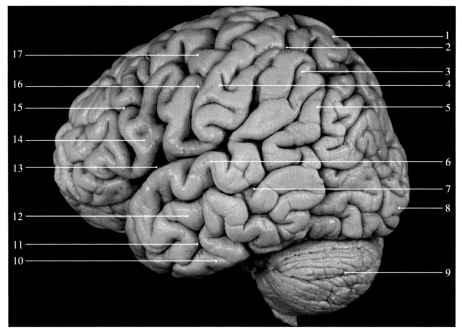

▲ 图556 脑外侧面(2)
Lateral surface of brain(2)

1. 顶上小叶 superior parietal lobule
2. 中央后沟 postcentral sulcus
3. 缘上回 supramarginal gyrus
4. 中央后回 postcentral gyrus
5. 角回 angular gyrus
6. 颞上回 superior temporal gyrus
7. 颞上沟 superior temporal sulcus
8. 枕极 occipital pole
9. 小脑 cerebellum
10. 颞下回 inferior temporal gyrus
11. 颞下沟 inferior temporal sulcus
12. 颞中回 middle temporal gyrus
13. 外侧沟 lateral sulcus
14. 额下回 inferior frontal gyrus
15. 额下沟 inferior frontal sulcus
16. 中央沟 central sulcus
17. 中央前回 precentral gyrus

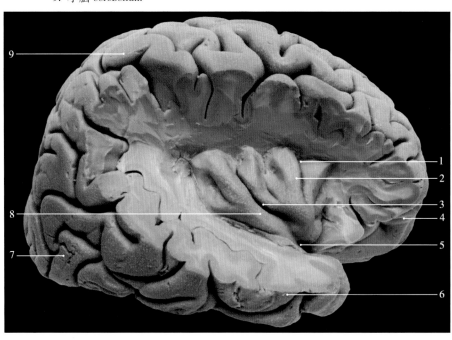

▲ 图557 岛叶
Insular lobe

1. 岛环状沟 circular sulcus of insula
2. 岛短回 short gyri of insula
3. 岛中央沟 central sulcus of insula
4. 额叶 frontal lobe
5. 岛阈 limen of insula
6. 颞叶 temporal lobe
7. 枕叶 occipital lobe
8. 岛长回 long gyrus of insula
9. 顶叶 parietal lobe

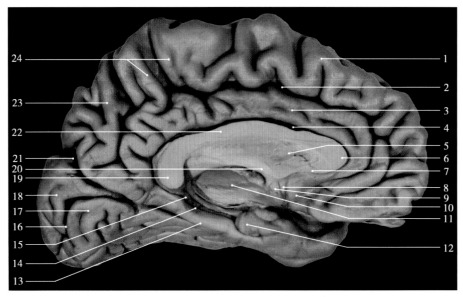

▲ 图 558　大脑半球内侧面
Medial surface of the cerebral hemisphere

1. 额上回 superior frontal gyrus
2. 扣带沟 cingulate sulcus
3. 扣带回 cingulate gyrus
4. 胼胝体沟 callosal sulcus
5. 透明隔 septum pellucidum
6. 胼胝体膝 genu of corpus callosum
7. 胼胝体嘴 rostrum of corpus callosum
8. 终板旁回 paraterminal gyrus
9. 前连合 anterior commissure
10. 胼胝体下区 subcallosal area
11. 背侧丘脑 dorsal thalamus
12. 钩 uncus
13. 海马旁回 parahippocampal gyrus
14. 海马沟 hippocampal sulcus
15. 齿状回 dentate gyrus
16. 距状沟 calcarine sulcus
17. 舌回 lingual gyrus
18. 楔叶 cuneus
19. 胼胝体压部 splenium of corpus callosum
20. 穹隆 fornix
21. 顶枕沟 parietooccipital sulcus
22. 胼胝体干 trunk of corpus callosum
23. 楔前叶 precuneus
24. 中央旁小叶 paracentral lobule

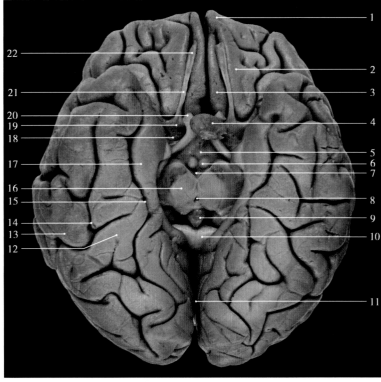

◀ 图 559

端脑底面
Basal surface of telencephalon

1. 额极 frontal pole
2. 眶回 orbital gyrus
3. 直回 gyrus rectus
4. 垂体 hypophysis
5. 灰结节 tuber cinereum
6. 乳头体 mamillary body
7. 脚间窝 interpeduncular fossa
8. 中脑水管 mesencephalic aqueduct
9. 松果体 pineal body
10. 胼胝体压部 splenium of corpus callosum
11. 大脑纵裂 cerebral longitudinal fissure
12. 枕颞内侧回 medial occipitotemporal gyrus
13. 枕颞外侧回 lateral occipitotemporal gyrus
14. 枕颞沟 occipitotemporal sulcus
15. 侧副沟 collateral sulcus
16. 中脑 midbrain
17. 海马旁回 parahippocampal gyrus
18. 前穿质 anterior perforated substance
19. 嗅三角 olfactory trigone
20. 视神经 optic n.
21. 嗅束 olfactory tract
22. 嗅球 olfactory bulb

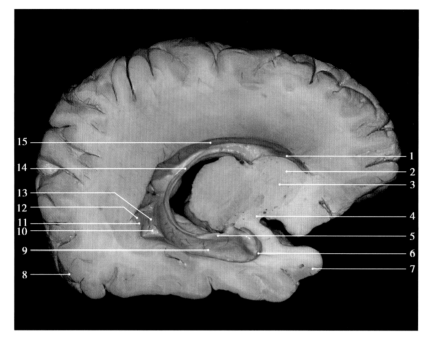

▲ 图 560　海马结构
Hippocampal formation

1. 侧脑室前角 anterior horn of lateral ventricle
2. 尾状核头 head of caudate nucleus
3. 内囊 internal capsule
4. 前连合 anterior commissure
5. 海马伞 fimbria of hippocampus
6. 侧脑室下角 inferior horn of lateral ventricle
7. 颞极 temporal pole
8. 枕极 occipital pole
9. 海马 hippocampus
10. 侧副三角 collateral trigone
11. 禽距 calcar avis
12. 后角球 bulb of posterior horn
13. 侧脑室后角 posterior horn of lateral ventricle
14. 穹隆体 body of fornix
15. 侧脑室中央部 central part of lateral ventricle

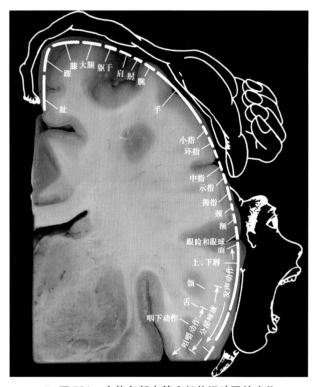

▲ 图 561　人体各部在第Ⅰ躯体运动区的定位
Localization of different parts of human body in primary somatomotor area

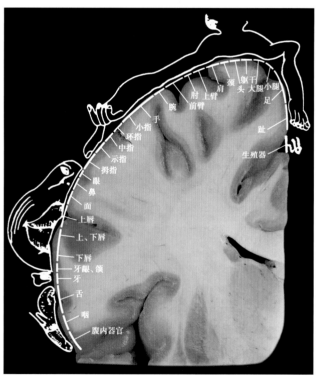

▲ 图 562　人体各部在第Ⅰ躯体感觉区的定位
Localization of different parts of human body in primary somesthetic area

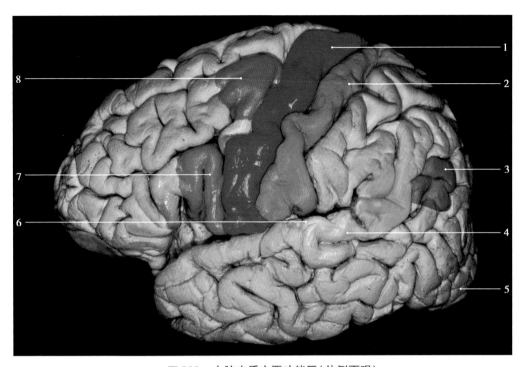

▲ 图 563　大脑皮质主要功能区（外侧面观）
Main functional areas of cerebral cortex. Lateral aspect

1. 第一躯体运动区 first somatic motor area
2. 第一躯体感觉区 first somathetic area (somatic sensory area)
3. 视觉性语言中枢 visual speech area
4. 听觉性语言中枢 auditory speech area
5. 视觉区 visual area
6. 听觉区 auditory area
7. 运动性语言中枢 motor speech area
8. 书写中枢 writing area

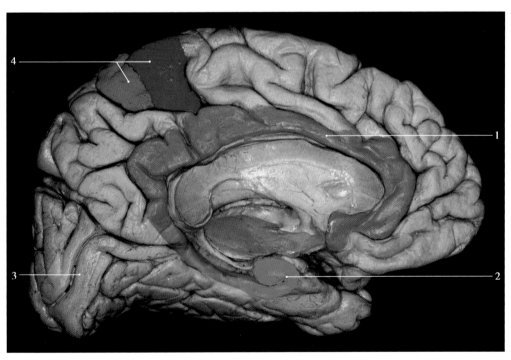

▲ 图 564　大脑皮质主要功能区（内侧面观）
Main functional areas of cerebral cortex. Medial aspect

1. 内脏调节中枢 visceral regulatory center
2. 钩 uncus
3. 视觉区 visual area
4. 中央旁小叶 paracentral lobule

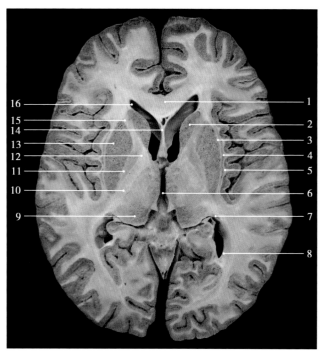

◀ 图 565
基底核、背侧丘脑和内囊
Basal nuclei , dorsal thalamus and internal capsule
1. 胼胝体膝 genu of corpus callosum
2. 尾状核 caudate nucleus
3. 外囊 external capsule
4. 屏状核 caudate nucleus
5. 最外囊 extreme capsule
6. 第三脑室 third ventricle
7. 尾状核尾 tail of caudate nucleus
8. 侧脑室后角 posterior horn of lateral ventricle
9. 背侧丘脑 dorsal thalamus
10. 内囊后肢 posterior limb of interal capsule
11. 苍白球 globus pallidus
12. 内囊膝 genu of internal capsule
13. 壳 putamen
14. 透明隔 septum pellucidum
15. 内囊前肢 anterior limb of interal capsule
16. 侧脑室前角 anterior horn of lateral ventricle

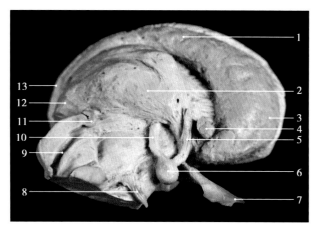

▲ 图 566 基底核(内侧面观)
Basal nuclei. Medial aspect
1. 尾状核 caudate nucleus
2. 背侧丘脑 dorsal thalamus
3. 尾状核头 head of caudate nucleus
4. 前连合 anterior commissure
5. 穹隆柱 column of fornix
6. 乳头体 mamillary body
7. 视神经 optic n.
8. 动眼神经 oculomotor n.
9. 中脑水管 mesencephalic aqueduct
10. 乳头丘脑束 mamillothalamic tract
11. 后连合 posterior commissure
12. 丘脑枕 pulvinar
13. 尾状核尾 tail of caudate nucleus

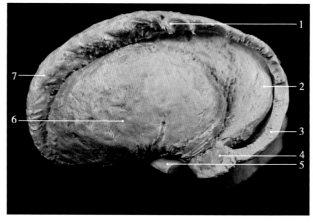

▲ 图 567 基底核(外侧面观)
Basal nuclei. Lateral aspect
1. 尾状核体 body caudate nucleus
2. 背侧丘脑 dorsal thalamus
3. 尾状核尾 tail of caudate nucleus
4. 杏仁体 amygdaloid body
5. 前连合 anterior commissure
6. 豆状核 lentiform nucleus
7. 尾状核头 head of caudate nucleus

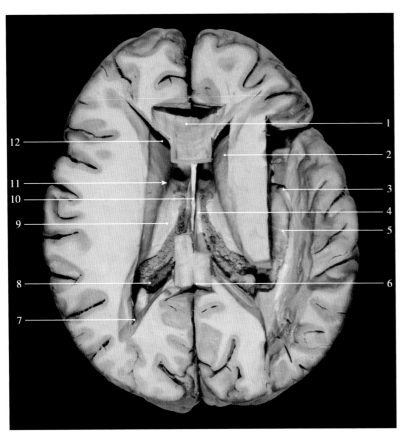

◀ 图568

侧脑室（上面观）
Lateral ventricle. Superior aspect
1. 胼胝体膝 genu of corpus callosum
2. 尾状核头 head of caudate nucleus
3. 侧脑室下角 inferior horn of lateral ventricle
4. 穹隆 fornix
5. 海马 hippocampus
6. 胼胝体压部 splenium of corpus callosum
7. 侧脑室后角 posterior horn of lateral ventricle
8. 侧脑室脉络丛 choroid plexus of lateral ventricle
9. 背侧丘脑 dorsal thalamus
10. 透明隔 septum pellucidum
11. 侧脑室中央部 central part of lateral ventricle
12. 侧脑室前角 anterior horn of lateral ventricle

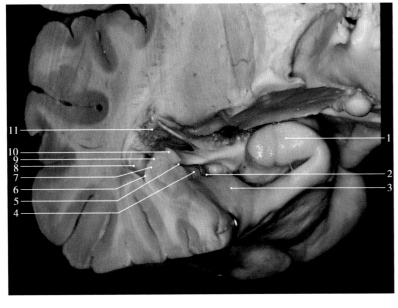

◀ 图569

海马旁回与海马结构的切面
Section through the parahippocampal gyrus and the hippocampal formation
1. 钩 uncus
2. 海马沟 hippocampal sulcus
3. 海马旁回 parahippocampal gyrus
4. 齿状回 dentate gyrus
5. 伞齿沟 fimbriodentate sulcus
6. 海马室床 hippocampal alveus
7. 海马槽 alveus of hippocampus
8. 下角 inferior horn
9. 海马 hippocampus
10. 海马伞 fimbria of hippocampus
11. 侧脑室脉络丛 choroids plexus of lateral ventricle

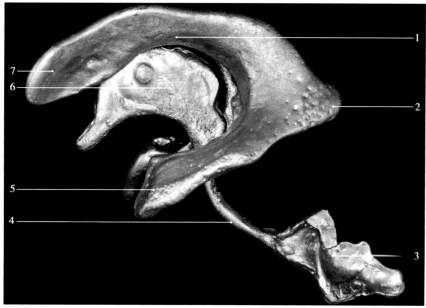

◀ 图 570

脑室铸型(侧面观)

Cast of ventricles of brain. Lateral aspect

1. 中央部 central part
2. 后角 posterior horn
3. 第四脑室 fourth ventricle
4. 中脑水管 mesencephalic aqueduct
5. 下角 inferior horn
6. 第三脑室 third ventricle
7. 前角 anterior horn

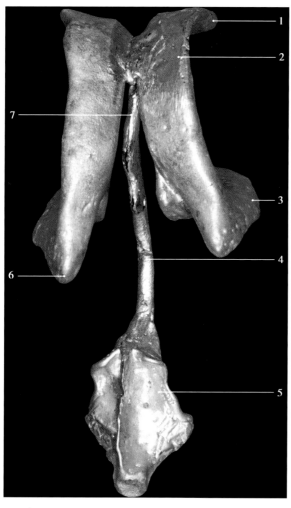

◀ 图 571

脑室铸型(后面观)

Cast of ventricles of brain. Posterior aspect

1. 前角 anterior horn
2. 中央部 central part
3. 下角 inferior horn
4. 中脑水管 mesencephalic aqueduct
5. 第四脑室 fourth ventricle
6. 后角 posterior horn
7. 第三脑室 third ventricle

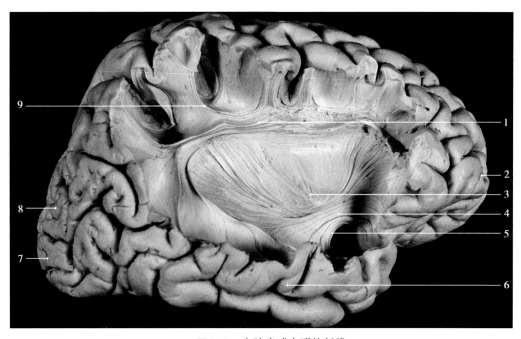

▲ 图 572　大脑半球内联络纤维
Association fibers in the cerebral hemisphere

1. 上纵束 superior longitudinal fasciculus　　6. 颞叶 temporal lobe
2. 额叶 frontal lobe　　　　　　　　　　　　7. 枕极 temporal pole
3. 外囊 external capsule　　　　　　　　　　8. 枕叶 occipital lobe
4. 额枕下束 inferior frontooccipital fasciculus　9. 弓状纤维 arcuate fibers
5. 钩束 uncinate fasciculus

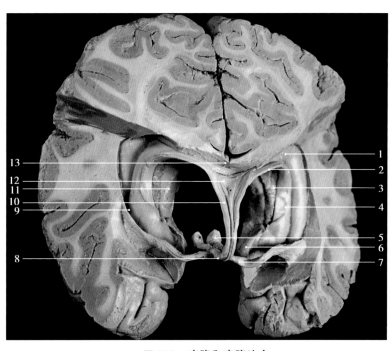

▲ 图 573　穹隆和穹隆连合
Fornix and the commissure of fornix

1. 侧副三角 collateral trigone　　6. 钩 uncus　　　　　　　　　　10. 穹隆体 body of fornix
2. 穹隆脚 crus of fornix　　　　　7. 前连合 anterior commissure　　11. 海马旁回 parahippocampal gyrus
3. 齿状回 dentate gyrus　　　　　8. 穹隆柱 column of fornix　　　　12. 穹隆连合 commissure of fornix
4. 海马 hippocampus　　　　　　　9. 侧脑室下角 inferior horn of lateral　13. 胼胝体 corpus callosum
5. 乳头体 mammillary body　　　　　　ventricle

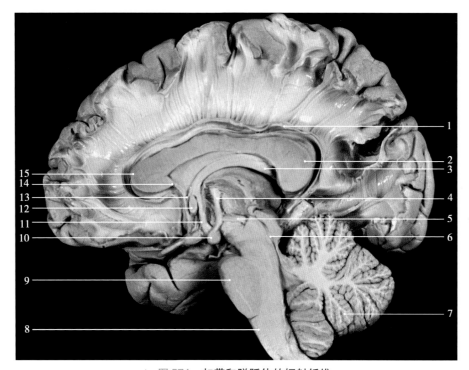

▲ 图574　扣带和胼胝体的辐射纤维
Fibers of cingulum and radiation of corpus callosum

1. 扣带 cingulum
2. 胼胝体压部 splenium of corpus callosum
3. 穹隆 fornix
4. 乳头丘脑束 mamillothalamic tract
5. 乳头被盖束 mamillotegmental tract
6. 中脑水管 mesencephalic aqueduct
7. 小脑 cerebellum
8. 延髓 medulla oblongata
9. 脑桥 pons
10. 乳头体 mamillary body
11. 连合后穹隆 retro-commissural fornix
12. 前连合 anterior commissure
13. 连合前穹隆 precommissural fornix
14. 胼胝体嘴 rostrum of corpus callosum
15. 胼胝体膝 genu of corpus callosum

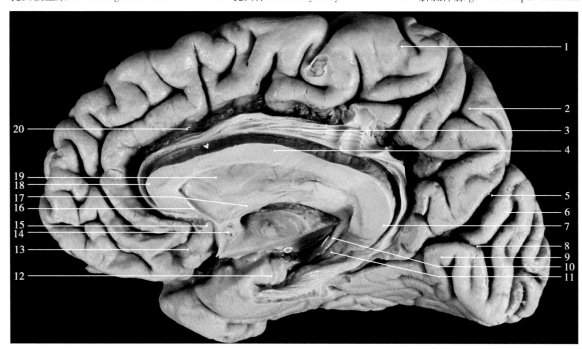

▲ 图575　扣带
Cingulum

1. 中央旁小叶 paracentral lobule
2. 楔前叶 precuneus
3. 扣带 cingulum
4. 胼胝体干 trunk of corpus callosum
5. 顶枕沟 parietooccipital sulcus
6. 楔叶 cuneus
7. 胼胝体压部 splenium of corpus callosum
8. 距状沟 calcarine sulcus
9. 舌回 lingual gyrus
10. 穹隆脚 crus of fornix
11. 齿状回 dentate gyrus
12. 钩 uncus
13. 胼胝体下区 subcallosal area
14. 前连合 anterior commissure
15. 终板旁回 paraterminal gyrus
16. 胼胝体嘴 rostrum of corpus callosum
17. 穹隆 fornix
18. 胼胝体膝 genu of corpus callosum
19. 透明隔 septum pellucidum
20. 扣带沟 cingulate sulcus

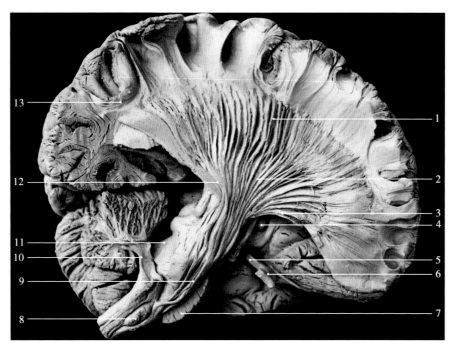

▲ 图576 **锥体束**
Pyramidal tract

1. 辐射冠 corona radiata
2. 内囊膝 genu of internal capsule
3. 内囊前肢 anterior limb of internal capsule
4. 前连合 anterior commissure
5. 视束 optic tract
6. 视交叉 optic chiasma
7. 脑桥 pons

8. 橄榄 olive
9. 锥体束 pyramidal tract
10. 小脑下脚 inferior cerebellar peduncle
11. 小脑上脚 superior cerebellar peduncle
12. 内囊后肢 posterior limb of internal capsule
13. 弓状纤维 arcuate fibers

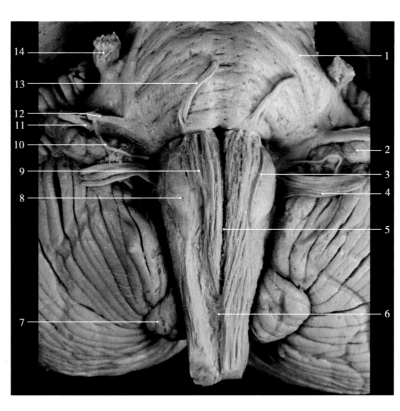

◀ 图577

锥体交叉
Decussation of pyramid

1. 脑桥 pons
2. 小脑绒球 flocculus of cerebellum
3. 前外侧沟 anterior lateral sulcus
4. 迷走神经 vagus n.
5. 前正中裂 anterior median fissure
6. 锥体交叉 decussation of pyramid
7. 小脑扁桃体 tonsil of cerebellum
8. 橄榄 olive
9. 锥体束 pyramidal tract
10. 舌咽神经 glossopharyngeal n.
11. 前庭蜗神经 vestibulocochlear n.
12. 面神经 facial n.
13. 展神经 abducent n.
14. 三叉神经 trigeminal n.

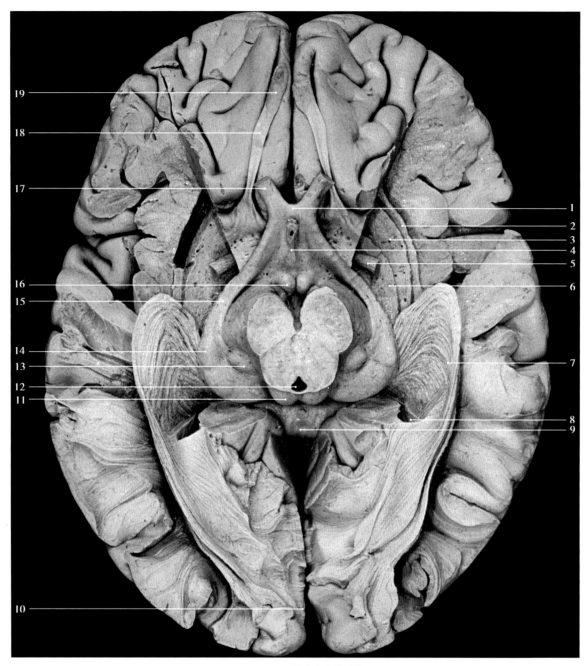

▲ 图 578　视束和视辐射
Optic tract and optic radiation

1. 视交叉 optic chiasma
2. 外囊 external capsule
3. 豆状核壳 putamen of lentiform nucleus
4. 灰结节 tuber cinereum
5. 前连合 anterior commissure
6. 苍白球 globus pallidus
7. 视辐射 optic radiation
8. 侧脑室下脚 inferior horn of lateral ventricle
9. 胼胝体压部 splenium of corpus callosum
10. 视觉区 visual area

11. 上丘 superior colliculus
12. 中脑水管 mesencephalic aqueduct
13. 内侧膝状体 medial geniculate body
14. 外侧膝状体 lateral geniculate body
15. 视束 optic tract
16. 乳头体 mamillary body
17. 视神经 optic n.
18. 嗅束 olfactory tract
19. 嗅球 olfactory bulb

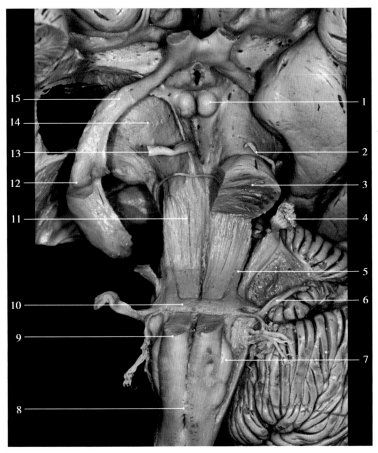

◀ 图 579

内、外侧丘系
Medial and lateral lemniscus
1. 乳头体 mamillary body
2. 滑车神经 trochlear n.
3. 脑桥 pons
4. 三叉神经 trigeminal n.
5. 外侧丘系 lateral lemniscus
6. 前庭蜗神经 vestibulocochlear n.
7. 橄榄 olive
8. 锥体交叉 decussation of pyramid
9. 锥体 pyramid
10. 斜方体 trapezoid body
11. 内侧丘系 medial lemniscus
12. 外侧膝状体 lateral geniculate body
13. 动眼神经 oculomotor n.
14. 大脑脚 cerebral peduncle
15. 视束 optic tract.

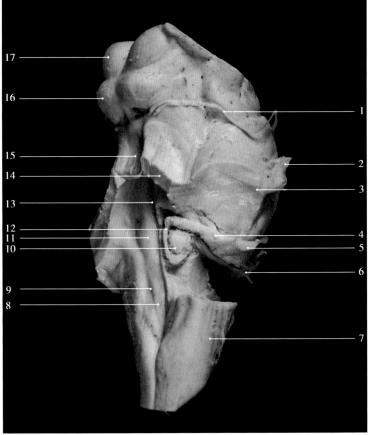

◀ 图 580

面神经在脑内的行路
Pathway of facial nerve in brain
1. 滑车神经 trochlear n.
2. 三叉神经 trigeminal n.
3. 小脑中脚 middle cerebellar peduncle
4. 面神经 facial n.
5. 前庭蜗神经 vestibulocochlear n.
6. 展神经 abducent n.
7. 延髓 medulla oblongata
8. 内侧隆起 medial eminence
9. 界沟 sulcus limitans
10. 展神经核 nucleus of abducent n.
11. 面神经丘 facial colliculus
12. 面神经膝 geniculum of facial n.
13. 正中沟 median sulcus
14. 小脑上脚 superior cerebellar peduncle
15. 上髓帆 superior medullary velum
16. 下丘 inferior colliculus
17. 上丘 superior colliculus

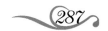

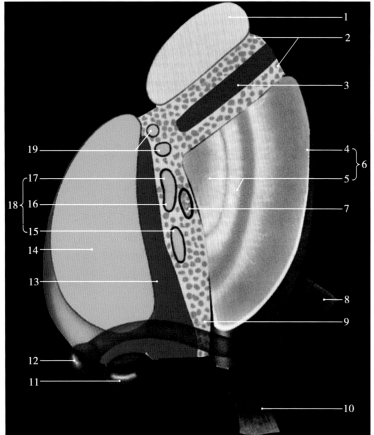

◀ 图 581

内囊主要结构（模式图）
Main structure of internal capsule. Diagram

1. 尾状核头 head of caudate nucleus
2. 额桥束 frontopontine tract
3. 丘脑前辐射 anterior thalamic radiations
4. 壳 putamen
5. 苍白球 globus pallidus
6. 豆状核 lenticular nucleus
7. 皮质红核束 corticorubral tract
8. 听辐射 acoustic radiation
9. 顶枕颞桥束 parictooccipitotemporopontine tract
10. 视辐射 optic radiation
11. 外侧膝状体 lateral geniculate body
12. 内侧膝状体 medial geniculate body
13. 丘脑中央辐射 central thalamic radiations
14. 背侧丘脑 dorsal thalamus
15. 下肢纤维束 fiber bundle of lower limb
16. 躯干纤维束 fiber bundle of trunk
17. 上肢纤维束 fiber bundle of upper limb
18. 皮质脊髓束 corticospinal tract
19. 皮质核束 corticonuclear tract

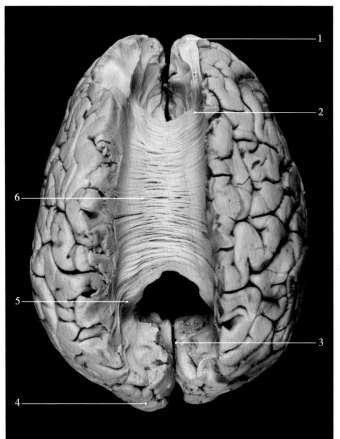

◀ 图 582

胼胝体（上面观）
Corpus callosum. Superior aspect

1. 额极 frontal pole
2. 额钳 frontal forceps
3. 大脑纵裂 cerebral longitudinal fissure
4. 枕极 occipital pole
5. 枕钳 occipital forceps
6. 胼胝体辐射 radiation of corpus callosum

第十四章 周围神经系统
Peripheral Nervous System

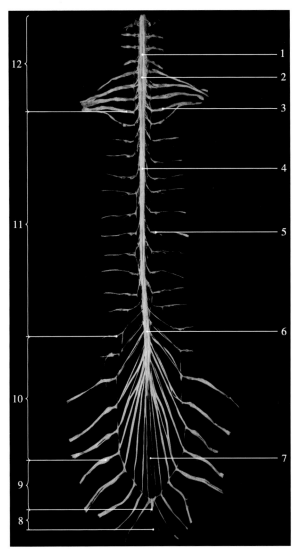

▲ 图583 脊神经
Spinal nerves
1. 颈段 cervical segments
2. 颈膨大 cervical enlargement
3. 脊神经 spinal nerve
4. 胸段 thoracic segments
5. 脊神经节 spinal ganglia
6. 腰骶膨大 lumbosacral enlargement
7. 终丝 filum terminale
8. 尾神经 coccygeal n.
9. 骶神经 sacral n
10. 腰神经 lumbar n.
11. 胸神经 thoracic n.
12. 颈神经 cervical n.

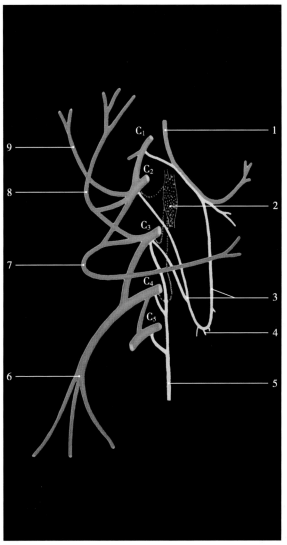

▲ 图584 颈丛的组成及颈襻
Formation of cervical plexus and
ansa cervicalis
1. 舌下神经 hypoglossal n.
2. 颈上神经节 superior cervical ganglion
3. 颈襻 ansa cervicalis
4. 肌支 muscular branch
5. 膈神经 phrenic n.
6. 锁骨上神经 supraclavicular n.
7. 颈横神经 transverse nerve of neck
8. 耳大神经 great auricular n.
9. 枕小神经 lesser occipital n.

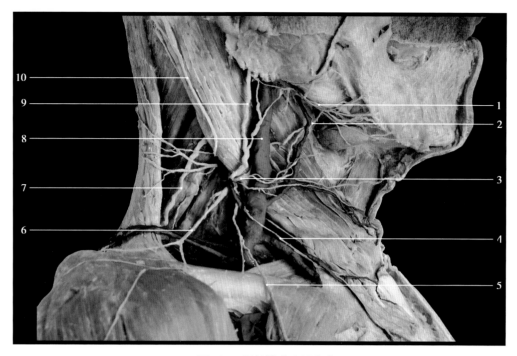

▲ 图 585　颈丛的皮支及分布
Distribution of cutaneous branches of cervical plexus

1. 下颌缘支 marginal mandibular branch
2. 颈支 cervical branch
3. 颈横神经 transverse nerve of neck
4. 锁骨上内侧神经 medial supraclavicular n.
5. 锁骨上中间神经 intermediate supraclavicular n.
6. 锁骨上外侧神经 lateral supraclavicular n.
7. 副神经 accessory n.
8. 颈外静脉 external jugular v.
9. 耳大神经 great auricular n.
10. 枕小神经 lesser occipital n.

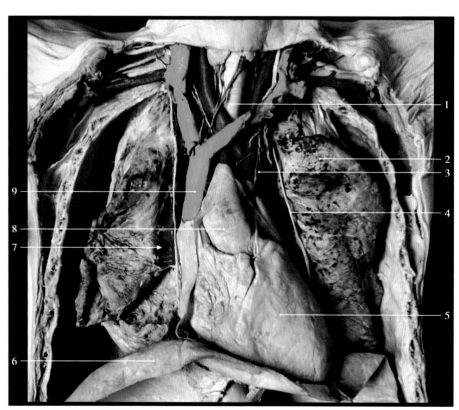

◀ 图 586

膈神经
Phrenic nerve
1. 气管 trachea
2. 左肺 left lung
3. 迷走神经心上支 superior cardiac branch of vagus n.
4. 膈神经 phrenic n.
5. 心 heart
6. 膈 diaphragm
7. 肺门 hilum of lung
8. 升主动脉 ascending aorta
9. 上腔静脉 superior vena cava

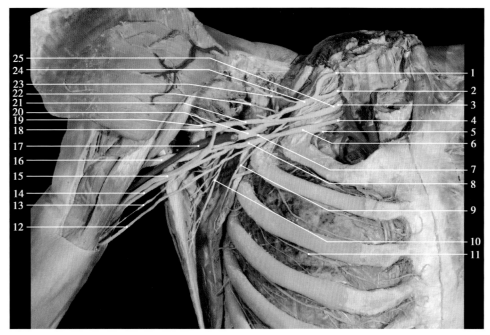

▲ 图 587 臂丛的组成
Formation of brachial plexus

1. 第 5 颈神经 5th cervical n.
2. 第 6 颈神经 6th cervical n.
3. 第 7 颈神经 7th cervical n.
4. 第 8 颈神经 8th cervical n.
5. 第 1 胸神经 1st thoracic n.
6. 下干 inferior trunk
7. 后股 posterior division
8. 内侧束 medial cord
9. 胸长神经 long thoracic n.
10. 胸背神经 thoracodorsal n.
11. 肋间神经 intercostal n.
12. 前臂内侧皮神经 medial antebrachial cutaneous n.
13. 臂内侧皮神经 medial brachial cutaneous n.
14. 尺神经 ulnar n.
15. 正中神经 median n.
16. 桡神经 radial n.
17. 腋动脉 axillary a.
18. 腋神经 axillary n.
19. 肌皮神经 musculocutaneous n.
20. 后束 posterior cord
21. 外侧束 lateral cord
22. 肩胛下神经 subscapular n.
23. 肩胛上神经 suprascapular n.
24. 上干 superior trunk
25. 中干 middle trunk

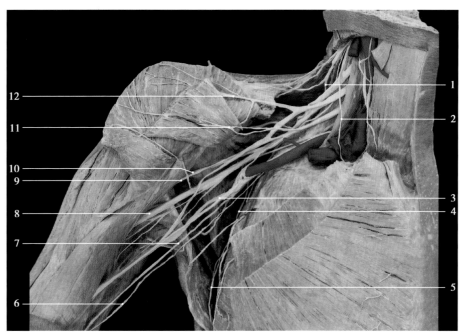

▲ 图 588 臂丛的主要分支
Main branches of brachial plexus

1. 肩胛背神经 dorsal scapular n.
2. 膈神经 phrenic n.
3. 正中神经 median n.
4. 胸长神经 long thoracic n.
5. 胸背神经 thoracodorsal n.
6. 前臂内侧皮神经 medial antebrachial cutaneous n.
7. 尺神经 ulnar n.
8. 桡神经 radial n.
9. 肌皮神经 musculocutaneous n.
10. 腋神经 axillary n.
11. 胸内侧神经 medial pectoral n.
12. 胸外侧神经 lateral pectoral n.

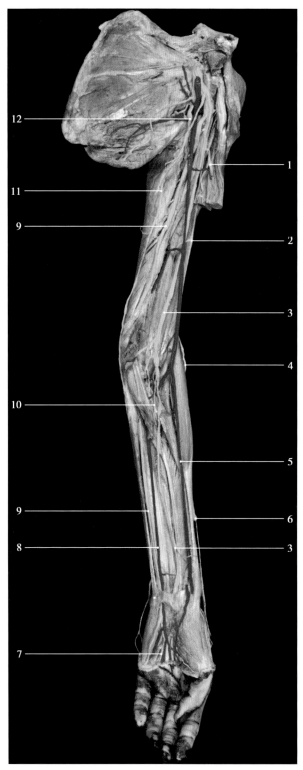

▲ 图 589　上肢的神经
Nerves of upper limb

1. 肱二头肌肌支 muscular branches of biceps brachii
2. 肌皮神经 musculocutaneous n.
3. 正中神经 median n.
4. 前臂外侧皮神经 lateral antebrachial cutaneous n.
5. 桡动脉 radial a.
6. 桡神经浅支 superficial branch of radial n.
7. 指掌侧总神经 common palmar digital n.
8. 尺动脉 ulnar a.
9. 尺神经 ulnar n.
10. 旋前圆肌肌支 muscular branches of pronator teres
11. 前臂内侧皮神经 medial antebrachial cutaneous n.
12. 桡神经 radial n.

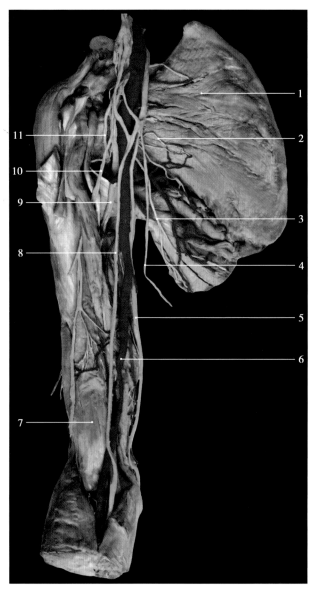

▲ 图 590 臂部的神经 (前面观)
Nerves of arm. Anterior aspect

1. 肩胛下肌 subscapularis
2. 上肩胛下神经 superior subscapular n.
3. 胸背神经 thoracodorsal n.
4. 前臂内侧皮神经 medial antebrachial cutaneous n.
5. 尺神经 ulnar n.
6. 肱动脉 brachial a.
7. 肱肌 brachialis
8. 正中神经 median n.
9. 桡神经 radial n.
10. 肌皮神经 musculocutaneous n.
11. 腋神经 axillary n.

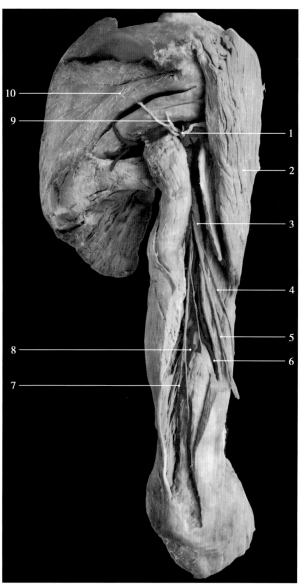

▲ 图 591 臂部的神经 (后面观)
Nerves of arm. Posterior aspect

1. 腋神经 axillary n.
2. 三角肌 deltoid
3. 桡神经 radial n.
4. 臂下外侧皮神经 inferior lateral brachial cutaneous n.
5. 前臂后皮神经 posterior antebrachial cutaneous n.
6. 桡侧副动脉 radial collateral a.
7. 肘肌神经 nerve of anconeus
8. 中副动脉 middle collateral a.
9. 小圆肌神经 never of teres minor
10. 冈下肌 infraspinatus

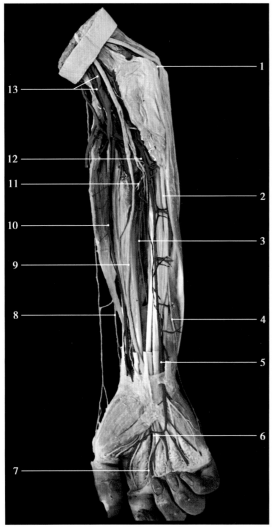

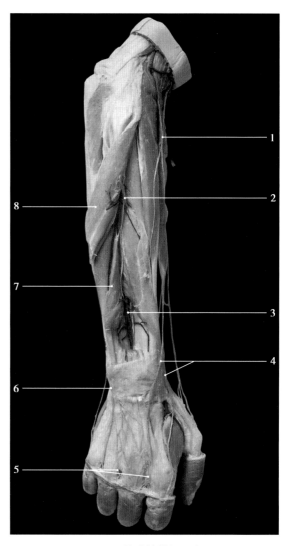

▲ 图 592　前臂的神经 (前面观)
Nerves of forearm. Anterior aspect

1. 尺神经沟 sulcus for ulnar n.
2. 尺神经 ulnar n.
3. 骨间前神经 anterior interosseous n.
4. 尺神经手背支 dorsal branch of ulnar n.
5. 尺动脉 ulnar a.
6. 指掌侧总神经 common palmar digital n.
7. 指掌侧固有神经 proper palmar digital n.
8. 桡神经浅支 superficial branch of radial n.
9. 正中神经 median n.
10. 桡动脉 radial a.
11. 肌支 muscular branch
12. 骨间总动脉 common interosseous a.
13. 肱动、静脉 brachial a. and v.

▲ 图 593　前臂的神经 (后面观)
Nerves of forearm. Posterior aspect

1. 前臂外侧皮神经 lateral antebrachial cutaneous n.
2. 骨间后神经 posterior interosseous n.
3. 骨间前动脉 anterior interosseous a.
4. 桡神经浅支 superficial branch of radial n.
5. 指背神经 dorsal digital n.
6. 尺神经手背支 dorsal branch of ulnar n.
7. 拇长伸肌 extensor pollicis longus
8. 指伸肌 extensor digitorum

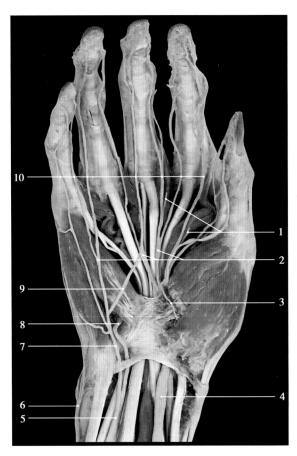

◀ 图 594

手的神经 (前面观 1)
Nerves of hand. Anterior aspect (1)

1. 蚓状肌神经 nerves of lumbricales
2. 指掌侧总侧神经 common palmar digital n.
3. 正中神经返支 recurrent branch of median n.
4. 正中神经 median n.
5. 尺神经 ulnar n.
6. 尺神经手背支 dorsal branch of ulnar n.
7. 尺神经浅支 superficial branch of ulnar n.
8. 尺神经深支 deep branch of ulnar n.
9. 尺神经交通支 communicating branch of ulnar n.
10. 指掌侧固有神经 proper palmar digital n.

图 595 ▶

手的神经 (前面观 2)
Nerves of hand. Anterior aspect (2)

1. 拇收肌 adductor pollicis
2. 拇收肌神经 nerve of adductor pollicis
3. 正中神经返支 recurrent branch of median n.
4. 屈肌支持带 flexor retinaculum
5. 正中神经 median n.
6. 尺神经手背支 dorsal branch of ulnar n.
7. 尺神经 ulnar n.
8. 尺神经浅支 superficial branch of ulnar n.
9. 尺神经深支 deep branch of ulnar n.
10. 小鱼际神经 nerves of hypothenar
11. 掌深弓 deep palmar arch
12. 第 4 蚓状肌神经 nerves of the 4th lumbricales
13. 第 3 蚓状肌神经 nerves of the 3rd lumbricales
14. 第 3、4 蚓状肌 3rd and the 4th lumbricales

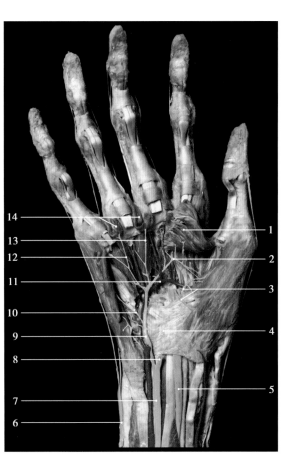

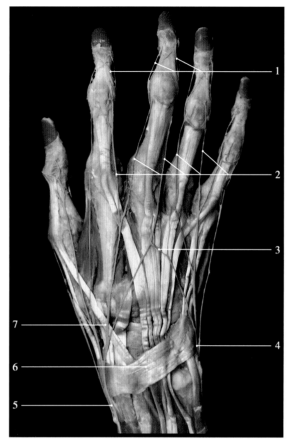

◄ 图 596

手的神经 (后面观)
Nerves of hand. Posterior aspect
1. 指掌侧固有神经 proper palmar digital n.
2. 指背神经 dorsal digital n.
3. 交通支 communicating branch
4. 尺神经手背支 dorsal branch of ulnar n.
5. 桡神经浅支 superficial branch of radial n.
6. 伸肌支持带 extensor retinaculum
7. 拇长伸肌腱 tendon of extensor pollicis longus

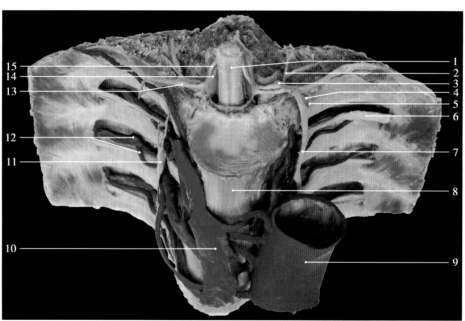

▲ 图 597　肋间神经
Intercostal nerve

1. 脊髓 spinal cord
2. 胸神经后支 posterior branch of thoracic n.
3. 脊神经节 spinal ganglia
4. 灰交通支 gray communicating branch
5. 白交通支 white communicating branch
6. 肋间神经 intercostal n.
7. 交感干 sympathetic trunk
8. 椎体 vertebral body
9. 胸主动脉 thoracic aorta
10. 奇静脉 azygos v.
11. 交感干神经节 ganglia of sympathetic trunk
12. 肋间动、静脉 posterior intercostal a. and v.
13. 胸神经前支 anterior branch of thoracic n.
14. 后根 posterior root
15. 前根 anterior root

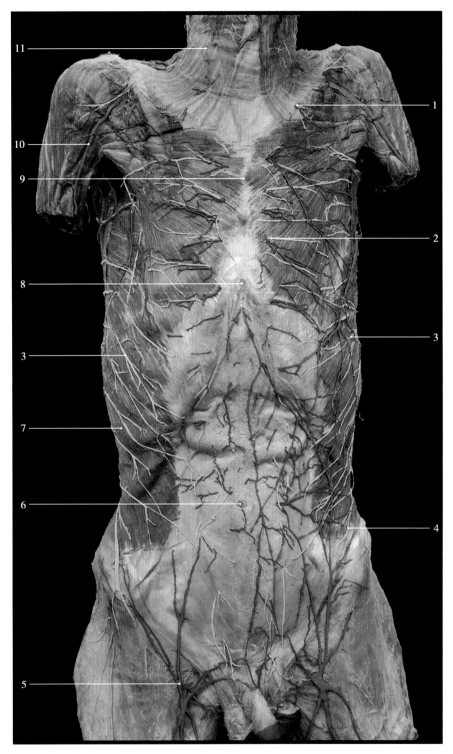

▲ 图 598　胸神经前支的分布（前面观）
Distribution of anterior branches of thoracic nerve. Anterior aspect

1. 锁骨上神经 supraclavicular n.
2. 肋间神经前皮支 anterior cutaneous branch of intercostal n.
3. 肋间神经外侧皮支 lateral cutaneous branch of intercostal n.
4. 髂腹下神经外侧皮支 lateral cutaneous branch of iliohypogastric n.
5. 腹壁浅静脉 superficial epigastric v.
6. 脐 umbilicus
7. 腹外斜肌 obliquus externus abdominis
8. 剑突 xiphoid process
9. 胸骨角 sternal angle
10. 头静脉 cephalic v.
11. 颈阔肌 platysma

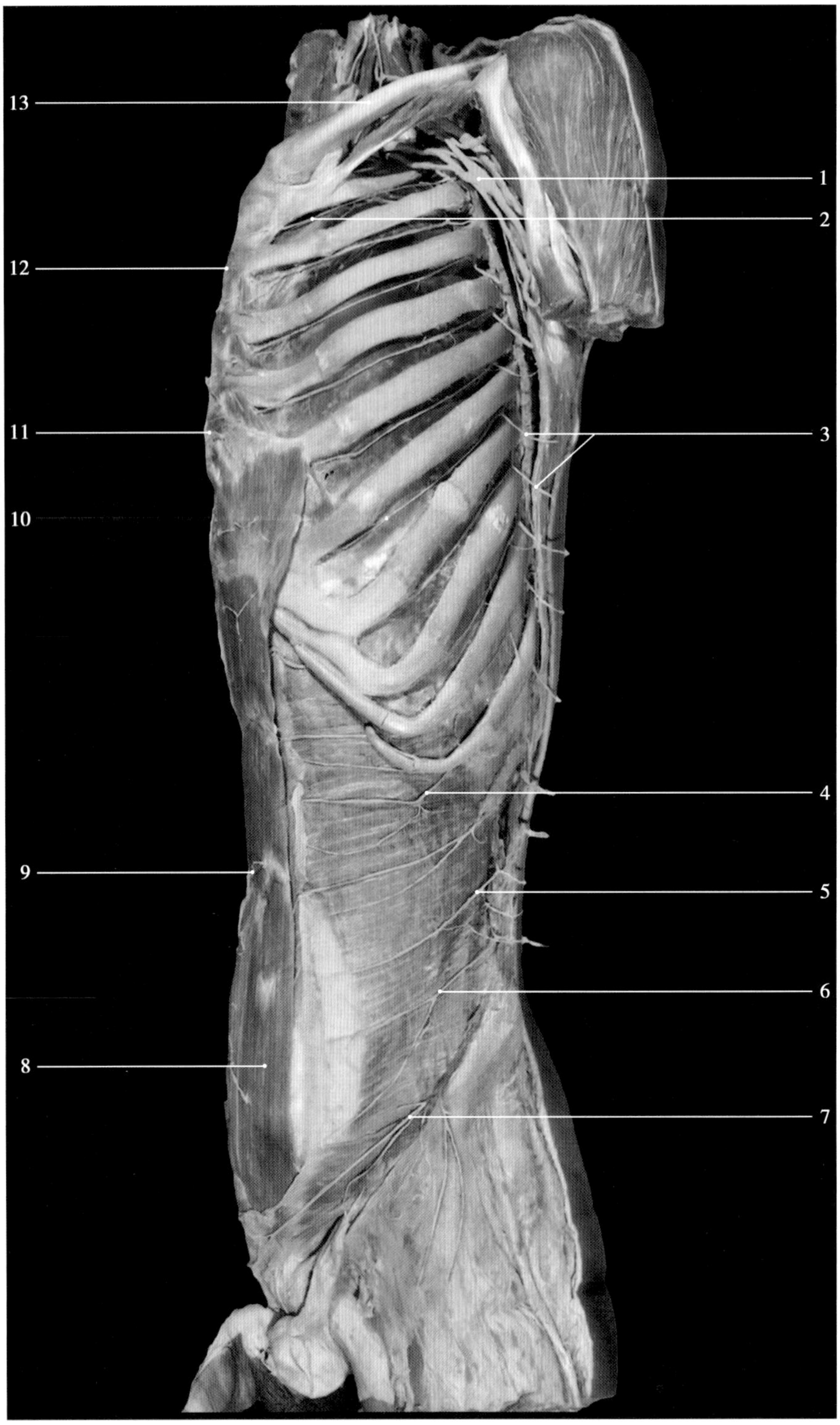

▲ 图 599 胸神经前支的分布（侧面观）
Distribution of anterior branches of thoracic nerve. Lateral aspect

1. 臂丛 brachial plexus
2. 第 1 肋间神经 1st intercostal n.
3. 肋间神经外侧皮支 lateral cutaneous branch of intercostal n.
4. 第 10 肋间神经 10th intercostal n.
5. 肋下神经 subcostal n.
6. 髂腹下神经 iliohypogastric n.
7. 髂腹股沟神经 ilioinguinal n.
8. 腹直肌 rectus abdominis
9. 脐 umbilicus
10. 第 6 肋间神经 6th intercostal n.
11. 肋间神经前皮支 anterior cutaneous branch of intercostal n.
12. 胸骨角 sternal angle
13. 锁骨 clavicle

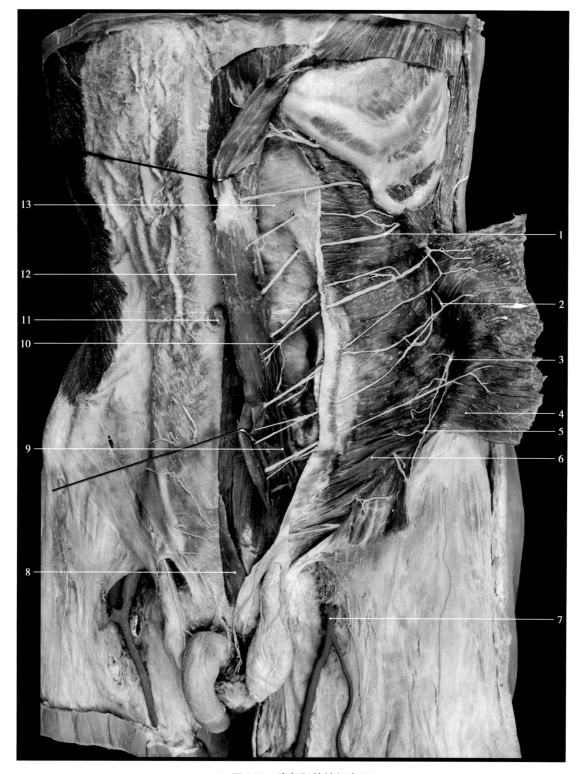

▲ 图 600　腹部肌的神经支配
Innervation of abdominal muscles

1. 第 10 肋间神经 10th intercostal n.
2. 肋下神经 subcostal n.
3. 髂腹下神经 iliohypogastric n.
4. 腹内斜肌 obliquus internus abdominis
5. 髂腹股沟神经 ilioinguinal n.
6. 腹横肌 transversus abdominis
7. 大隐静脉 great saphenous v.
8. 锥状肌 pyramidalis
9. 腹壁下动脉 inferior epigastric a.
10. 腹直肌肌支 muscular branch of rectus abdominis
11. 脐 umbilicus
12. 腹直肌 rectus abdominis
13. 腹直肌鞘后层 posterior layer of rectus abdominis

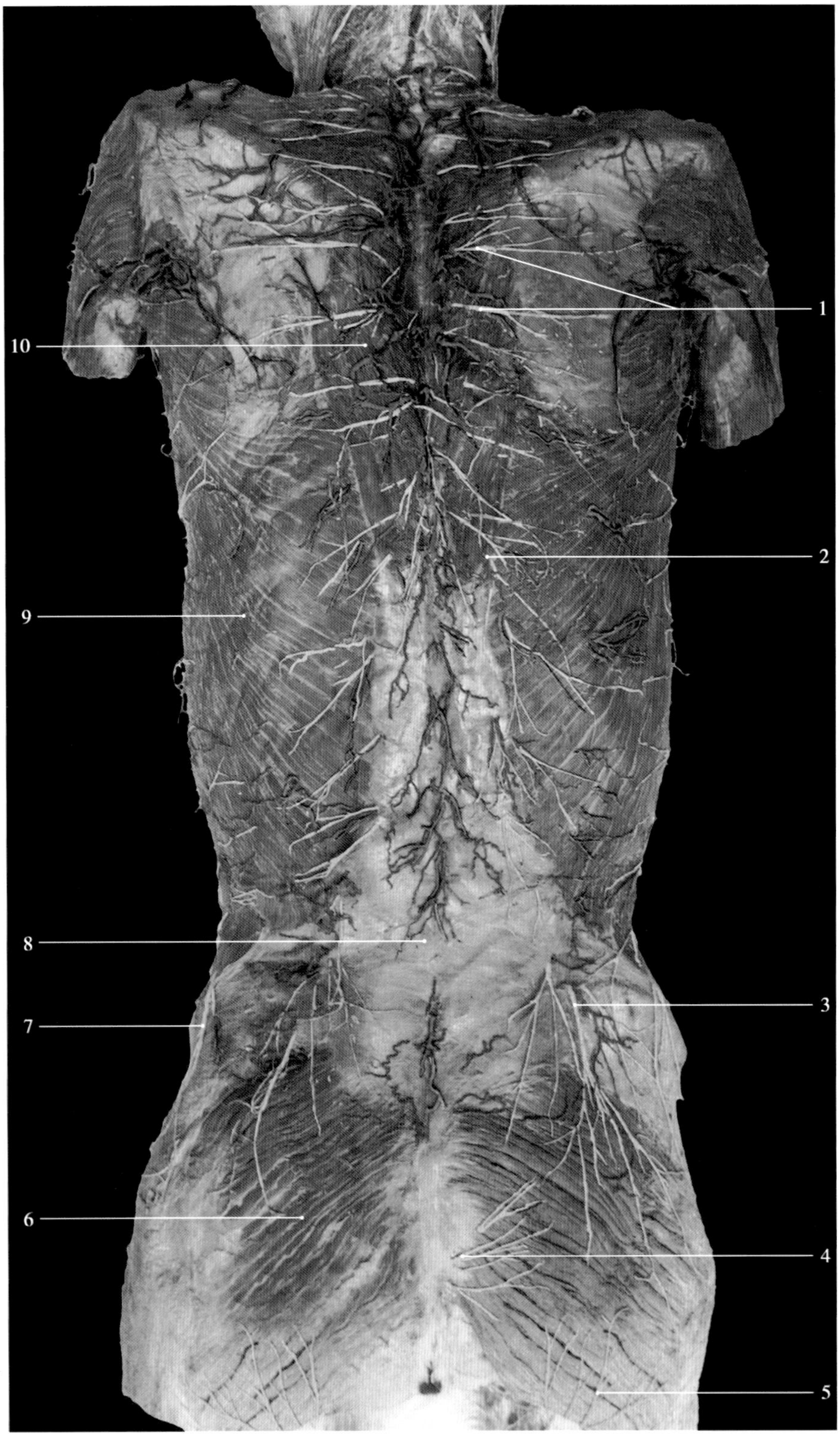

▲ 图 601　背部皮神经的分布
Distribution of dorsal cutaneous nerves

1. 肋间神经后支 posterior branch of intercostal n.
2. 肋间后动脉后支 posterior branch of posterior intercostal a.
3. 臀上皮神经 superior clunial n.
4. 臀内侧皮神经 medial cluneal n.
5. 臀下皮神经 inferior clunial n.
6. 臀大肌 gluteus maximus
7. 髂腹下神经外侧皮支 lateral cutaneous branch of iliohypogastric n.
8. 胸腰筋膜 thoracolumbar fascia
9. 背阔肌 latissimus dorsi
10. 斜方肌 trapezius

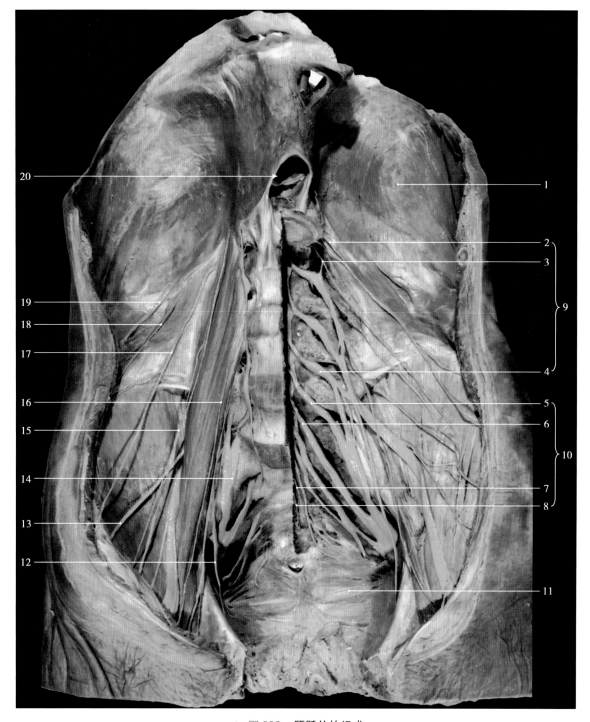

▲ 图 602 腰骶丛的组成
Formation of lumbar and sacral plexus

1. 膈 diaphragm
2. 第 12 胸神经前支 anterior branch of the 12th thoracic n.
3. 第 1 腰神经前支 anterior branch of the 1st lumbar n.
4. 第 4 腰神经前支 anterior branch of the 4th lumbar n.
5. 第 5 腰神经前支 anterior branch of the 5th lumbar n.
6. 第 1 骶神经前支 anterior branch of the 1st sacral n.
7. 第 5 骶神经前支 anterior branch of the 5th sacral n.
8. 尾神经前支 anterior branch of coccygeal n.
9. 腰丛 lumbar plexus
10. 骶丛 sacral plexus
11. 盆膈 pelvic diaphragm
12. 闭孔神经 obturator n.
13. 股外侧皮神经 lateral femoral cutaneous n.
14. 腰骶干 lumbosacral trunk
15. 生殖支 genital branch
16. 股支 femoral branch
17. 髂腹股沟神经 ilioinguinal n.
18. 髂腹下神经 iliohypogastric n.
19. 肋下神经 subcostal n.
20. 主动脉裂孔 aortic hiatus

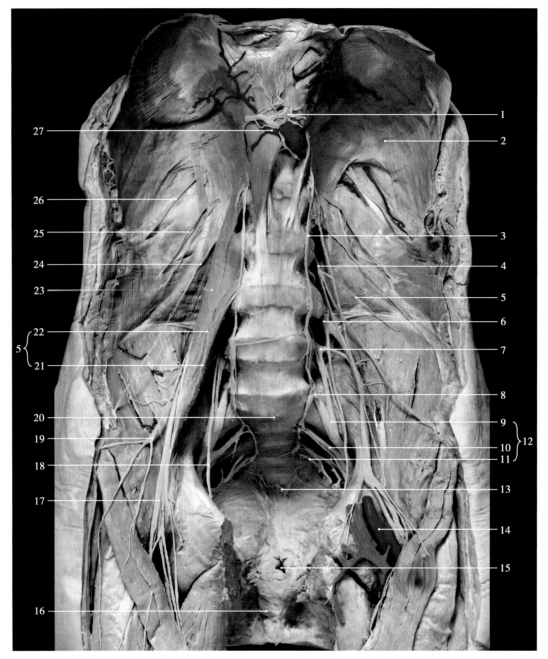

▲ 图 603　**腰骶丛**
Lumbar and sacral plexus

1. 腹腔神经节 celiac ganglia
2. 膈 diaphragm
3. 交感干 sympathetic trunk
4. 第 2 腰神经前支 anterior branch of the 2nd lumbar n.
5. 生殖股神经 genitofemoral n.
6. 第 3 腰神经前支 anterior branch of the 3rd lumbar n.
7. 第 4 腰神经前支 anterior branch of the 4th lumbar n.
8. 第 5 腰神经前支 anterior branch of the 5th lumbar n.
9. 腰骶干 lumbosacral trunk
10. 第 1 骶神经 1st sacral n.
11. 第 3 骶神经 3rd sacral n.
12. 骶丛 sacral plexus
13. 奇神经节 ganglion impar
14. 股动脉 femoral a.

15. 直肠 rectum
16. 肛门括约肌 anal sphincter
17. 股神经 femoral n.
18. 闭孔神经 obturator n.
19. 股外侧皮神经 lateral femoral cutaneous n.
20. 岬 promontory
21. 股支 femoral branch
22. 生殖支 genital branch
23. 腰大肌 psoas major
24. 髂腹股沟神经 ilioinguinal n.
25. 髂腹下神经 iliohypogastric n.
26. 肋下神经 subcostal n.
27. 膈下动脉 inferior phrenic a.

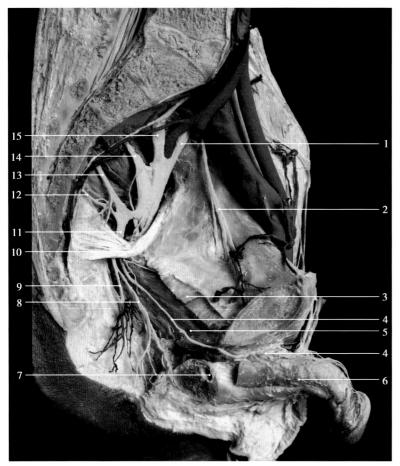

◀ 图 604
男性阴部神经
Male pudendal nerve
1. 腰骶干 lumbosacral trunk
2. 闭孔神经 obturator n.
3. 肛提肌 levator ani
4. 阴茎背神经 dorsal nerve of penis
5. 闭孔内肌 obturator internus
6. 阴茎 penis
7. 尿道 urethra
8. 会阴神经 perineal n.
9. 肛神经 anal n.
10. 坐骨棘 ischial spine
11. 阴部神经 pudendal n.
12. 第 4 骶神经 4th sacral n.
13. 第 3 骶神经 3rd sacral n.
14. 第 2 骶神经 2nd sacral n.
15. 第 1 骶神经 1st sacral n.

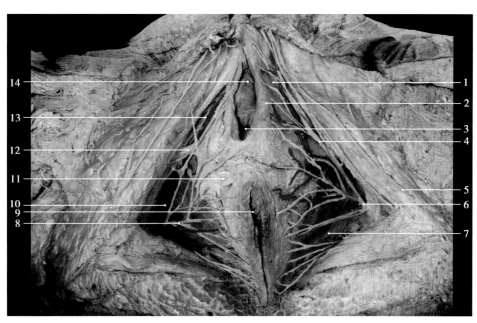

▲ 图 605 **女性会阴部的神经**
Nerves of female perineum

1. 坐骨海绵体肌 ischiocavernosus	7. 肛提肌 levator ani
2. 球海绵体肌 bulbocavernosus	8. 肛神经 anal n.
3. 阴道口 vaginal orifice	9. 肛门 anus
4. 阴唇后神经 posterior labial n.	10. 阴部内动脉 internal pudendal a.
5. 会阴支 perineal branch	11. 会阴浅横肌 superficial transverse muscle of perineum
6. 会阴神经 perineal n.	

12. 尿生殖膈下筋膜 inferior fascia of urogenital diaphragm
13. 阴蒂背神经 dorsal nerve of clitoris
14. 尿道外口 external orifice of urethra

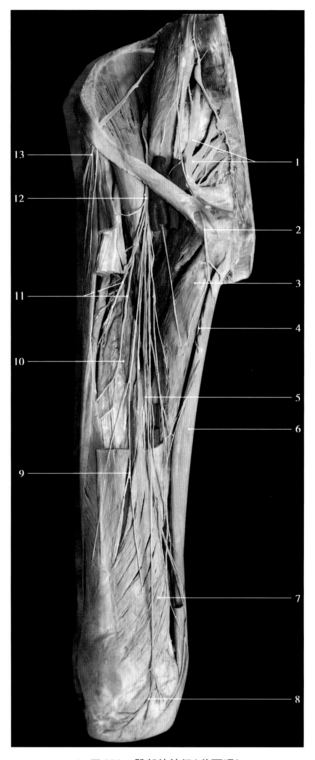

▲ 图606　股部的神经（前面观）
Nerves of thigh. Anterior aspect

1. 骶丛 sacral plexus
2. 生殖股神经生殖支 genital branch of genitofemoral n.
3. 长收肌 adductor longus
4. 闭孔神经皮支 cutaneous branch of obturator n.
5. 隐神经 saphenous n.
6. 股薄肌 gracilis
7. 股内侧肌 vastus medialis
8. 髌下支 infrapatellar branch
9. 股神经前皮支 anterior cutaneous branches of femoral n.
10. 股中间肌 vastus intermedius
11. 肌支 muscular branch
12. 股神经 femoral n.
13. 股外侧皮神经 lateral femoral cutaneous n.

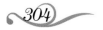

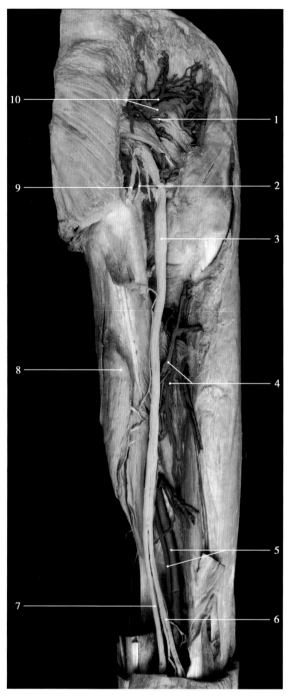

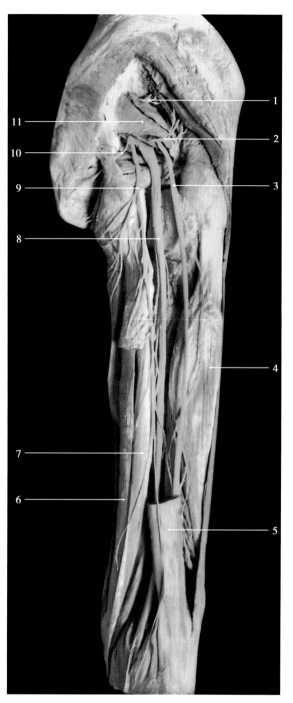

▲ 图 607　股部的神经（后面观 1）
Nerves of thigh. Posterior aspect（1）

1. 臀上神经 superior gluteal n.
2. 臀下神经 inferior gluteal n.
3. 坐骨神经 sciatic n.
4. 穿动、静脉 perforating a. and v.
5. 腘动、静脉 popliteal a. and v.
6. 腓总神经 common peroneal n.
7. 胫神经 tibial n.
8. 大收肌 adductor magnus
9. 股后皮神经 posterior femoral cutaneous n.
10. 臀上动、静脉 superior gluteal a. and v.

▲ 图 608　股部的神经（后面观 2）
Nerves of thigh. Posterior aspect（2）

1. 臀上神经 superior gluteal n.
2. 臀下神经 inferior gluteal n.
3. 腓总神经 common peroneal n.
4. 股外侧肌 vastus lateralis
5. 股二头肌 biceps femoris
6. 半膜肌 semimembranosus
7. 半腱肌 semitendinosus
8. 胫神经 tibial n.
9. 股后皮神经 posterior femoral cutaneous n.
10. 股后皮神经会阴支 perineal branches of posterior
    femoral cutaneous n.
11. 梨状肌 piriformis

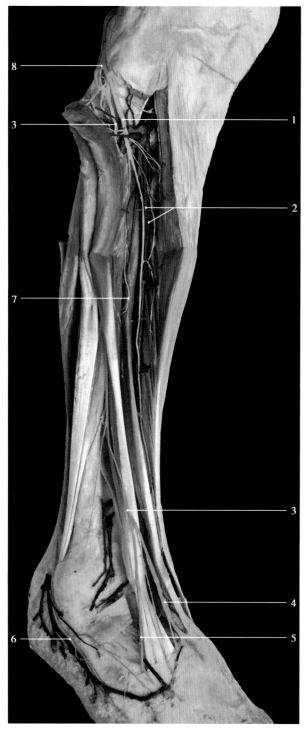

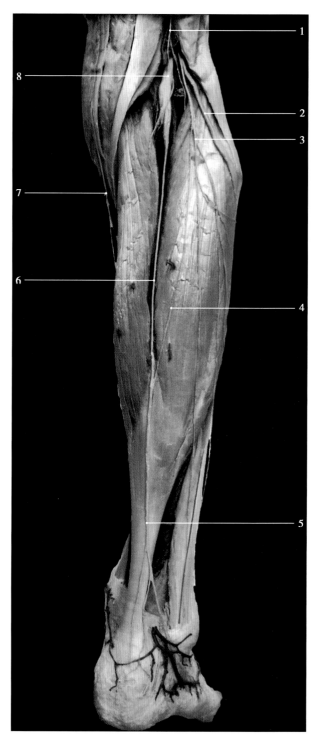

▲ 图609　小腿的神经(前面观)
Nerves of leg. Anterior aspect
1. 腓深神经 deep peroneal n.
2. 胫前动、静脉 anterior tibial a. and v.
3. 腓浅神经 superficial peroneal n.
4. 足背内侧皮神经 medial dorsal cutaneous nerve of foot
5. 足背中间皮神经 intermediate dorsal cutaneous nerve of foot
6. 足背外侧皮神经 lateral dorsal cutaneous nerve of foot
7. 肌支 muscular branch;
8. 腓总神经 common peroneal n.

▲ 图610　小腿的神经(后面观1)
Nerves of leg. Posterior aspect(1)
1. 股后皮神经 posterior femoral cutaneous n.
2. 腓总神经 common peroneal n.
3. 腓肠外侧皮神经 lateral sural cutaneous n.
4. 腓神经交通支 communicating branch of peroneal n.
5. 腓肠神经 sural n.
6. 腓肠内侧皮神经 medial sural cutaneous n.
7. 隐神经 saphenous n.
8. 胫神经 tibial n.

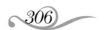

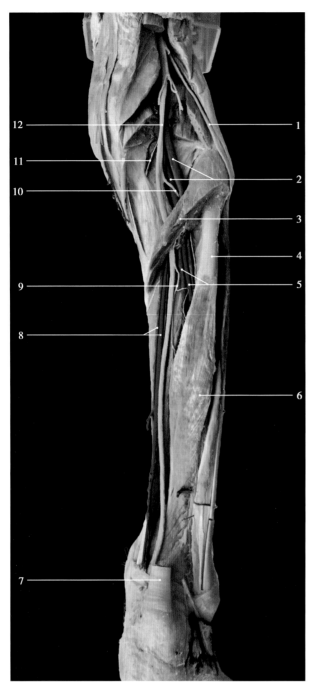

▲ 图 611　小腿的神经（后面观 2）
Nerves of leg. Posterior aspect（2）

1. 腓总神经 common peroneal n.
2. 腘动、静脉 popliteal a. and v.
3. 比目鱼肌 soleus
4. 腓骨 fibula
5. 腓动、静脉 fibular a. and v.
6. 𧿹长屈肌 flexor hallucis longus
7. 跟腱 tendo calcaneus
8. 胫后动、静脉 posterior tibial a. and v.
9. 𧿹长屈肌肌支 muscular branch of flexor hallucis longus
10. 比目鱼肌肌支 muscular branch of soleus
11. 腘肌肌支 muscular branch of popliteus
12. 胫神经 tibial n.

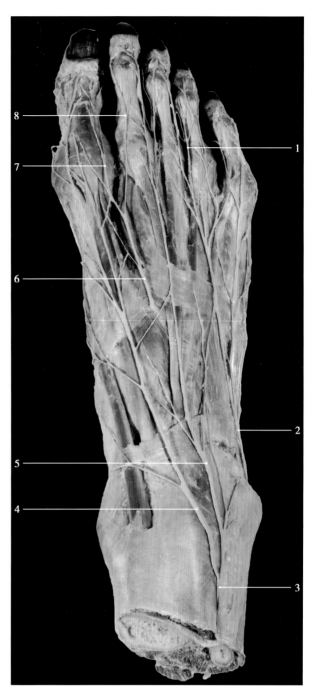

▲ 图 612　足背的神经
Dorsal nerves of foot

1. 趾背神经 dorsal digital nerve of foot
2. 足背外侧皮神经 lateral dorsal cutaneous nerve of foot
3. 腓浅神经 superficial peroneal n.
4. 足背内侧皮神经 medial dorsal cutaneous nerve of foot
5. 足背中间皮神经 intermediate dorsal cutaneous nerve of foot
6. 腓深神经 deep peroneal n.
7. 𧿹趾背外侧神经 dorsal lateral nerve of great toe
8. 第 2 趾背内侧神经 dorsal medial nerve of second toe

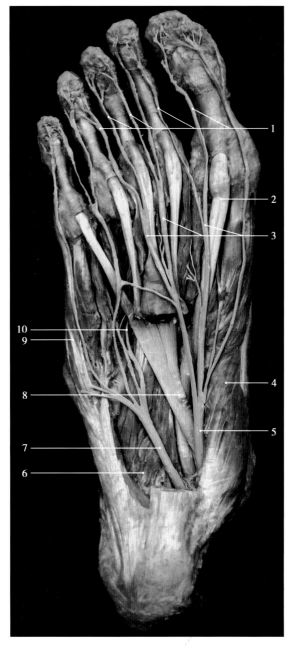

◀ 图 613
足底的神经(1)
Plantar nerves of foot(1)
1. 趾足底固有神经 proper plantar digital n.
2. 姆长屈肌腱 tendon of flexor hallucis longus
3. 趾足底总神经 common plantar digital n.
4. 姆短展肌 abductor pollicis brevis
5. 足底内侧神经 medial plantar n.
6. 足底方肌 quadratus plantae
7. 足底外侧神经 lateral plantar n.
8. 趾长屈肌腱 tendon of flexor digitorum longus
9. 小趾展肌 abductor digiti minimi
10. 足底外侧神经深支 deep branch of plantar
    nerves of foot

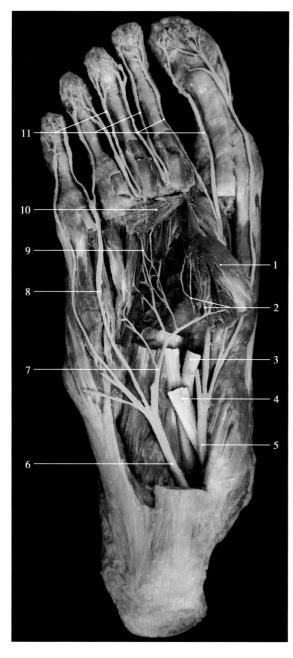

图 614 ▶
足底的神经(2)
Plantar nerves of foot(2)
1. 姆收肌斜头 oblique head of adductor hallucis
2. 姆收肌斜头神经 nerve of oblique head of adductor hallucis
3. 姆长屈肌腱 tendon of flexor hallucis longus
4. 趾长屈肌腱 tendon of flexor digitorum longus
5. 足底内侧神经 medial plantar n.
6. 足底外侧神经 lateral plantar n.
7. 足底外侧神经深支 deep branch of lateral plantar n.
8. 趾足底总神经 common plantar digital n.
9. 姆收肌横头神经 nerve of transverse head of adductor hallucis
10. 姆收肌横头 transverse head of adductor hallucis
11. 趾足底固有神经 proper plantar digital n.

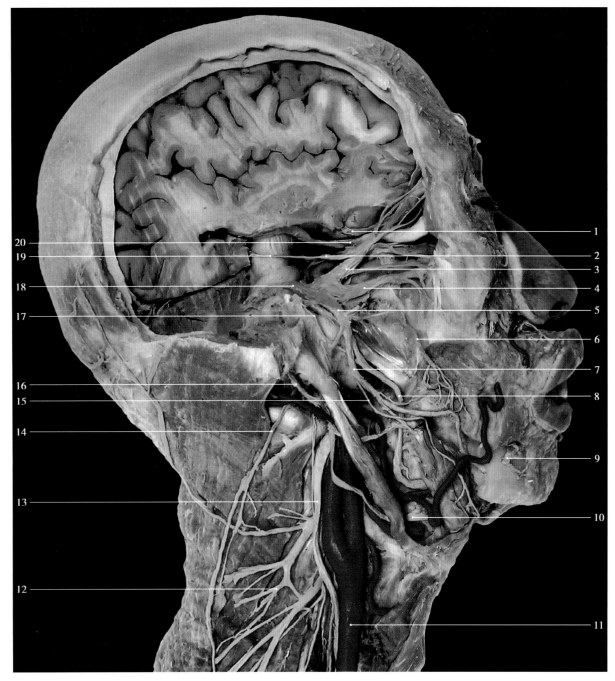

▲ 图615 脑神经(外侧面观1)
Cranial nerves. Lateral aspect(1)

1. 嗅束 olfactory tract
2. 动眼神经 oculomotor n.
3. 眼神经 ophthalmic n.
4. 上颌神经 maxillary n.
5. 下颌神经 mandibular n.
6. 颊神经 buccal n.
7. 下牙槽神经 inferior alveolar n.
8. 舌神经 lingual n.
9. 颏神经 mental n.
10. 舌下神经 hypoglossal n.
11. 颈总动脉 common carotid a.
12. 颈丛 cervical plexus
13. 迷走神经 vagus n.
14. 副神经 accessory n.
15. 下颌舌骨肌神经 mylohyoid n.
16. 面神经 facial n.
17. 鼓索 chorda tympani
18. 三叉神经 trigeminal n.
19. 滑车神经 trochlear n.
20. 视神经 optic n.

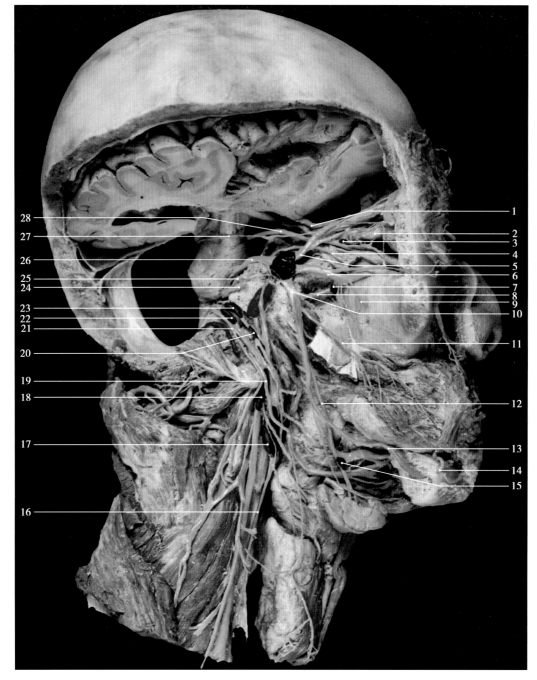

▲ 图616 脑神经(外侧面观2)
Cranial nerves. Lateral aspect(2)

1. 嗅束 olfactory tract
2. 视神经 optic n.
3. 睫状神经节 ciliary ganglion
4. 展神经 abducent n.
5. 眼神经 ophthalmic n.
6. 上颌神经 maxillary n.
7. 翼腭神经节 pterygopalatine ganglion
8. 翼管神经 nerve of pterygoid canal
9. 上牙槽神经 superior alveolar n.
10. 下颌神经 mandibular n.
11. 颊神经 buccal n.

12. 舌神经 lingual n.
13. 下牙槽神经 inferior alveolar n.
14. 颏神经 mental n.
15. 下颌下神经节 submandibular ganglion
16. 颈交感干 cervical sympathetic trunk
17. 颈上神经节 superior cervical ganglion
18. 迷走神经下神经节 inferior ganglion of vagus n.
19. 舌下神经 hypoglossal n.
20. 舌咽神经下神经节 inferior ganglion of glossopharyngeal n.
21. 副神经 accessory n.

22. 迷走神经上神经节 superior ganglion of vagus n.
23. 舌咽神经上神经节 superior ganglion of glossopharyngeal n.
24. 前庭蜗神经 vestibulocochlear n.
25. 面神经 facial n.
26. 三叉神经 trigeminal n.
27. 滑车神经 trochlear n.
28. 动眼神经 oculomotor n.

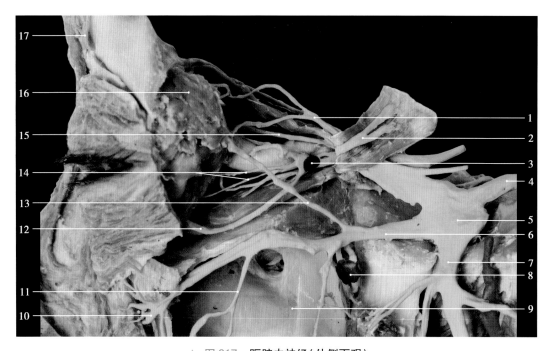

▲ 图 617　眶腔内神经 (外侧面观)
Nerves in the orbital cavity. Lateral aspect

1. 泪腺神经 lacrimal n.
2. 展神经 abducent n.
3. 睫状神经节 ciliary ganglion
4. 三叉神经 trigeminal n.
5. 三叉神经节 trigeminal ganglion
6. 上颌神经 maxillary n.
7. 下颌神经 mandibular n.
8. 翼腭神经节 pterygopalatine ganglion
9. 上颌窦 maxillary sinus

10. 眶下神经 infraorbital n.
11. 上牙槽神经 superior alveolar n.
12. 动眼神经下支 inferior branch of oculomotor n.
13. 颧神经 zygomatic n.
14. 睫状短神经 short ciliary n.
15. 鼻睫神经 nasociliary n.
16. 泪腺 lacrimal gland
17. 眶上神经 supraorbital n.

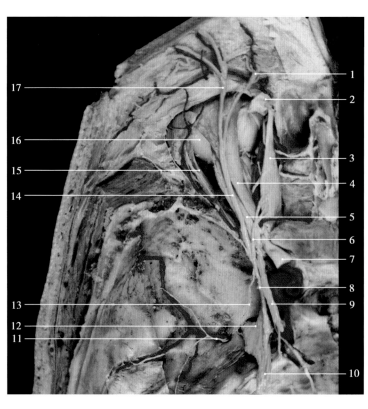

◀ 图 618
眶腔内神经 (上面观)
Nerves in the orbital cavity. Superior aspect

1. 滑车上神经 supratrochlear n.
2. 滑车 trochlea
3. 上斜肌 superior obliquus
4. 上睑提肌 levator palpebrae superioris
5. 上直肌 superior rectus
6. 滑车神经 trochlear n.
7. 视神经 optical n.
8. 眼神经 ophthalmic n.
9. 动眼神经 oculomotor n.
10. 三叉神经 trigeminal n.
11. 棘神经 nervus spinosus
12. 三叉神经节 trigeminal ganglion
13. 小脑幕支 tentorial branch
14. 额神经 frontal n.
15. 外直肌 lateral rectus
16. 眼球 eyeball
17. 眶上神经 supraorbital n.

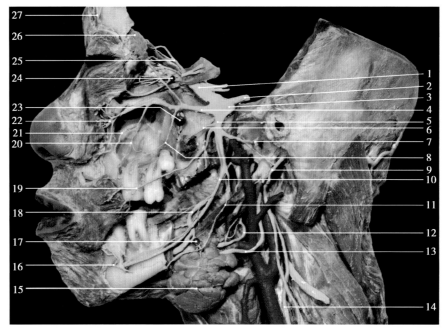

▲ 图619 三叉神经
Trigeminal nerve

1. 眼神经 ophthalmic n.
2. 三叉神经 trigeminal n.
3. 三叉神经节 trigeminal ganglion
4. 上颌神经 maxillary n.
5. 下颌神经 mandibular n.
6. 咬肌神经 masseteric n.
7. 耳颞神经 auriculotemporal n.
8. 上牙槽后支 posterior superior alveolar branches
9. 面神经 facial n.
10. 下牙槽神经 inferior alveolar n.
11. 下颌舌骨肌神经 mylohyoid n.
12. 舌咽神经 glossopharyngeal n.
13. 舌下神经 hypoglossal n.
14. 迷走神经 vagus n.
15. 下颌下腺 submandibular gland
16. 颏神经 mental n.
17. 下颌下神经节 submandibular ganglion
18. 舌神经 lingual n.
19. 颊神经 buccal n.
20. 上牙槽中支 middle superior alveolar branches
21. 上牙槽前支 anterior superior alveolar branches
22. 眶下神经 infraorbital n.
23. 翼腭神经节 pterygopalatine ganglion
24. 睫状神经节 ciliary ganglion
25. 泪腺神经 lacrimal n.
26. 泪腺 lacrimal gland
27. 眶上神经 supraorbital n.

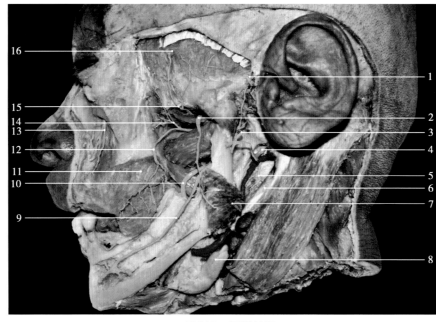

▲ 图620 下颌神经
Maxillary nerve

1. 耳颞神经 auriculotemporal n.
2. 咬肌神经 masseteric n.
3. 吻合支 ramus anastomoticus
4. 面神经 facial n.
5. 二腹肌后腹肌支 muscular branch to the posterior belly of digastric
6. 二腹肌 digastric
7. 咬肌 masseter
8. 下颌下腺 submandibular gland
9. 下牙槽神经 inferior alveolar n.
10. 舌神经 lingual n.
11. 颊肌 buccinator
12. 颊神经 buccal n.
13. 眶下神经 infraorbital n.
14. 颞深前神经 deep anterior temporal n.
15. 颞深后神经 deep posterior temporal n.
16. 颞肌 temporalis

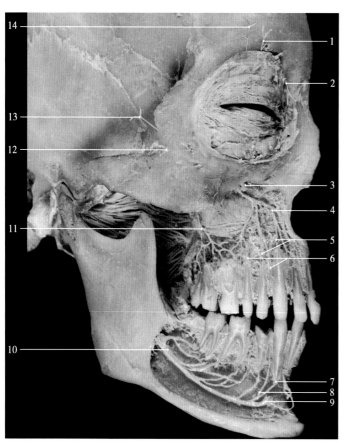

◀ 图 621

上、下牙槽神经
Superior and inferior alveolar nerves

1. 滑车上神经 supratrochlear n.
2. 滑车下神经 infratrochlear n.
3. 眶下神经 infraorbital n.
4. 上牙槽前支 anterior superior alveolar branch
5. 上牙支 superior dental branches
6. 上牙龈支 superior gingival branches
7. 下牙支 inferior dental branches
8. 下牙龈支 inferior gingival branches
9. 颏神经 mental n.
10. 下牙槽神经 inferior alveolar n.
11. 上牙槽后支 posterior superior alveolar branch
12. 颧面支 zygomaticofacial branch
13. 颧颞支 zygomaticotemporal branch
14. 眶上神经 supraorbital n.

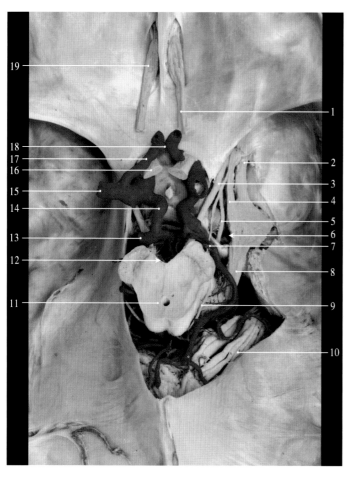

◀ 图 622

眼外肌的神经与海绵窦
Cavernous sinus and nerves of extraocular muscles

1. 嗅束 olfactory tract
2. 上颌神经 maxillary n.
3. 动眼神经 oculomotor n.
4. 眼神经 ophthalmic n.
5. 展神经 abducent n.
6. 海绵窦 cavernous sinus
7. 小脑上动脉 superior cerebellar a.
8. 三叉神经 trigeminal n.
9. 滑车神经 trochlear n.
10. 小脑 cerebellum
11. 中脑 midbrain
12. 脚间窝 interpeduncular fossa
13. 大脑后动脉 posterior cerebral a.
14. 后交通动脉 posterior communicating a.
15. 大脑中动脉 middle cerebral a.
16. 视神经 optic n.
17. 大脑前动脉 anterior cerebral a.
18. 前交通动脉 anterior communicating a.
19. 嗅球 olfactory bulb

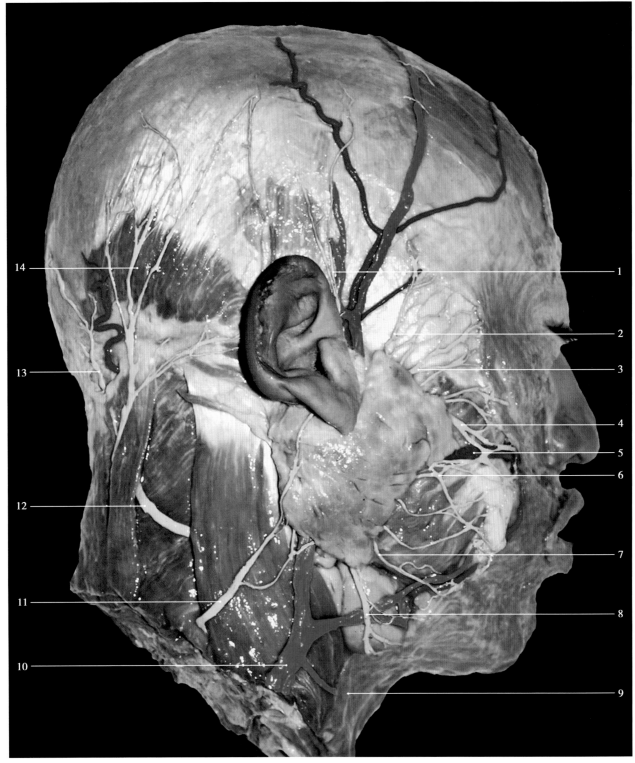

▲ 图 623　面神经分支(1)
Branches of facial nerve(1)

1. 耳颞神经 auriculotemporal n.
2. 颞支 temporal branch
3. 颧支 zygomatic branches
4. 上颊支 superior buccal branch
5. 腮腺管 parotid duct
6. 下颊支 inferior buccal branch
7. 下颌缘支 marginal mandibular branch
8. 颈支 cervical branch
9. 颈阔肌 platysma
10. 颈外静脉 external jugular v.
11. 耳大神经 great auricular n.
12. 枕小神经 lesser occipital n.
13. 枕大神经 greater occipital n.
14. 枕腹 occipital belly

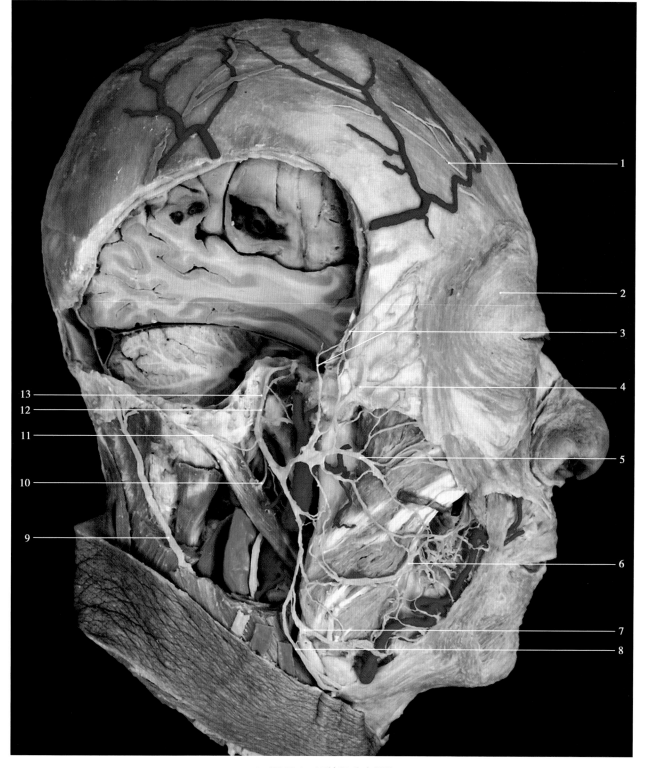

▲ 图624　面神经分支（2）
Branches of facial nerve（2）

1. 眶上神经 supraorbital n.
2. 眼轮匝肌 orbicularis oculi
3. 颞支 temporal branches
4. 颧支 zygomatic branches
5. 上颊支 superior buccal branch
6. 下颊支 inferior buccal branch
7. 下颌缘支 marginal mandibular branch

8. 颈支 cervical branch
9. 枕小神经 lesser occipital n.
10. 二腹肌后腹肌支 muscular branch of posterior belly of digastric
11. 耳后神经 posterior auricular n.
12. 面神经 facial n.
13. 茎乳孔 stylomastoid foramen

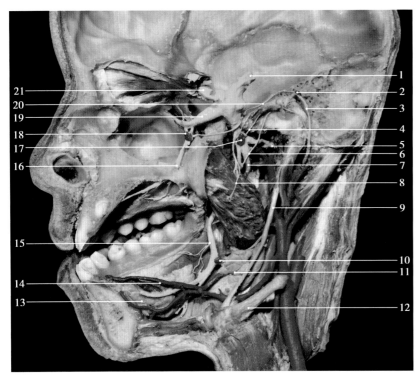

◀ 图 625

鼓索、翼腭神经节与耳神经节
Chorda tympani, pterygopalatine ganglion and otic ganglion
1. 三叉神经 trigeminal n.
2. 膝神经节 geniculate ganglion
3. 面神经 facial n.
4. 岩小神经 petrosal n.
5. 耳颞神经 auriculotemporal n.
6. 鼓索 chorda tympani
7. 下牙槽神经 inferior alveolar n.
8. 翼内肌神经 pterygoid n.
9. 茎突 styloid process
10. 下颌下神经节 submandibular ganglion
11. 下颌下腺 submandibular gland
12. 舌骨 hyoid bone
13. 舌下腺 sublingual gland
14. 下颌下腺管 submandibular duct
15. 舌神经 lingual n.
16. 腭大神经 greater palatine n.
17. 耳神经节 otic ganglion
18. 翼腭神经节 pterygopalatine ganglion
19. 上颌神经 maxillary n.
20. 岩大神经 greater petrosal n.
21. 眼神经 ophthalmic n.

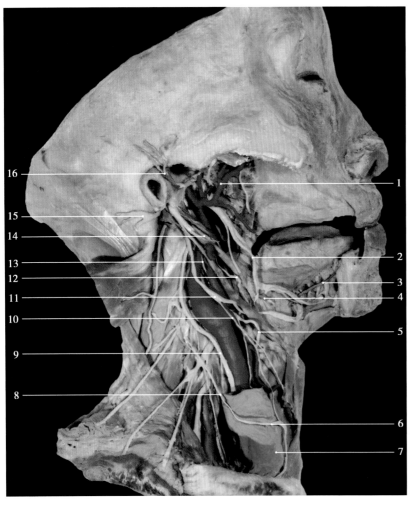

◀ 图 626

舌咽神经和舌下神经
Glossopharyngeal and hypoglossal nerves
1. 上颌动脉 maxillary a.
2. 舌神经 lingual n.
3. 下颌下腺管 submandibular duct
4. 下颌下神经节 submandibular ganglion
5. 喉上神经内支 internal branch of superior laryngeal n.
6. 颈袢 ansa cervicalis
7. 颈内静脉 internal carotid v.
8. 下根 inferior root
9. 迷走神经 vagus n.
10. 上根 superior root
11. 舌下神经 hypoglossal n.
12. 舌咽神经咽支 pharyngeal branches of glossopharyngeal n.
13. 窦神经 sinus n.
14. 舌咽神经 glossopharyngeal n.
15. 面神经 facial n.
16. 耳颞神经 auriculotemporal n.

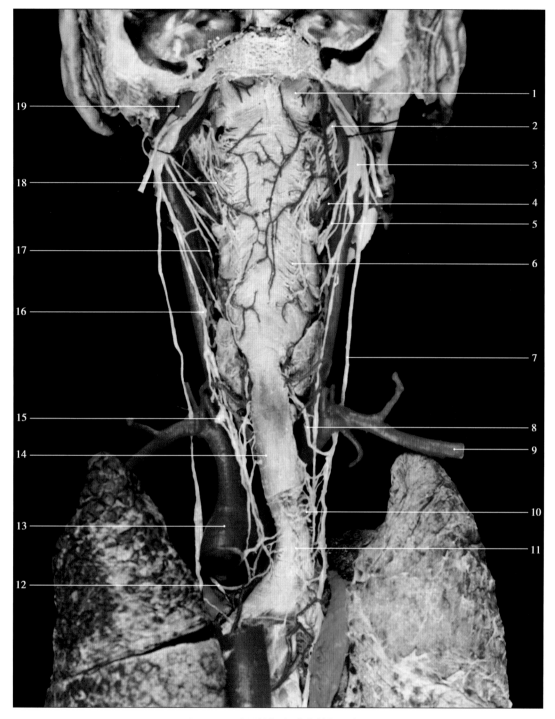

▲ 图 627 舌咽神经和迷走神经(后面观)
Glossopharyngeal and vagus nerves. Posterior aspect

1. 咽颅底筋膜 pharyngobasilar fascia
2. 舌咽神经 glossopharyngeal n.
3. 颈上神经节 superior cervical ganglion
4. 舌动脉 lingual a.
5. 喉上神经内支 internal branch of superior laryngeal n.
6. 咽下缩肌 inferior constrictor of pharynx
7. 迷走神经 vagus n.
8. 右喉返神经 right recurrent laryngeal n.
9. 锁骨下动脉 subclavian a.
10. 气管支 tracheal branches

11. 气管 trachea
12. 左喉返神经 left recurrent laryngeal n.
13. 主动脉弓 aortic arch
14. 食管 esophagus
15. 颈下神经节 inferior cervical ganglion
16. 颈中神经节 middle cervical ganglion
17. 喉上神经外支 external branch of superior laryngeal n.
18. 舌咽神经咽支 pharyngeal branches of glossopharyngeal n.
19. 颈内静脉 internal carotid v.

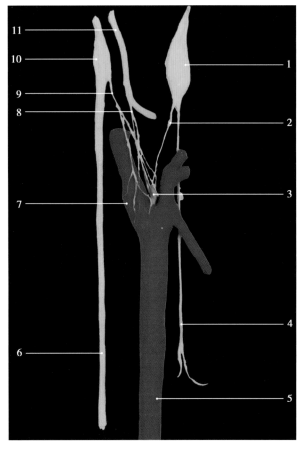

◀ 图 628

舌咽神经的颈动脉窦支
Carotid sinus branch of glossopharyngeal nerve

1. 颈上神经节 superior cervical ganglion
2. 交感支 sympathetic branch
3. 颈动脉小球 carotid glomus
4. 交感干 sympathetic trunk
5. 颈总动脉 common carotid a.
6. 迷走神经 vagus n.
7. 颈动脉窦 carotid sinus
8. 颈动脉窦支 carotid sinus branch
9. 迷走神经支 branch of vagus n.
10. 迷走神经下神经节 inferior ganglion of vagus n.
11. 舌咽神经 glossopharyngeal n.

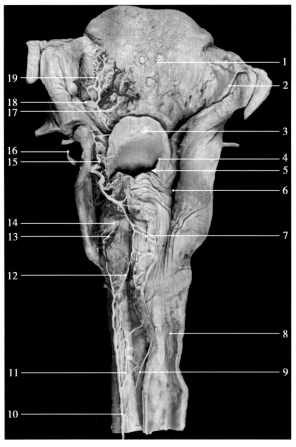

◀ 图 629

喉部的神经(后面观)
Nerves of the laryngeal cavity.
Posterior aspect

1. 舌根 root of tongue
2. 腭扁桃体 palatine tonsil
3. 会厌 epiglottis
4. 杓状会厌襞 aryepiglottic fold
5. 喉口 apertura of larynx
6. 梨状隐窝 piriform recess
7. 咽支(喉上神经)pharyngeal branches
8. 食管 esophagus
9. 喉下神经食管支 esophageal branches of inferior laryngeal n.
10. 喉返神经 recurrent laryngeal n.
11. 喉下神经气管支 tracheal branches of inferior laryngeal n.
12. 喉下神经交通支 communicating branch with inferior laryngeal n.
13. 环杓后肌支 muscular branch of posterior cricoarytenoid
14. 杓横肌支 muscular branch of transverse arytenoid
15. 会厌支 epiglottic branch
16. 喉上神经内支 internal branch of superior laryngeal n.
17. 舌咽神经舌支 lingual branch of glossopharyngeal n.
18. 舌咽神经 glossopharyngeal n.
19. 舌咽神经扁桃体支 tonsillar branch of glossopharyngeal n.

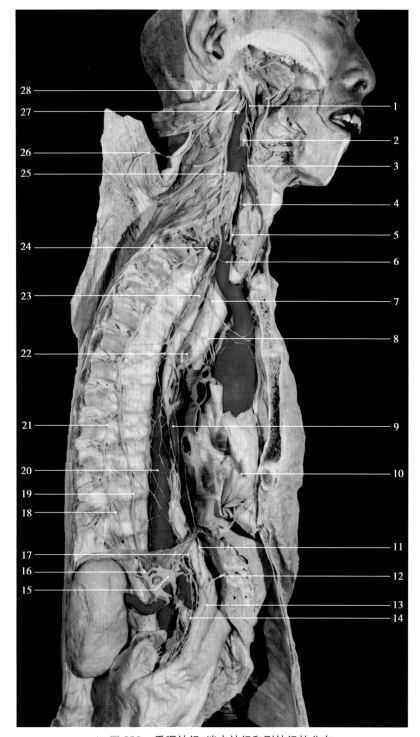

▲ 图630 舌咽神经、迷走神经和副神经的分布
Distribution of glossopharyngeal, vagus and accessory nerves

1. 舌咽神经 glossopharyngeal n.
2. 颈上神经节 superior cervical ganglion
3. 喉上神经内支 internal branch of superior laryngeal n.
4. 喉上神经外支 external branch of superior laryngeal n.
5. 喉返神经 recurrent laryngeal n.
6. 锁骨下襻 ansa subclavia
7. 颈上心神经 superior cervical cardiac n.
8. 心丛 cardiac plexus
9. 食管 esophagus
10. 心 heart
11. 迷走神经前干 anterior vagal trunk
12. 肝支 hepatic branches
13. 胃前支 anterior gastric branches
14. 胃后支 posterior gastric branches
15. 腹腔神经节 celiac ganglia
16. 主动脉肾神经节 aorticorenal ganglia
17. 迷走神经后干 posterior vagal trunk
18. 内脏小神经 lesser splanchnic n.
19. 内脏大神经 greater splanchnic n.
20. 胸主动脉 thoracic aorta
21. 胸交感干 thoracic sympathetic trunk
22. 右主支气管 right principal bronchus
23. 食管丛 esophageal plexus
24. 颈胸神经节 cervicothoracic ganglion
25. 迷走神经 vagus n.
26. 斜方肌肌支 muscular branch of trapezius
27. 舌下神经 sublingual n.
28. 副神经 accessory n.

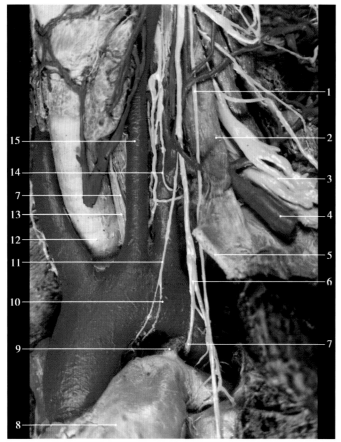

◀ 图 631

左侧喉返神经

Left recurrent laryngeal nerve

1. 左膈神经 left phrenic n.
2. 前斜角肌 scalenus anterior
3. 左臂丛 left brachial plexus
4. 左锁骨下动脉 left subclavian a.
5. 第 1 肋 1st rib
6. 左迷走神经 left vagus n.
7. 左喉返神经 left recurrent laryngeal n.
8. 肺动脉干 pulmonary trunk
9. 动脉韧带 arterial lig.
10. 主动脉弓 aortic arch
11. 左迷走神经心上支 superior cardiac branches of left vagus n.
12. 气管 trachea
13. 食管 esophagus
14. 左锁骨下襻 left ansa subclavia
15. 左颈总动脉 left common carotid a.

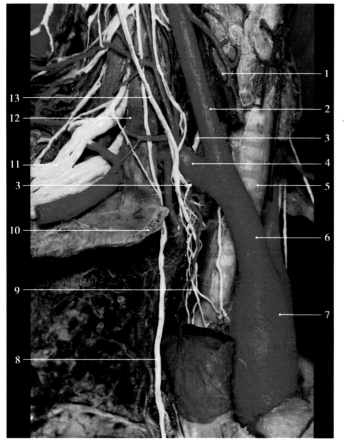

◀ 图 632

右侧喉返神经

Right recurrent laryngeal nerve

1. 甲状腺右叶 right lobe of thyroid gland
2. 右颈总动脉 right common carotid a.
3. 右喉返神经 right recurrent laryngeal n.
4. 锁骨下动脉 subclavian a.
5. 气管 trachea
6. 头臂干 brachiocephalic trunk
7. 主动脉弓 aortic arch
8. 右膈神经 right phrenic n.
9. 右迷走神经心下支 inferior cardiac branches of right vagus n.
10. 第 1 肋骨 1st rib
11. 臂丛 brachial plexus
12. 前斜角肌 scalenus anterior
13. 右迷走神经 right vagus n.

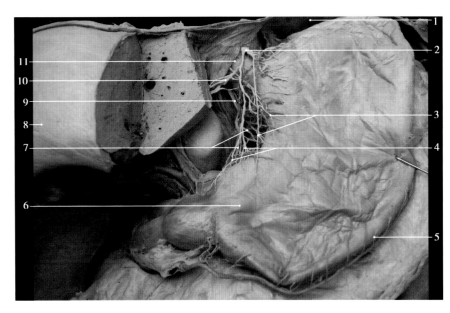

◀ 图 633
迷走神经的胃部分支（1）
Gastric branches of vagus nerve
（1）
1. 膈 diaphragm
2. 迷走神经前干 anterior vagal trunk
3. 前胃壁支 branches of anterior wall of stomach
4. "鸦爪"形分支 "Grows" claw branch
5. 胃大弯 greater curvature of stomach
6. 幽门部 pyloric part
7. 后胃壁支 branches of posterior wall of stomach
8. 肝 liver
9. 迷走神经后干 posterior vagal trunk
10. 肝支 hepatic branches
11. 食管 esophagus

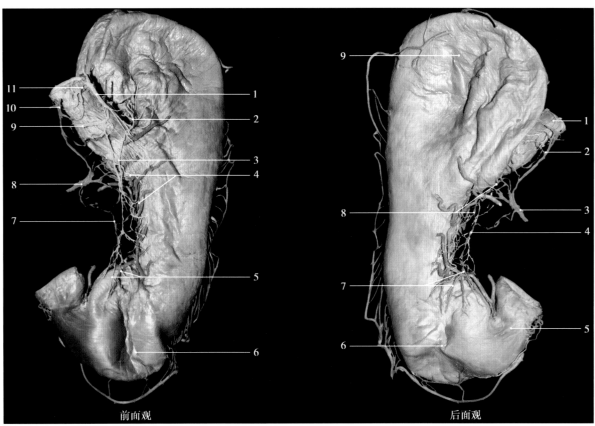

前面观　　　　　　后面观

▲ 图 634　迷走神经的胃部分支（2）
Gastric branches of vagus nerve（2）

1. 迷走神经前干 anterior vagal trunk
2. 贲门支 cardial branch
3. 胃前支 anterior gastric branches
4. 前胃壁支 branches of anterior wall of stomach
5. "鸦爪"形分支 "Grows"claw branch
6. 幽门部 pyloric part
7. 胃后支 posterior gastric branches
8. 腹腔支 celiac branches
9. 肝支 hepatic branches
10. 迷走神经后干 posterior vagal trunk
11. 食管丛 esophageal plexus

1. 食管 esophagus
2. 迷走神经后干 posterior vagal trunk
3. 腹腔支 celiac branches
4. 胃后支 posterior gastric branches
5. 幽门 pylorus
6. 幽门部 pyloric part
7. "鸦爪"形分支 "Grows" claw branch
8. 后胃壁支 branches of posterior wall of stomach
9. 胃底 fundus of stomach

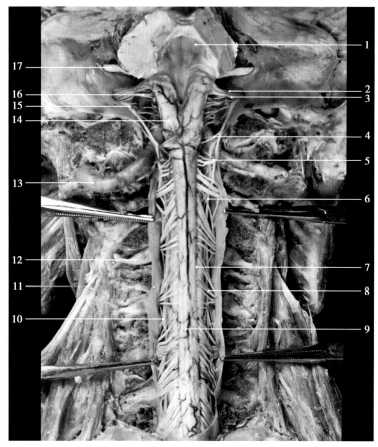

◀ 图 635

舌咽神经、迷走神经和副神经(后面观)
Glossopharyngeal, vagus and accessory nerves. Posterior aspect

1. 菱形窝 rhomboid fossa
2. 舌咽神经 glossopharyngeal n.
3. 迷走神经 vagus n.
4. 副神经脑根 cranial roots of accessory n.
5. 第 1 颈神经后根 posterior root of the 1st cervical n.
6. 副神经脊髓根 spinal roots of accessory n.
7. 后外侧沟 posterolateral sulcus
8. 后根丝 posterior rootlets
9. 脊髓 spinal cord
10. 齿状韧带 denticulate lig.
11. 硬脊膜 spinal dura mater
12. 脊神经节 spinal ganglion
13. 椎动脉 vertebral a.
14. 延髓 medulla oblongata
15. 副神经 accessory n.
16. 舌下神经 hypoglossal n.
17. 前庭蜗神经 vestibulocochlear n.

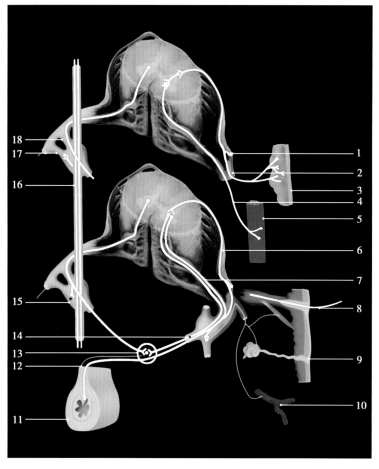

◀ 图 636

交感神经纤维走行(模式图)
Course of sympathetic nerve. Diagram

1. 脊神经节 spinal ganglion
2. 脊神经 spinal n.
3. 皮 skin
4. 躯体运动神经纤维 fibers of somatomotor n.
5. 骨骼肌 skeletal muscles
6. 内脏感觉神经纤维 fibers of viscerosensory n.
7. 内脏运动神经纤维 fibers of visceromotor n.
8. 毛 hair
9. 汗腺 sweat gland
10. 血管 blood vessel
11. 肠 intestines
12. 节后纤维 postganglionic fiber
13. 椎前神经节 prevertebral ganglia
14. 节前纤维 preganglionic fiber
15. 交感干神经节 ganglia of sympathetic trunk
16. 交感干 sympathetic trunk
17. 灰交通支 gray communicating branch
18. 白交通支 white communicating branch

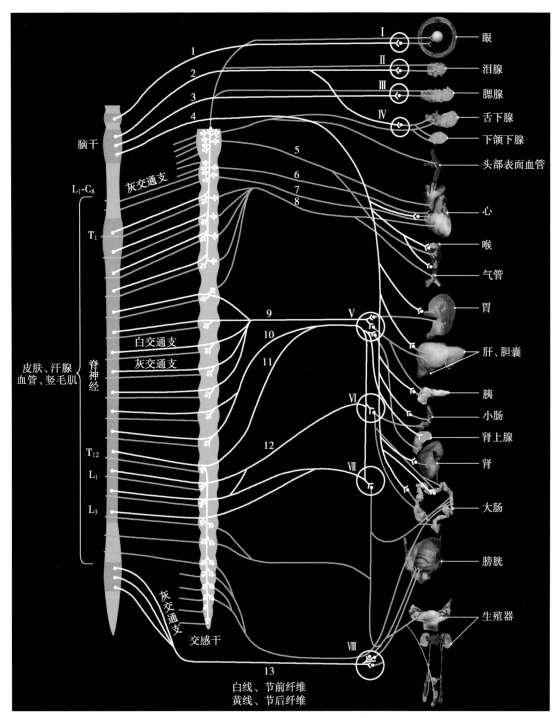

▲ 图 637　内脏运动神经（模式图）
Diagram of viscera motor nerves

1. 动眼神经 oculomotor n.
2. 面神经 facial n.
3. 舌咽神经 glossopharyngeal n.
4. 迷走神经 vagus n.
5. 颈上心神经 superior cervical cardiac n.
6. 颈中心神经 middle cervical cardiac n.
7. 颈下心神经 inferior cervical cardiac n.
8. 胸心神经 thoracic cardiac n.
9. 内脏大神经 greater splanchnic n.
10. 内脏小神经 lesser splanchnic n.
11. 内脏最下神经 lowest splanchnic n.
12. 腰内脏神经 lumbar splanchnic n.
13. 盆内脏神经 pelvic splanchnic n.
Ⅰ睫状神经节 ciliary ganglion
Ⅱ翼腭神经节 pterygopalatine ganglion
Ⅲ耳神经节 otic ganglion
Ⅳ下颌下神经节 submandibular ganglion
Ⅴ腹腔神经节 celiac ganglion
Ⅵ肠系膜上神经节 superior mesenteric ganglion
Ⅶ肠系膜下神经节 inferior mesenteric ganglion
Ⅷ盆神经节 pelvic ganglion

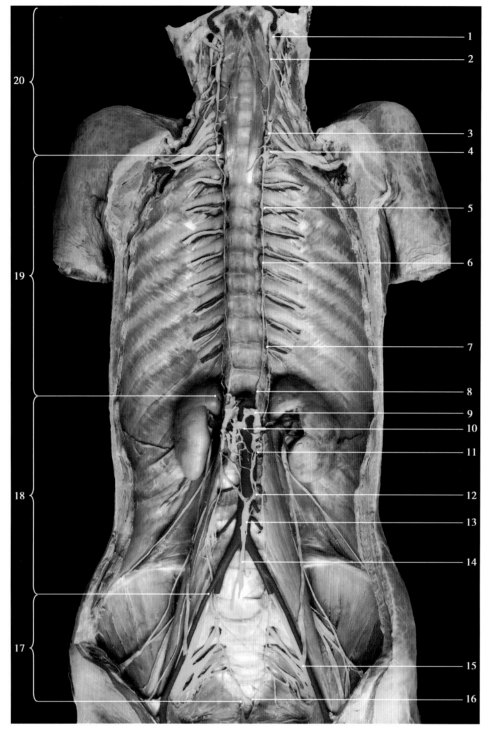

▲ 图 638　交感干和交感干神经节
Sympathetic trunk and ganglia

1. 颈内动脉神经 internal carotid n.
2. 颈上神经节 superior cervical ganglion
3. 颈中神经节 middle cervical ganglion
4. 颈下神经节 inferior cervical ganglion
5. 胸神经节 thoracic ganglia
6. 交感干 sympathetic trunk
7. 内脏小神经 lesser splanchnic n.
8. 内脏大神经 greater splanchnic n.
9. 腹腔神经节 celiac ganglia
10. 肠系膜上神经节 superior mesenteric ganglion

11. 主动脉肾神经节 aorticorenal ganglia
12. 肠系膜下神经节 inferior mesenteric ganglion
13. 腹主动脉丛 abdominal aortic plexus
14. 上腹下丛 superior hypogastric plexus
15. 骶丛 sacral plexus
16. 奇神经节 ganglion impar
17. 交感神经盆部 sympathetic nerve of pelvic part
18. 交感神经腰部 sympathetic nerve of lumbar part
19. 交感神经胸部 sympathetic nerve of thoracic part
20. 交感神经颈部 sympathetic nerve of cervical part

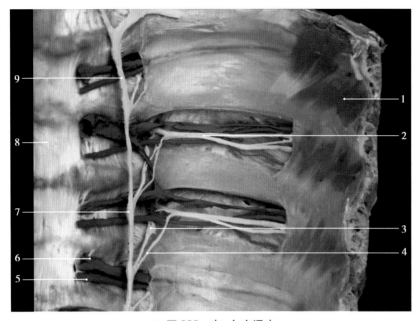

▲ 图 639 灰、白交通支
Grey and white communicating branches

1. 肋间内肌 intercostales interni
2. 肋间神经 intercostal n.
3. 灰交通支 gray communicating branch
4. 白交通支 white communicating branch
5. 肋间后动脉 posterior intercostal a.
6. 肋间后静脉 posterior intercostal v.
7. 交感干神经节 ganglia of sympathetic trunk
8. 胸椎 thoracic vertebrae
9. 胸交感干 thoracic sympathetic trunk

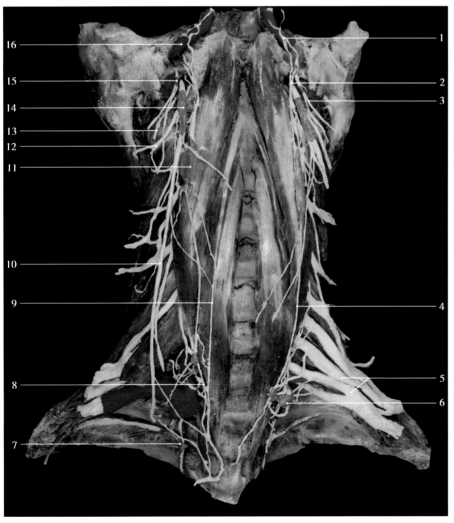

◀ 图 640

颈交感干和颈神经节
Cervical sympathetic trunk and cervical ganglia

1. 颈内动脉丛 internal carotid plexus
2. 颈内动脉神经 internal carotid n.
3. 舌咽神经 glossopharyngeal n.
4. 颈交感干 cervical sympathetic trunk
5. 臂丛 brachial plexus
6. 颈胸神经节 cervicothoracic ganglion
7. 胸神经节 thoracic ganglia
8. 颈中心神经 middle cervical cardiac n.
9. 颈上心神经 superior cervical cardiac n.
10. 迷走神经 vagus n.
11. 颈上神经节 superior cervical ganglion
12. 舌下神经 hypoglossal n.
13. 副神经 accessory n.
14. 迷走神经下神经节 inferior ganglion of vagus n.
15. 舌咽神经下神经节 inferior ganglion of glossopharyngeal n.
16. 颈内动脉 internal carotid a.

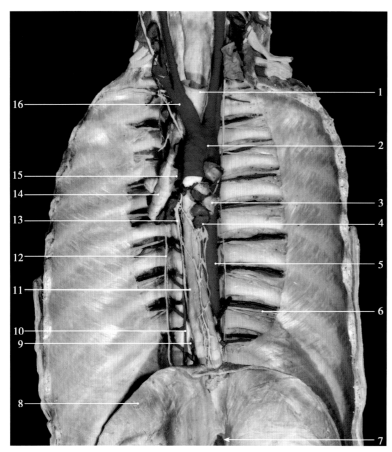

◀ 图 641

胸交感干和胸神经节
Thoracic sympathetic trunk and thoracic ganglia
1. 气管 trachea
2. 主动脉弓 aortic arch
3. 左主支气管 left principal bronchus
4. 淋巴结 lymphoid node
5. 胸主动脉 thoracic aorta
6. 肋间神经 intercostal n.
7. 主动脉裂孔 aortic hiatus
8. 膈 diaphragm
9. 胸导管 thoracic duct
10. 奇静脉 azygous v.
11. 食管 esophagus
12. 胸交感干 thoracic sympathetic trunk
13. 迷走神经 vagus n.
14. 右主支气管 right principal bronchus
15. 气管杈 bifurcation of trachea
16. 头臂干 brachiocephalic trunk

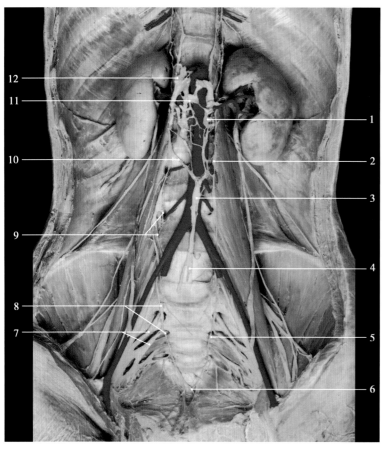

◀ 图 642

腰交感干和腰神经节
Lumbar sympathetic trunk and lumbar ganglia
1. 主动脉肾神经节 aorticorenal ganglia
2. 腰神经节 lumbar ganglia
3. 腹主动脉丛 abdominal aortic plexus
4. 上腹下丛 superior hypogastric plexus
5. 骶交感干 sacral sympathetic trunk
6. 奇神经节 ganglion impar
7. 骶神经 sacral n.
8. 骶神经节 sacral ganglia
9. 灰交通支 gray communicating branches
10. 腰内脏神经 lumbar splanchnic n.
11. 肠系膜上神经节 superior mesenteric ganglion
12. 腹腔神经节 celiac ganglia

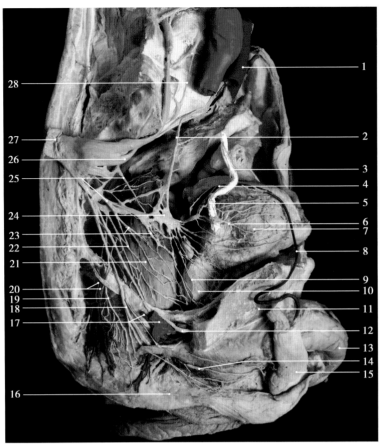

◀ 图 643

盆部内脏神经丛
Splanchnic plexus of pelvic part
1. 右髂总动脉 right common iliac a.
2. 右腹下神经 right hypogastric n.
3. 输尿管 ureter
4. 输精管丛 deferential plexus
5. 输尿管丛 ureteric plexus
6. 膀胱丛 vesical plexus
7. 膀胱 urinary bladder
8. 输精管 ductus deferens
9. 前列腺丛 prostatic plexus
10. 前列腺 prostate
11. 耻骨 pubis
12. 阴茎背神经 dorsal nerve of penis
13. 阴茎 penis
14. 阴囊后神经 posterior scrotal n.
15. 睾丸 testis
16. 股后皮神经会阴支 perineal branch of posterior femoral cutaneous n.
17. 阴部内动、静脉 internal pudendal a. and v.
18. 阴部神经 pudendal n.
19. 肛神经 anal n.
20. 肛动、静脉 anal a. and v.
21. 直肠 rectum
22. 直肠丛 rectal plexus
23. 下腹下丛 inferior hypogastric plexus
24. 盆神经节 pelvic ganglia
25. 盆内脏神经 pelvic splanchnic n.
26. 第 1 骶神经前支 anterior branch of the 1st sacral n.
27. 坐骨神经 sciatic n.
28. 交感干 sympathetic trunk

图 644 ▶

副交感神经的分布
Distribution of parasympathetic nerves
1. 中脑 midbrain
2. 脑桥 pons
3. 延髓 medulla oblongata
4. 脊髓 spinal cord；
5. 腰骶膨大 lumbosacral enlargement
6. 男性生殖器 male genital organ
7. 女性生殖器 female genital organ
8. 直肠 rectum
9. 膀胱 urinary bladder
10. 肾 kidney
11. 小肠 small intestine
12. 大肠 large intestine
13. 肝 liver
14. 胃 stomach
15. 肺 lung
16. 心 heart
17. 腮腺 parotid gland
18. 下颌下腺 submandibular gland
19. 舌下腺 sublingual gland
20. 泪腺 lacrimal gland
21. 瞳孔括约肌 sphincter pupillae
① 睫状神经节 ciliary ganglion
② 翼腭神经节 pterygopalatine ganglion
③ 下颌下神经节 submandibular ganglion
④ 耳神经节 otic ganglion
⑤ 胸部副交感神经节 parasympathetic ganglion of thoracic part
⑥ 腹部副交感神经节 parasympathetic ganglion of abdominal part
⑦ 盆部副交感神经节 parasympathetic ganglion of pelvic part

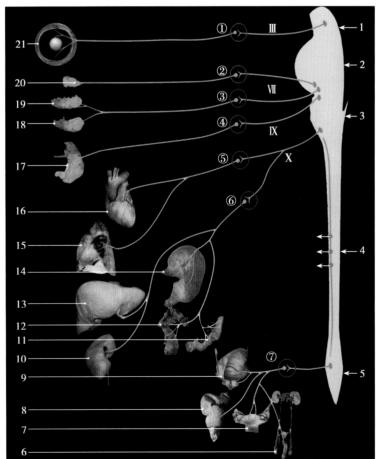

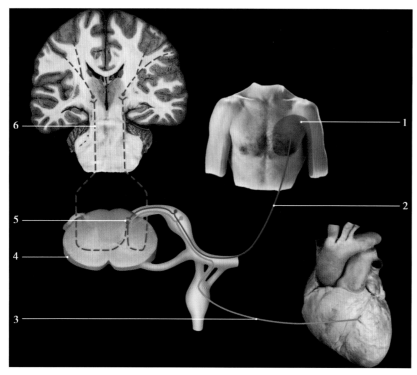

◀ 图 645

心传入神经与皮肤传入神经中枢投射关系
Project relationship of the centers between heart and skin afferent nerves

1. 皮肤感觉区 skin sensation region
2. 胸 1~5 感觉区皮肤传入纤维 $T_{1~5}$ afferent fibers of skin sensory region
3. 胸 1~5 内脏传入纤维 $T_{1~5}$ visceral afferent fiber
4. 胸 1~5 脊髓节段 $T_{1~5}$ spinal segment
5. 后角固有核 nucleus proprius
6. 脊髓丘脑束 spinothalamic tract

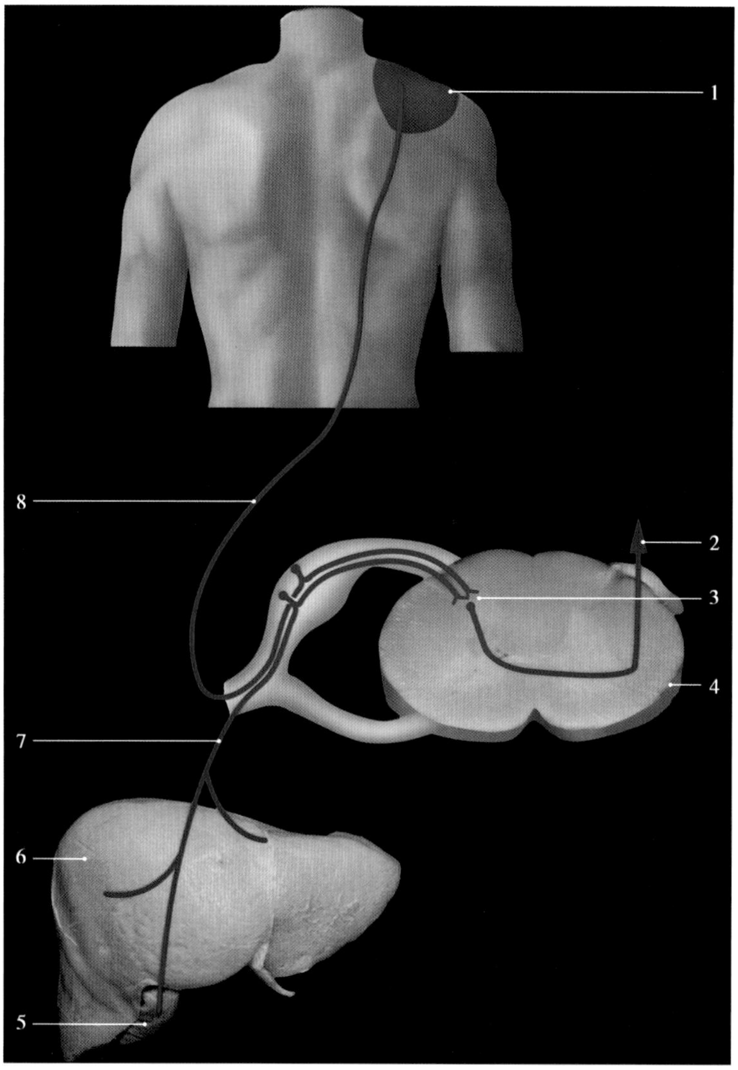

◀ 图 646

肝胆牵涉性痛
Referred pain of liver and gallbladder

1. 皮肤感觉区 skin sensation region
2. 脊髓丘脑侧束 lateral spinothalamic tract
3. 胶状质 substantia gelatinosa
4. 第 4 颈段 4th cervical segment
5. 胆囊 gallbladder
6. 肝 liver
7. 内脏传入纤维(第 4 颈段) visceral afferent fiber(C_4)
8. 皮肤传入纤维(第 4 颈段) dermatic afferent fiber(C_4)

第十五章　神经的传导通路
Nervous Pathways

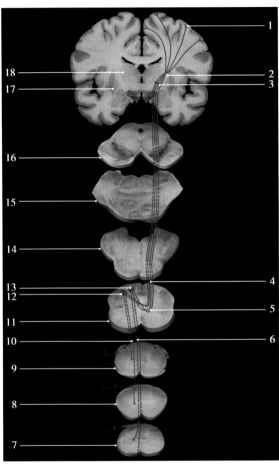

▲ 图647　躯干和四肢意识性本体感觉传导通路
Conscious proprioceptive pathway of
trunk and limbs

1. 中央后回 posterior central gyrus
2. 内囊 internal capsule
3. 腹后外侧核 lateral ventral posterior nucleus
4. 内侧丘系 medial lemniscus
5. 内侧丘系交叉 decussation of medial lemniscus
6. 薄束 fasciculus gracilis
7. 第3腰段 3rd lumbar segment
8. 第4胸段 4th thoracic segment
9. 第5颈段 5th cervical segment
10. 楔束 fasciculus cuneatus
11. 延髓(下段) medulla oblongata(inferior segment)
12. 楔束核 cuneate nucleus
13. 薄束核 gracile nucleus
14. 延髓(上段) medulla oblongata(superior segment)
15. 脑桥 pons
16. 中脑 midbrain
17. 豆状核 lenticular nucleus
18. 背侧丘脑 dorsal thalamus

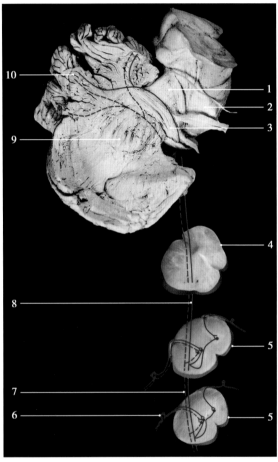

▲ 图648　躯干和四肢非意识性本体感觉传导通路
Unconscious proprioceptive pathway of
trunk and limbs

1. 小脑上脚 superior cerebellar peduncle
2. 小脑中脚 middle cerebellar peduncle
3. 小脑下脚 inferior cerebellar peduncle
4. 延髓 medulla oblongata
5. 脊髓 spinal cord
6. 脊神经节 spinal ganglia
7. 脊髓小脑后束 posterior spinocerebellar tract
8. 脊髓小脑前束 anterior spinocerebellar tract
9. 齿状核 dental nucleus
10. 小脑皮质 cerebellar cortex

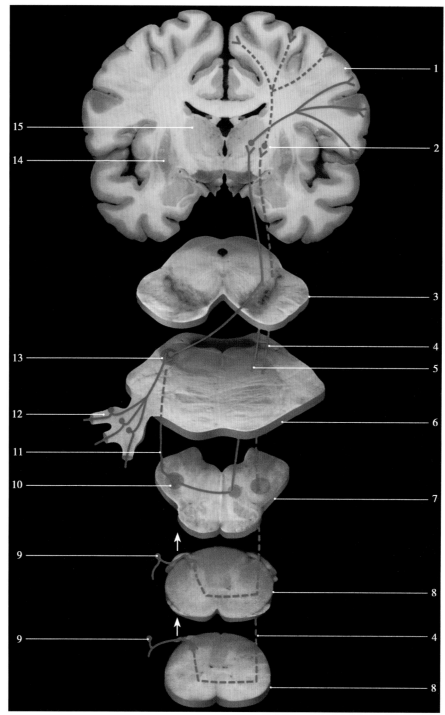

▲ 图649　痛温觉、粗略触觉和压觉传导通路
Pain, thermal, rude tactile and pressure sensation pathways

1. 中央后回 posterior central gyrus
2. 腹后核 ventral posterior nucleus
3. 中脑 midbrain
4. 脊髓丘脑束 spinothalamic tract
5. 三叉丘系 trigeminal lemniscus
6. 脑桥 pons
7. 延髓 medulla oblongata
8. 脊髓 spinal cord
9. 脊神经节(躯干、四肢) spinal ganglia(trunk and extremities)
10. 三叉神经脊束核 spinal nucleus of trigeminal n.
11. 三叉神经脊束 spinal tract of trigeminal n.
12. 三叉神经节(头面部) trigeminal ganglion(head and face part)
13. 三叉神经脑桥核 pontine nucleus of trigeminal n.
14. 豆状核 lenticular nucleus
15. 背侧丘脑 dorsal thalamus

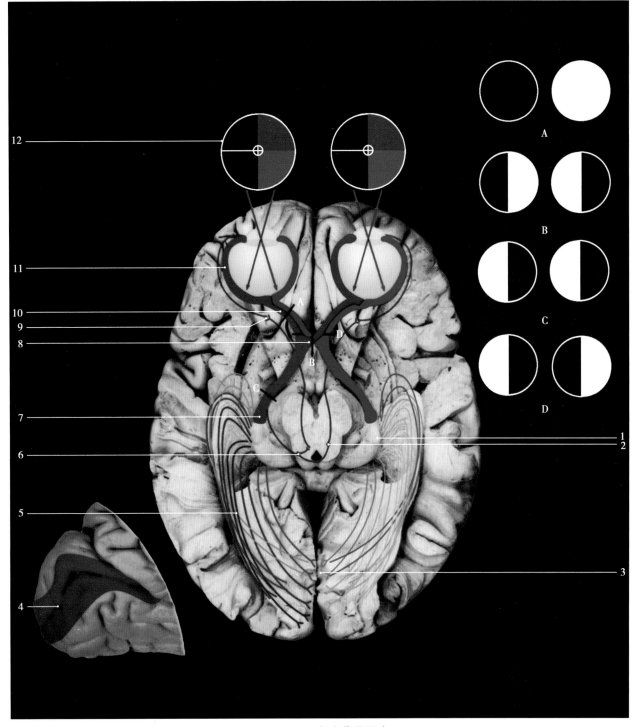

▲ 图 650　视觉传导通路
Visual pathway

1. 外侧膝状体 lateral geniculate body
2. 动眼神经副核 accessory nucleus of oculomotor n.
3. 枕叶视区 occipital eye field
4. 距状沟 calcarine sulcus
5. 视辐射 optic radiation
6. 顶盖前区 pretectal region

7. 视束 optic tract
8. 视交叉 optic chiasm
9. 睫状神经节 ciliary ganglion
10. 视神经 optic n.
11. 视网膜 retina
12. 视野 visual field
A. 左眼全盲 total blindness of left eye

B. 双眼颞侧偏盲 double temporal hemianopsia in both eyes
C. 左眼鼻侧、右眼颞侧偏盲 nasal hemianopsia in left eye and temporal hemianopsia in right eye
D. 双眼鼻侧偏盲 nasal hemianopsia in both eyes

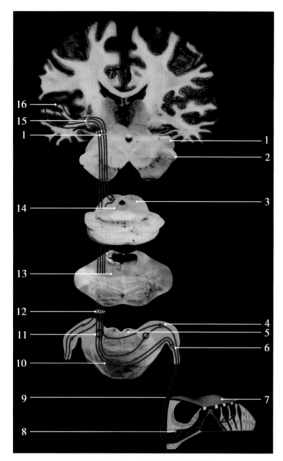
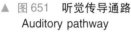
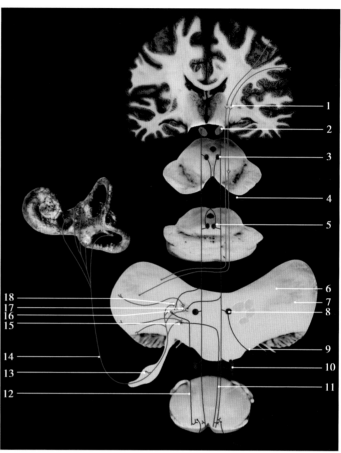

▲ 图651　听觉传导通路
Auditory pathway

1. 内侧膝状体 medial geniculate body
2. 外侧膝状体 lateral geniculate body
3. 下丘核 nucleus of inferior colliculus
4. 蜗神经后核 posterior cochlear nucleus
5. 展神经核 nucleus of abducent n.
6. 蜗神经前核 anterior cochlear nucleus
7. 内耳螺旋器 spiral organ of internal ear
8. 蜗神经节 cochlear ganglion
9. 蜗神经 cochleae n.
10. 斜方体 trapezoid body
11. 上橄榄核 superior olivary nucleus
12. 外侧丘系 lateral lemniscus
13. 内侧丘系 medial lemniscus
14. 滑车神经核 trochlear nucleus
15. 听辐射 acoustic radiation
16. 颞横回 transverse temporal gyrus

▲ 图652　平衡觉传导通路
Equilibratory sensation pathway

1. 背侧丘脑 dorsal thalamus
2. 间位核 interstitial nucleus
3. 动眼神经核 nucleus of oculomotor n.
4. 动眼神经 oculomotor n.
5. 滑车神经核 nucleus of trochlear n.
6. 球状核 globose nucleus
7. 齿状核 dental nucleus
8. 展神经核 nucleus of abducent n.
9. 展神经 abducent n.
10. 副神经核 nucleus of accessory n.
11. 内侧纵束 medial longitudinal fasciculus
12. 前庭脊髓束 vestibulospinal tract
13. 前庭神经节 vestibular ganglion
14. 前庭蜗神经 vestibulocochlear n.
15. 前庭下核 inferior vestibular nucleus
16. 前庭外侧核 lateral vestibular nucleus
17. 前庭内侧核 medial vestibular nucleus
18. 前庭上核 superior vestibular nucleus

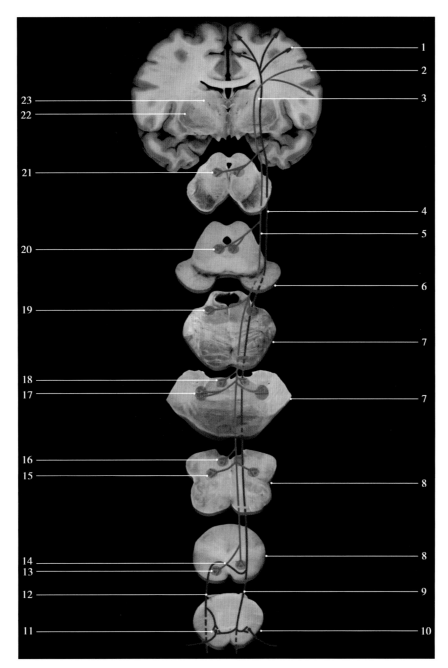

▲ 图 653 **皮质脊髓束与皮质核束**
Corticospinal tract and corticonuclear tract

1. 锥体细胞 pyramidal cell
2. 中央前回 anterior central gyrus
3. 内囊 internalcapsule
4. 皮质脊髓束 corticospinal tract
5. 皮质核束 corticonuclear tract
6. 中脑 midbrain
7. 脑桥 pons
8. 延髓 medulla oblongata
9. 皮质脊髓前束 anterior corticospinal tract
10. 脊髓 spinal cord
11. 前角运动神经元 motor neuron of anterior horn
12. 皮质脊髓侧束 lateral corticospinal tract
13. 副神经核 accessory nucleus
14. 锥体交叉 decussation of pyramid
15. 疑核 nucleus ambiguus
16. 舌下神经核 nucleus of hypoglossal n.
17. 面神经核 nucleus of facial n.
18. 展神经核 nucleus of abducent n.
19. 三叉神经运动核 motor nucleus of trigeminal n.
20. 滑车神经核 nucleus of trochlear n.
21. 动眼神经核 nucleus of oculomotor n.
22. 豆状核 lentiform nucleus
23. 背侧丘脑 dorsal thalamus

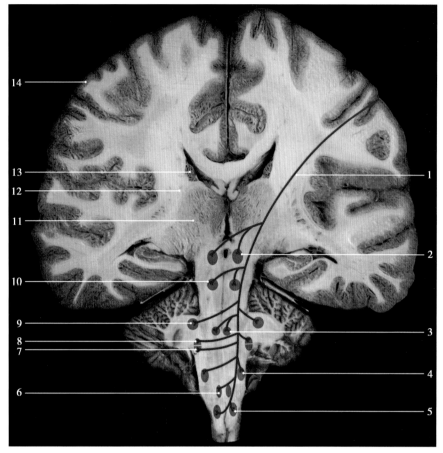

◀ 图 654

皮质核束
Corticonuclear tract

1. 皮质核束 corticonuclear tracts
2. 动眼神经核 nucleus of oculomotor n.
3. 展神经核 nucleus of abducent n.
4. 疑核 nucleus ambiguus
5. 副神经核 accessory nucleus
6. 舌下神经核 hypoglossal nucleus
7. 面神经核（下半）nucleus of facial n.
8. 面神经核（上半）nucleus of facial n.
9. 三叉神经运动核 motor nucleus of trigeminal n.
10. 滑车神经核 nucleus of trochlear n.
11. 丘脑 thalamus
12. 内囊 internal capsule
13. 尾状核 caudate nucleus
14. 中央前回 anterior central gyrus

图 655 ▶

皮质-脑桥-小脑-皮质环路
Corticoponto-cerebellar-cortex circuit

1. 背侧丘脑 dorsal thalamus
2. 红核 red nucleus
3. 齿状丘脑束 dentatothalamic tract
4. 齿状红核束 dentatorubral tract
5. 齿状核 dentate nucleus
6. 脑桥小脑纤维 pontocerebellar fibers
7. 小脑皮质 cerebellar cortex
8. 脊髓小脑后束 posterior spinocerebellar tract
9. 脊髓前角 anterior horn of spinal cord
10. 红核脊髓束 rubrospinal tract
11. 脑桥核 pontine nucleus
12. 皮质脑桥束 corticopontine tract
13. 屏状核 claustrum
14. 内囊 internal capsule
15. 大脑皮质 cerebral cortex

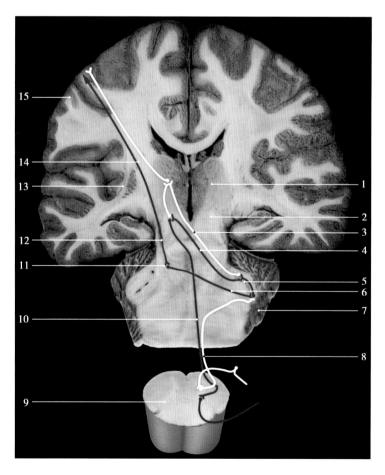

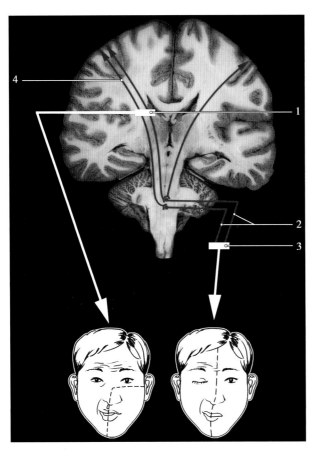

◀ 图 656

面神经瘫
Paralysis of the facial nerve
1. 核上瘫 supranuclear paralysis
2. 面神经 facial n.
3. 核下瘫 infranuclear paralysis
4. 皮质核束 corticonuclear tract

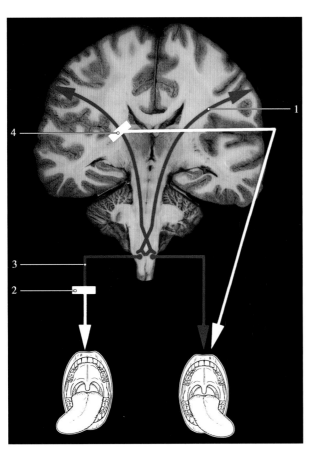

◀ 图 657

舌下神经瘫
Paralysis of the hypoglossal nerve
1. 皮质核束 corticonuclear tract
2. 核下瘫 infranuclear paralysis
3. 舌下神经 hypoglossal n.
4. 核上瘫 supranuclear paralysis

第十六章 脑和脊髓的被膜、血管及脑脊液循环
Meninges, Blood Vessels and Cerebrospinal Fluid Circulation of Brain and Spinal Cord

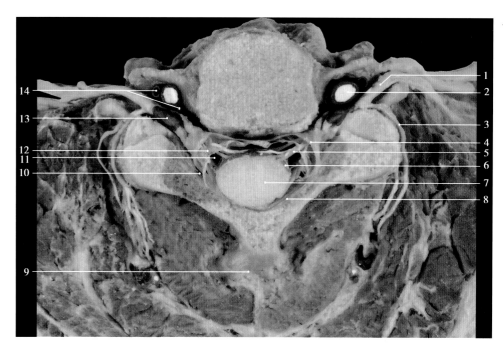

◀ 图 658

脊髓的被膜
Coverings of spinal cord
1. 前支 anterior branch
2. 椎动脉 vertebral a.
3. 后支 posterior branch
4. 硬脊膜 spinal dura mater
5. 前根 anterior root
6. 软脊膜 spinal pia mater
7. 脊髓 spinal cord
8. 黄韧带 ligamenta flava
9. 棘突 spinal process
10. 硬膜外隙 epidural space
11. 蛛网膜下隙 subarachnoid space
12. 脊髓蛛网膜 spinal arachnoid mater
13. 脊神经节 spinal ganglion
14. 椎静脉 vertebral v.

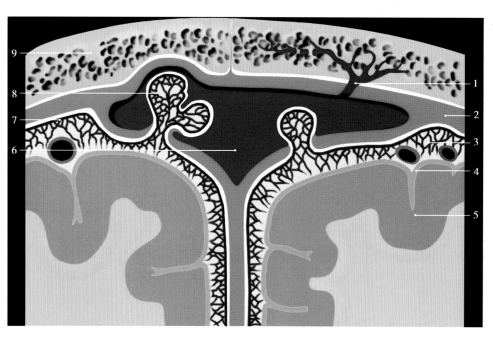

◀ 图 659

脑的被膜、蛛网膜粒和硬脑膜窦
Meninges of brain, arachnoid granulation and sinuses of dura mater
1. 顶导静脉 parietal emissary v.
2. 硬脑膜 cerebral dura mater
3. 蛛网膜下隙 subarachnoid space
4. 软脑膜 cerebral pia mater
5. 大脑皮质 cerebral cortex
6. 上矢状窦 superior sagittal sinus
7. 脑蛛网膜 cerebral arachnoid mater
8. 蛛网膜粒 arachnoid granulations
9. 顶骨 parietal bone

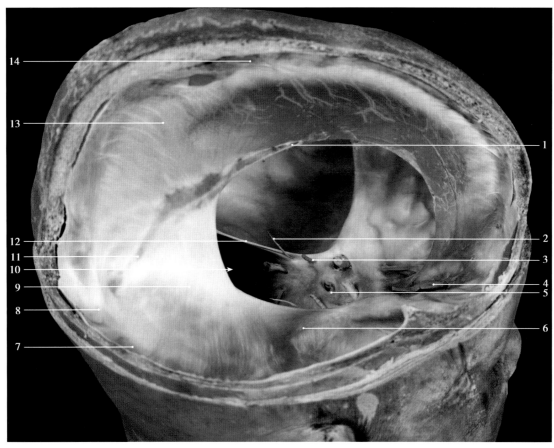

▲ 图 660　硬脑膜及硬脑膜窦
Cerebral dura mater and sinuses of dura mater

1. 下矢状窦 inferior sagittal sinus
2. 滑车神经 trochlear n.
3. 动眼神经 oculomotor n.
4. 嗅球 olfactory bulb
5. 鞍膈 diaphragma sellae
6. 岩上窦 superior petrosal sinus
7. 横窦 transverse sinus
8. 窦汇 confluence of sinuses
9. 小脑幕 tentorium of cerebellum
10. 小脑幕裂孔 hiatus of tentorium of cerebellum
11. 直窦 straight sinus
12. 幕切迹 tentorial incisure
13. 大脑镰 cerebral falx
14. 上矢状窦 superior sagittal sinus

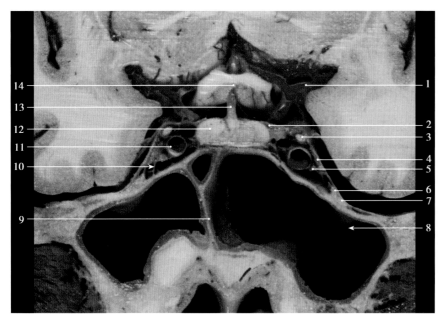

◀ 图 661

海绵窦（冠状切面）
Cavernous sinus.
Coronal section

1. 大脑中动脉 middle cerebral a.
2. 鞍膈 diaphragma sellae
3. 动眼神经 oculomotor n.
4. 滑车神经 trochlear n.
5. 展神经 abducent n.
6. 眼神经 ophthalmic n.
7. 上颌神经 maxillary n.
8. 蝶窦 sphenoidal sinus
9. 蝶窦中隔 septum of sphenoidal sinus
10. 海绵窦 cavernous sinus
11. 颈内动脉 internal carotid a.
12. 垂体 hypophysis
13. 垂体柄 stalk hypophysial
14. 视交叉 optic chiasma

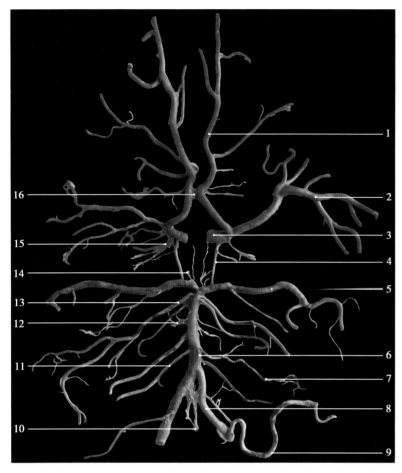

◀ 图 662

脑动脉
Cerebral arteries

1. 大脑前动脉 anterior cerebral a.
2. 大脑中动脉 middle cerebral a.
3. 颈内动脉 internal carotid a.
4. 后交通动脉 posterior communicating a.
5. 大脑后动脉 posterior cerebral a.
6. 基底动脉 basilar a.
7. 迷路动脉 labyrinthine a.
8. 椎动脉 vertebral a.
9. 小脑下后动脉 posterior inferior cerebellar a.
10. 脊髓前动脉 anterior spinal a.
11. 小脑下前动脉 anterior inferior cerebellar a.
12. 脑桥动脉 pontine a.
13. 小脑上动脉 superior cerebellar a.
14. 后内侧中央动脉 posteromedial central a.
15. 脉络丛前动脉 anterior choroidal a.
16. 前交通动脉 anterior communicating a.

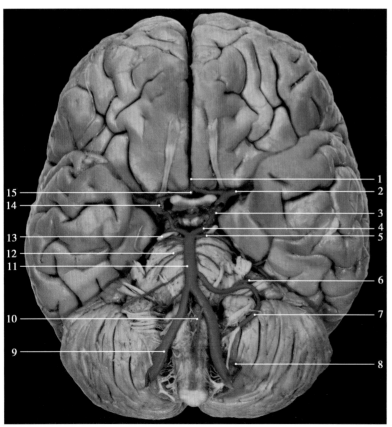

◀ 图 663

脑底动脉
Arteries at the base of brain

1. 大脑前动脉 anterior cerebral a.
2. 大脑中动脉 middle cerebral a.
3. 后交通动脉 posterior communicating a.
4. 大脑后动脉 posterior cerebral a.
5. 小脑上动脉 superior cerebellar a.
6. 迷路动脉 labyrinthine a.
7. 小脑下前动脉 anterior inferior cerebellar a.
8. 小脑下后动脉 posterior inferior cerebellar a.
9. 椎动脉 vertebral a.
10. 脊髓前动脉 anterior spinal a.
11. 基底动脉 basilar a.
12. 脑桥动脉 pontine a.
13. 动眼神经 oculomotor n.
14. 颈内动脉 internal carotid a.
15. 前交通动脉 anterior communicating a.

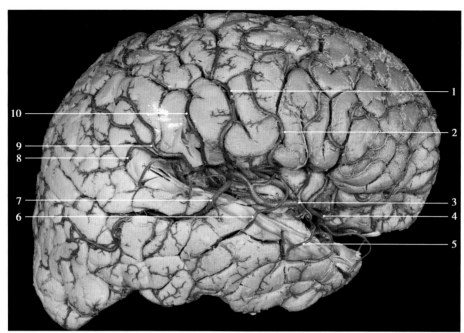

▲ 图 664 大脑外侧面的动脉
Arteries of lateral surface of cerebrum

1. 中央沟动脉 artery of central sulcus
2. 中央前沟动脉 artery of precentral sulcus
3. 大脑中动脉 middle cerebral a.
4. 额叶底外侧动脉 lateral frontobasal a.
5. 颞叶前动脉 anterior temporal a.
6. 颞叶中动脉 middle temporal a.
7. 颞叶后动脉 posterior temporal a.
8. 角回动脉 artery of angular gyrus
9. 顶叶后动脉 posterior parietal a.
10. 中央后沟动脉 artery of postcentral sulcus

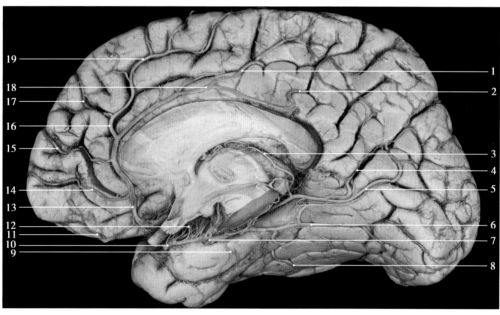

▲ 图 665 大脑内侧面的动脉
Arteries of medial surface of cerebrum

1. 旁中央动脉 paracentral a.
2. 楔前动脉 precuneal a.
3. 脉络膜后内侧支 posterior medial choroidal branches
4. 顶枕支 parietooccipital branch
5. 距状沟支 calcarine branch
6. 颞叶后支 posterior temporal branch
7. 大脑后动脉 posterior cerebral a.
8. 颞叶中间支 intermediate temporal branches
9. 颞叶前支 anterior temporal branches
10. 颈内动脉 internal carotid a.
11. 额叶底内侧动脉 medial frontobasal a.
12. 后交通动脉中央支 central branches of posterior communicating a.
13. 大脑前动脉 anterior cerebral a.
14. 额极动脉 frontopolar a.
15. 额叶前内侧支 anteromedial frontal branch
16. 胼胝体缘动脉 callosomarginal a.
17. 额叶中内侧支 mediomedial frontal branch
18. 胼胝体周围动脉 pericallosal a.
19. 额叶后内侧支 posteromedial frontal branch

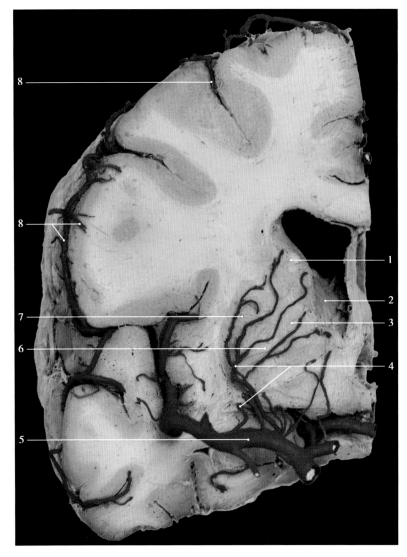

◀ 图 666

大脑中动脉的皮质支和中央支
Central branches and cortical branches
of middle cerebral arteries

1. 尾状核头 head of caudate nucleus
2. 背侧丘脑 dorsal thalamus
3. 内囊 internal capsule
4. 中央支 central branches
5. 大脑中动脉 middle cerebral a.
6. 苍白球 globus pallidus
7. 壳 putamen
8. 皮质支 cortical branches

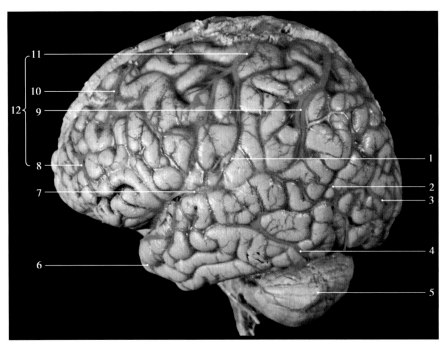

◀ 图 667

大脑浅静脉(外侧面观)
Superficial veins of
cerebrum. Lateral aspect

1. 上吻合静脉 superior
   anastomotic v.
2. 下吻合静脉 inferior
   anastomotic v.
3. 枕静脉 occipital v.
4. 大脑下静脉 inferior cerebral v.
5. 小脑 cerebellum
6. 颞极 temporal pole
7. 大脑中浅静脉 superficial
   middle cerebral v.
8. 额前静脉 prefrontal v.
9. 顶静脉 parietal v.
10. 额静脉 frontal v.
11. 中央静脉 central v.
12. 大脑上静脉 superior cerebral v.

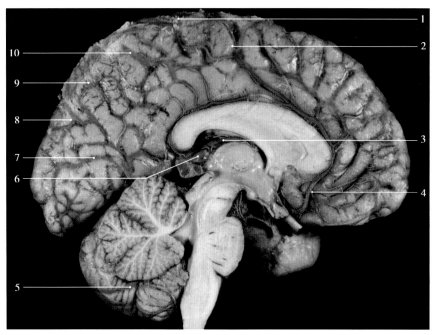

▲ 图 668　**大脑的静脉（内侧面观）**
Veins of the cerebrum. Medial aspect

1. 蛛网膜颗粒 arachnoid granulations
2. 蛛网膜 arachnoid mater
3. 大脑内静脉 internal cerebral v.
4. 大脑前动脉 anterior cerebral a.
5. 蚓下静脉 inferior vein of vermis

6. 大脑大静脉 great cerebral v.
7. 枕内侧静脉 internal occipital v.
8. 顶枕内侧静脉 medial parietooccipital v.
9. 顶内侧静脉 medial parietal v.
10. 中央内侧静脉 medial central v.

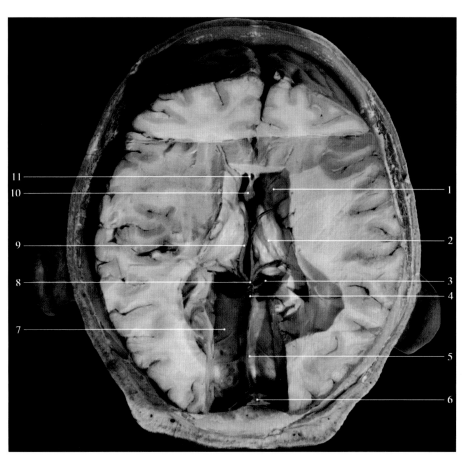

◀ 图 669

大脑大静脉及其属支
Great cerebral vein and its tributaries

1. 尾状核 caudate nucleus
2. 背侧丘脑 dorsal thalamus
3. 基底静脉 basal v.
4. 下矢状窦 inferior sagittal sinus
5. 直窦 straight sinus
6. 上矢状窦 superior sagittal sinus
7. 小脑幕 tentorium of cerebellum
8. 大脑大静脉 great cerebral v.
9. 大脑内静脉 internal cerebral v.
10. 穹隆 fornix
11. 透明隔 septum pellucidum

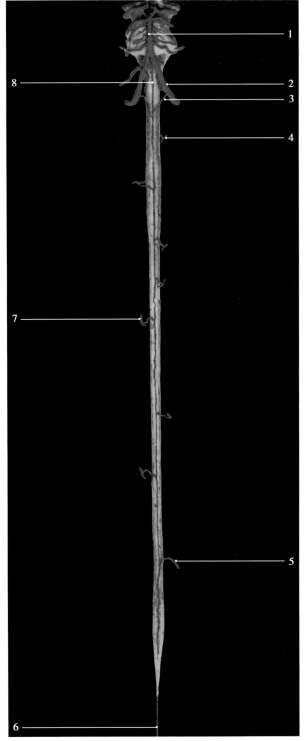

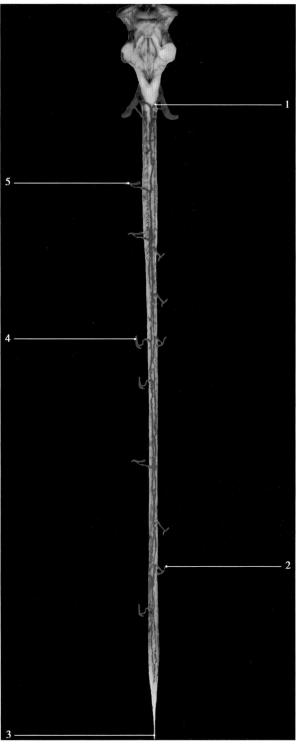

▲ 图 670　脊髓动脉（前面观）
Spinal arteries. Anterior aspect

1. 基底动脉 basilar a.
2. 椎动脉 vertebral a.
3. 椎动脉脊支 spinal branches of vertebral a.
4. 颈升动脉 ascending cervical a.
5. 腰动脉 lumbar a.
6. 终丝 filum terminale
7. 肋间后动脉 posterior intercostal a.
8. 脊髓前动脉 anterior spinal a.

▲ 图 671　脊髓动脉（后面观）
Spinal arteries. Posterior aspect

1. 脊髓后动脉 posterior spinal a.
2. 腰动脉 lumbar a.
3. 终丝 filum terminale
4. 肋间后动脉 posterior intercostal a.
5. 颈升动脉 ascending cervical a.

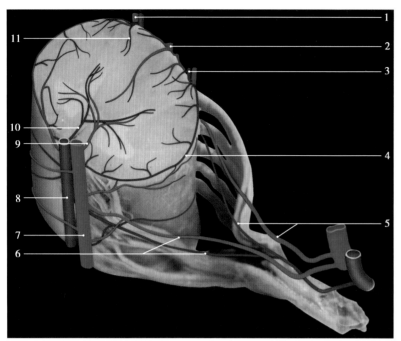

◀ 图 672

脊髓内部的血管分布
Distribution of vessels in spinal cord

1. 右脊髓后外侧静脉 right spinal external posterior v.
2. 脊髓后静脉 posterior spinal v.
3. 左脊髓后动脉 left posterior spinal a.
4. 动脉冠 vasocorona
5. 后根动、静脉 posterior radicular a. and v.
6. 前根动、静脉 anterior radicular a. and v.
7. 脊髓前静脉 anterior spinal v.
8. 脊髓前动脉 anterior spinal a.
9. 沟连合静脉 sulcocommissural v.
10. 沟连合动脉 sulcocommissural a.
11. 周围支 peripheral branch

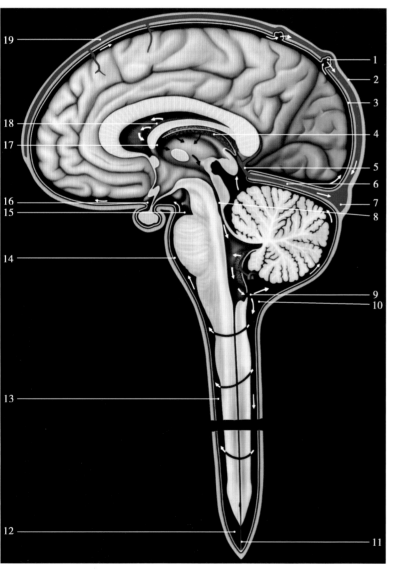

◀ 图 673

脑脊液循环
Circulation of cerebrospinal fluid

1. 蛛网膜粒 arachnoid granulation
2. 硬脑膜 cerebral dura mater
3. 脑蛛网膜 cerebral arachnoid mater
4. 第三脑室脉络丛 choroid plexus of the third ventricle
5. 大脑大静脉 great cerebral v.
6. 直窦 sinus rectus
7. 窦汇 confluence of sinuses
8. 中脑水管 mesencephalic aqueduct
9. 第四脑室正中孔 median aperture of the fourth ventricle
10. 小脑延髓池 cerebellomedullary cistern
11. 终丝 filum terminale
12. 终池 terminal cistern
13. 蛛网膜下隙 subarachnoid space
14. 桥池 pontine cistern
15. 脚间池 interpeduncular cistern
16. 交叉池 chiasmatic cistern
17. 室间孔 interventricular foramen
18. 侧脑室脉络丛 choroid plexus of lateral ventricle
19. 上矢状窦 superior sagittal sinus

第十七章　内分泌系统
Endocrine System

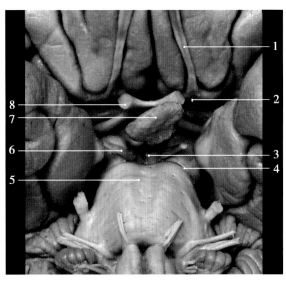

◀ 图 674
垂体
Hypophysis
1. 嗅束 olfactory tract
2. 嗅三角 olfactory trigone
3. 脚间窝 interpeduncle fossa
4. 滑车神经 trochlear n.
5. 脑桥 pons
6. 动眼神经 oculomotor n.
7. 垂体 hypophysis
8. 视神经 optic n.

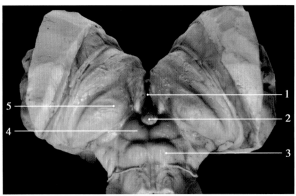

◀ 图 675
松果体
Pineal body
1. 第三脑室 third ventricle
2. 松果体 pineal body
3. 下丘 inferior colliculus
4. 上丘 superior colliculus
5. 背侧丘脑 dorsal thalamus

图 676 ▶
胸腺
Thymus
1. 气管 trachea
2. 左头臂静脉 left brachiocephalic v.
3. 胸腺左叶 left lobe of thymus
4. 左肺 left lung
5. 心包 pericardium
6. 右肺 right lung
7. 胸腺右叶 right lobe of thymus
8. 右头臂静脉 right brachiocephalic v.

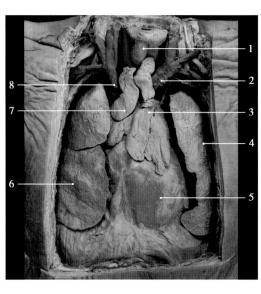

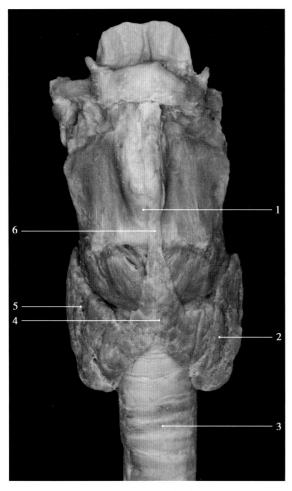

▲ 图 677 甲状腺
Thyroid gland
1. 喉结 laryngeal prominence
2. 甲状腺左叶 left lobe of thyroid gland
3. 气管 trachea
4. 甲状腺峡 isthmus of thyroid gland
5. 甲状腺右叶 right lobe of thyroid gland
6. 甲状腺锥状叶 pyramidal lobe of thyroid gland

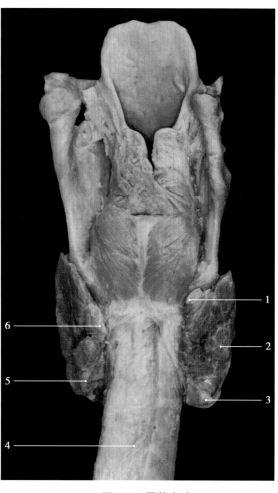

▲ 图 678 甲状旁腺
Parathyroid gland
1. 右上甲状旁腺 right superior parathyroid gland
2. 甲状腺右叶 right lobe of thyroid gland
3. 右下甲状旁腺 right inferior parathyroid gland
4. 气管 trachea
5. 左下甲状旁腺 left inferior parathyroid gland
6. 左上甲状旁腺 left superior parathyroid gland

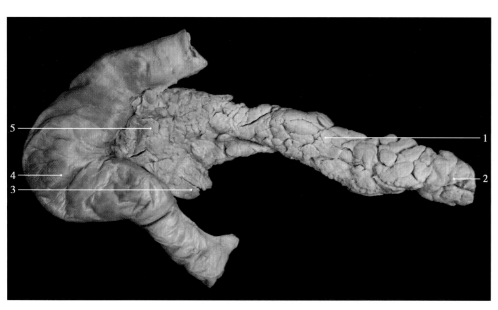

◀ 图 679 胰
Pancreas
1. 胰体 body of pancreas
2. 胰尾 tail of pancreas
3. 钩突 uncinate process
4. 十二指肠 duodenum
5. 胰头 head of pancreas

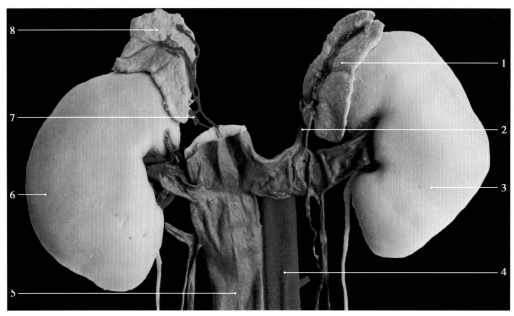

▲ 图 680　肾上腺
Suprarenal gland

1. 左肾上腺 left suprarenal gland
2. 肾上腺静脉 suprarenal v.
3. 左肾 left kidney
4. 腹主动脉 abdominal aorta
5. 下腔静脉 inferior caval v.
6. 右肾 right kidney
7. 肾上腺动脉 suprarenal a.
8. 右肾上腺 right suprarenal gland

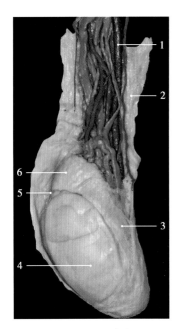

▲ 图 681　睾丸
Testis

1. 输精管 ductus deferens
2. 提睾肌筋膜 cremasteric fascia
3. 附睾体 body of epididymis
4. 睾丸 testis
5. 睾丸附件 appendage of testis
6. 附睾头 head of epididymis

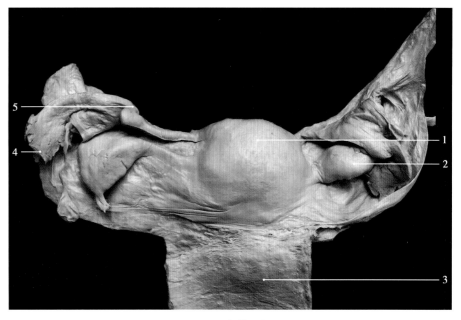

▲ 图 682　卵巢（后面观）
Ovary. Posterior aspect

1. 子宫 uterus
2. 卵巢 ovary
3. 阴道 vagina
4. 输卵管伞 fimbriae of uterine tube
5. 输卵管 uterine tube

06检